CANCER ETIOLOGY, DIAGNOSIS AND TREATMENTS

ENDOMETRIAL CANCER

PREVENTION, DIAGNOSIS AND TREATMENT

Cancer Etiology, Diagnosis and Treatments

Additional books in this series can be found on Nova's website under the Series tab.

Additional E-books in this series can be found on Nova's website under the E-book tab.

Obstetrics and Gynecology Advances

Additional books in this series can be found on Nova's website under the Series tab.

Additional E-books in this series can be found on Nova's website under the E-book tab.

CANCER ETIOLOGY, DIAGNOSIS AND TREATMENTS

ENDOMETRIAL CANCER

PREVENTION, DIAGNOSIS AND TREATMENT

STEFANO GREGGI
EDITOR

New York

For permission to use material from this book please contact us:
Telephone 631-231-7269; Fax 631-231-8175
Web Site: http://www.novapublishers.com

Library of Congress Cataloging-in-Publication Data

Library of Congress Control Number: 2012945373

ISBN: 978-1-62257-740-8

Published by Nova Science Publishers, Inc. † New York

Contents

Preface

A book devoted to endometrial cancer is very appropriate at this time. Endometrial malignancies have risen in incidence to become the most common gynecologic cancer in industrialized nations. In the United Sates the incidence has doubled in the last twenty years and the American Cancer Society is predicting that there will be 47,000 new cases in 2012 in the United States. An explanation of this dramatic increase in incidence usually is associated with a discussion of the rise in obesity, life expectancy in general and maybe the use of post menopausal estrogen therapy. However when these potential explanations are carefully studied there appears to be other unknown factors underlying the increase in this disease.

No practical screening tool exists and post menopausal bleeding continues to be the earliest signal for diagnosis and intervention. The use of pelvic ultrasound for calculation of "the endometrial stripe" is not always reliable and may create excess surgery. Most clinicians are satisfied with the statement that "any post menopausal bleeding is endometrial cancer until proven otherwise". This combined with the fact that twenty-five percent of endometrial cancer cases occur in women in the age group under 50 makes early diagnosis somewhat elusive.

The clinical pathologic behavior of endometrial malignancies is much better understood today in great part due to some of the early studies of the Gynecologic Oncology Group in the 1970's and 1980's. These studies brought out several key aspects of the malignancy and its behavior. Pelvic lymph node involvement was confirmed where previously there had been doubt. The concept of early metastasis directly from the fundus to the para-arotic area was thought to be the principal route of spread. The depth of myometrial invasion was determined to be the most predictive of extrauterine spread of the disease. The importance of cervical involvement was brought to light. Grade and size of lesion became secondary predictors of metastasis and poor outcome. Utilizing these pathological features, the clinician was now able to define the high risk group and consider this subset for adjuvant therapy. This permitted more than 50% of the patients to avoid adjuvant therapy entirely, even patients with Grade 3 lesions. The result was a diminished morbidity for patients afflicted with this disease without loss of curability. The clinician was able to tailor post operative therapy to the findings at surgery. This was particularly important to young patients with so called "type I" lesions of the endometrium which are in great part supported by endogenous and exogenous estrogen in excess. These type I lesions are often low-grade endometrioid adenocarcinoma and they carry a very favorable prognosis. "Type II" lesions can occur in any patient and are defined primarily as high grade lesions including clear cell, serous and mixed Mullerian pathology of the endometrium. This category of lesions behaves in a much more aggressive manner and carries a poorer prognosis.

In the last decade the use of adjuvant chemotherapy has improved. Drug combinations that are effective which may be superior to radiation therapy are now commonly used post operatively and will be discussed in this text. Ongoing research utilizing biologic agents in combination with radiation and/or chemotherapy may become the best therapy of the future.

In summary, much has been learned about the behavior and the treatment of this disease. Therefore a textbook devoted to this disease is timely and should be in the library of all individuals who treat gynecologic cancer.

Philip J. DiSaia, MD
The Dorothy Marsh Chair in Reproductive Biology
Professor, Department of Obstetrics and Gynecology
Division of Gynecologic Oncology,
University of California, Irvine, CA, US

In: Endometrial Cancer: Prevention, Diagnosis and Treatment ISBN: 978-1-62257-740-8
Editor: Stefano Greggi

Chapter I

Epidemiology and Risk Factors

Sonia Cipriani[1,2], Elena Ricci[2], Francesca Chiaffarino[2], Mirella Di Martino[2], Francesca Bravi[1] and Fabio Parazzini[2*]

[1]Istituto di Ricerche Farmacologiche "Mario Negri," Milan, Italy
[2]Obstetrics and Gynecology, Fondazione IRCCS "Cà Granda," Ospedale Maggiore Policlinico, University of Milan, Italy

Abstract

Endometrial cancer (EC) is the seventh most common female cancer in the world and the fourth in developed countries, where the age-standardised incidence rates are more than twice that of developing countries. About 290,000 new cases of EC are diagnosed every year worldwide, 90% in women older than 50. About 74,000 women die every year for EC. Because of its favourable prognosis, it is considered a cause of morbidity rather than mortality. Increasing incidence trends observed in last decades are related to characteristics linked to Westernisation of lifestyles. The etiopathogenesis of EC has been linked, at least in part, to high and prolonged estrogen levels.

Obesity is considered responsible for 40% of incidence. Other well recognised risk factors are: early age at menarche, nulliparity, late age at menopause, unopposed estrogen hormone replacement therapy use, never oral contraceptives use, history of diabetes and metabolic syndrome. Other risk factors have a more limited and/or controversial role, and do not help to identify a high risk population.

Introduction

Endometrial cancer (EC) is the seventh most common female cancer in the world and the fourth in developed countries [1]. About 290,000 new cases of EC are diagnosed every year

[*] E-mail address: fabio.parazzini@unimi.it.

worldwide [2] (90% diagnosed in women older than 50 [1]) and about 74,000 women die every year of EC [2]. Because of its favourable prognosis, it is considered a cause of morbidity rather than mortality.

In the last few decades, age-standardised EC rates have been rising in several countries, thus suggesting that some risk factors are increasing. Well recognised risk factors are related to high and prolonged estrogen levels such as early age at menarche, nulliparity, late age at menopause, unopposed estrogen hormone replacement therapy (HRT), never oral contraceptives (OC) use, obesity and history of diabetes [3-5]. Obesity, that increases estrogen level, is the most important risk factor for EC worldwide and has been estimated to explain 40% of EC incidence [1].

In the recent years, some studies has distinguished two type of EC: type I and type II. However, the majority of the literature considered the two types together. Thus, in this paper we review the main epidemiological characteristics of EC, without distinction between type I and II if not otherwise specified.

Descriptive Epidemiology

Tables 1 and 2 show the EC incidence and mortality age-standardised rates (ASR) in different regions.

The areas characterised by the highest incidences are Northern America (16.4), Europe (10.4 to 14.6), Australia/New Zealand (11.5) and China (11.1). Incidence is low in Africa (2.5) and Asia (6.6). In the United States, incidence rates are higher in white than in black or Asian women. However, the higher incidence in "Westernised" populations suggests environmental rather than genetic risk factors [1,3-7]. Difficulty in distinguishing between cancer of the corpus and cervix uteri, in the developing countries, where the latter is very common, should be considered in the interpretation of these data.

Trend in Endometrial Cancer Incidence

From early 1960s till mid 1970s EC incidence rates increased, in high-risk areas, because of the widespread use of unopposed estrogen by postmenopausal women; then they fall to previous levels in the early 1980s [8]. In the same period, in low- and middle-risk areas, the trends were generally increasing but differences in diagnostic and registration accuracy should be taken into account, when interpreting geographical and temporal trend [8]. Further, it is necessary to consider the change in hysterectomy rates decreasing in the USA and Canada but increasing in Southern European Countries.

During the 1990s, in the USA the incidence increased by 0.5 per year whereas mortality decreased by 0.6 per year; in the 1999-2006 period an increasing trend was observed for type I EC incidence whereas type II incidence remained stable [9].

Between 1980 and 2000, in Northern and Western Europe, age-standardised EC rates decreased among pre- and peri-menopausal women whereas increased among post-menopausal women with the exception of Denmark, France and Switzerland that showed decreasing trends [10].

In India, an increasing trend emerged during the 1998-2005 period, presumably as a result both of higher prevalence of risk factors and also of the improvement in diagnostic procedures [11].

Information available on incidence trend in other developing countries is sparse.

Table 1. Corpus uteri - Incidence and mortality, all ages. Globocan 2008 - IARC [2]

	Incidence		Mortality	
Population	n	ASR	n	ASR
World	288,387	8.2	73,854	2.0
More developed regions	143,518	13.0	32,689	2.3
Less developed regions	144,869	5.9	41,165	1.7

Legend. ASR: age-standardised rate.

Table 2. Corpus uteri - Incidence and mortality, all ages. Globocan 2008 - IARC [2]

	Incidence (ASR)	Mortality (ASR)
Africa	2.5	0.9
Sub-saharian Africa	2.6	0.9
Eastern Africa	2.4	0.8
Middle Africa	1.9	0.7
Northern Africa	2.2	0.7
Southern Africa	6.9	2.1
Western Africa	1.9	0.7
America		
Central America	6.1	2.5
South America	4.4	1.7
Northern America	16.4	2.4
Asia	6.6	1.7
Eastern Asia	10.3	2.2
South-Eastern Asia	5.7	2.0
South-Central Asia	2.1	1.1
Western Asia	5.6	1.5
Australia/New Zealand	11.5	1.6
Europe	12.8	2.5
Central and Eastern Europe	14.6	3.4
Northern Europe	13.8	2.2
Southern Europe	10.4	1.9
Western Europe	11.2	1.8

Legend. ASR: age-standardised rate.

Risk Factors

A summary of risk or protective factors is shown in table 3.

Table 3. Risk factors for endometrial cancer

Risk / protective factors	Effect on endometrial cancer risk
Demographic and lifestyle	
Family history	↑
Education	↑
Obesity	↑
Smoking	↓
Physical activity	↓
Menstrual and reproductive factors	
Late age at menarche	↓
Early age at menopause	↓
Parity	↓
Fertility	Non directly related
Medical history	
Diabetes	↑
High GI	No effect
High GL	↑
IGF-I	↓
IGF-II	↑
Metabolic syndrome	↑
Large waist circumference	↑
Hypertension	↑
High fasting blood glucose	↑
Drug use	
Oral Contraceptive use	↓
Unopposed HRT	↑
Tamoxifen	↑
Therapy for infertility	↑
Dietary factors	
Coffee	↓
Tea	No effect
Isoflavone-containing food	↓

GI Glycemic index, GL Glycemic load, IGF Insulin-like growth factors
HRT Hormone replacement therapy.

Family History

Some studies have found an increased risk of EC in women with a family history of cancer. The Swedish Family-Cancer Database found a standardized incidence ratio (SIR) of EC in women with mother or sisters with history of EC of 2.9 and 4.0 respectively [12]. The SIR was also higher for a family history of colorectal and urinary bladder cancers.

In a case-control study conducted in Italy on 726 women, a 50% increased risk of developing EC was estimated in women with first-degree relatives with EC history [13]. Further, the risk seemed to be higher in younger women: in a case-control study conducted in Denmark on 237 cancer cases and 538 controls aged less than 50 years, women with a family history had a two-fold risk as compared to women without family history [14]. In another case-control study conducted in the USA on 455 women aged 20-54 years the OR was 2.8 [15]. In a more recent case-control study, conducted in Italy on 454 cancer cases and 908 controls, family history of uterine cancer (first-degree) was estimated to double the EC risk; the estimated risk was higher (OR=2.6) for women younger than 55 years [16].

Family history of colorectal cancer was recognised to increase the EC risk in young women [15] but no association emerged with a family history of breast or ovarian cancer [13].

Similarly, in a cohort study from the United States, no familial association was detected between family history of breast cancer and risk of developing EC [17]. Finally, the Iowa Women's Health Study cohort of postmenopausal women showed no association between risk of EC and family history of uterine, other female genital tract, breast or colon cancer in first-degree relatives [18].

Socioeconomic Indicators

Epidemiological studies have recognised that education was directly related with EC risk. However, part of the association seemed to be explained by other risk factors for EC, as the more frequent use of HRT among higher social class women or differences in overweight and obesity frequency in social classes in different areas [19-21].

Obesity

Obesity is the most important risk factor for EC worldwide and has been estimated to explain the 40% of the EC incidence [1]. A recent meta-analysis including 19 prospective observational studies conducted in Northern America, Europe, Australia and Asia, found a relative risk to develop EC of 1.59 (95%CI: 1.5-1.7) for a 5 kg/m^2 increase in body mass index (BMI) [22]. Further, this risk concerned both pre-menopausal and post-menopausal women [23].

Obesity is often associated with irregular menstrual period, characterized by low serum progesterone level [24]. Further, obesity implies an increased availability of unopposed peripheral estrogens and a lower concentration of sex hormone-binding globulin (SHBG), leading to an increased availability of peripheral estrogens to hormone responsive tissues such as endometrium [25]. For these reasons obesity leads to an increased risk of EC.

Obesity is also recognised to decrease life-expectancy, specifically in cancer patients. Some studies suggested that women with EC had a greater potential to die from obesity-related disease, in particular women with BMI higher than 40.0, but no relation was found between obesity and risk of EC recurrence [7, 26].

Smoking

Smoking habit has been suggested to decrease the risk of post-menopausal EC in relation to its anti-estrogenic effect [27]. This effect, linked with decreased urinary estrogens in smokers, is supposed to be mediated by the induction of hepatic microsomal enzymes [28-30].

Usually, smokers have an early menopause [7,31-34], so the observed protective effect could be due to the anticipation of age at menopause. Further, smokers tend to be leaner than non-smokers [29], but this did not seem to totally explain the inverse association.

Physical Activity

EC is more common in Westernised countries in relation to behaviours like sedentary lifestyle [35]. A recent meta-analysis, including 9 prospective cohort studies, suggested that recreational physical activity reduced the risk of EC of about 30% [36].

Furthermore, the lack of physical exercise affected blood lipids and proteins, and SHBG, with a negative effect on the menstrual cycle pattern [37, 38].

Menstrual and Reproductive Factors

Menstrual Factors

Late age at menarche has been suggested to reduce EC risk [19,39,40]. In a large multicenter prospective study (EPIC cohort) conducted in Europe, a significant inverse linear association between age at menarche and EC risk emerged [41]. The same study suggested that menarche at 15 years or more (versus ≤ 12 years) reduced EC risk of about 30% [41].

This finding has plausible biological correlates in the likely late-stage (promotional) effect of hormonally-mediated menstrual factors [19]. Women with long menstrual cycles [42] or amenorrhea are at increased risk of EC. In biological terms this association may be explained by the fact that amenorrhea or irregular (long) menstrual cycles are associated with anovulation and unopposed estrogen stimulation.

An association between EC and late age at menopause is commonly reported. The menstrual cycles before menopause are generally without ovulation, thus characterized by unopposed estrogen stimulation. Many studies reported relative risks between 1.5 and 2.5 for women with menopause at 52-53 years vs. 45 years or less [19,21,39,43-45]. Consistently, in the EPIC cohort [41], a late menopause (age > 55 years) versus a menopause at 50 years or less was suggested to double the risk of EC.

Pregnancy and Fertility

Parity has been consistently recognised to reduce EC risk of about 40-50% [14, 41, 46]. A decrease in risk with increasing number of birth has also been reported [41, 44, 46-50];

further, risk reduction was greater in women younger than 55 years [46,49]. Some studies suggested that age at first birth was inversely associated with EC risk [14,51] but not other [41,46,49]. A recent review suggested that infertile women had an increased risk of EC [52]. However, in a recent study on a large cohort of Danish women with primary or secondary infertility, the increase in risk (29%) was not significant when results were adjusted for parity [53].

Medical History

Diabetes

The relation between diabetes and EC risk is well recognised [7,16,54-63]. However, it is important to take into account that obesity, which is the most important risk factor for EC, is also the major determinant of diabetes. Thus, the association between diabetes and EC may be at least partially explained by higher body weight of women with EC.

To define this point, some studies investigated if the role of diabetes was independent from obesity, and consistently found a residual risk of EC after adjustment for BMI [54,55,57,58,62,63]. Other studies investigated the combined role of BMI and diabetes and reported a higher risk of EC among obese diabetic women [56,58,61-63] and the same studies, except that of Anderson [61], suggested that diabetic women of normal weight had a higher risk of EC compared to non-diabetic women of normal weight.

A meta-analysis, which included 16 studies and 7,596 cases of EC, suggested that diabetes (mainly type II) doubled the risk of EC and the risk was 3.2 for type I diabetes (meta-analysis based on three studies) [63].

Glycemic Index, Glycemic Load and Insulin-Like Growth Factors

High glycemic index (GI) and glycemic load (GL) diet, which rises glucose, insulin and insulin-like growth factors (IGF) levels have been suggested to increase the risk of several chronic disease [64] such as diabetes, coronary heart disease, obesity and also several malignancies including cervical [65], lung [66], prostate [66-68] and breast cancer [69].

A recent meta-analysis which included 5 cohort studies and 2 case-control studies conducted in Europe, Canada and USA, reported an increased risk for high dietary GL (overall RR=1.19, 95%CI 1.1-1.3) but not for high dietary GI (overall RR=1.09, 95%CI 0.9-1.3) [70].

A case-control study including 84 cases conducted in Greece [71] suggested that EC was inversely associated with IGF-I and directly associated with IGF-II.

Metabolic Syndrome

Two recent case-control studies from Canada [72] and Italy [73] have investigated the effect of metabolic syndrome (MS) on EC risk. Both found an increased risk (OR=2.77 and

OR=1.53, respectively) of EC among women with MS. An increased risk was also found for some components of MS including waist circumference (threshold 88 cm) (OR=1.57 and 1.90, respectively), hypertension (OR=1.57 and 1.77, respectively), and fasting blood glucose ≥100 mg/dl (OR=1.31 in Canadian study).

Arthritis and Thyroid Diseases

Other diseases suggested to be associated with EC risk are arthritis and thyroid diseases but the data are scanty and controversial [21,48,74,75].

Drug Use

Oral contraceptive

Oral contraceptives have been consistently indicated as protective against EC [8, 41, 76]. In ever OC users versus non-users, the risk was about halved [45] and it decreased with duration of use [41, 77, 78]. The reduced risk seemed to persist after OC discontinuation: a study conducted in Swiss suggested a RR=0.4 for 10-19 years after OC interruption and RR=0.8 after 20 years or more [79].

Hormonal Replacement Therapy

Unopposed estrogen therapy has been suggested to double the risk of EC [1,80,81]. This effect increased with duration of use and lasted after discontinuation. In a meta-analysis including 30 cohort and case-control studies, the combined RR was 2.3 (95%CI: 2.1-2.5) for unopposed estrogen users versus non-users; the RR was 9.5 for 10 years use or more [81]. Regarding estrogen plus progestin replacement therapy the finding were controversial: the same study estimated a combined RR=0.4 from cohort studies but a RR=1.8 from case-control studies [81].

In a recent population-based case-control study conducted in the USA a lower EC risk was found (OR=0.6) among combined HRT users versus non-users; the OR was 0.8 (not significant) for long-term (≥ 6 years) users [82].

Few data are available on the relation between EC risk and different dosage and route of HRT administration (oral, transdermal, intranasal).

Tamoxifen

Tamoxifen is a non-steroidal hormone widely used in the treatment of breast cancer; it is also considered a chemopreventive agent.

It has been suggested to increase EC risk, effect that is biologically plausible since tamoxifen, alone or in combination with estradiol, stimulates growth of endometrial tumor in athymic mouse [83, 84].

Three clinical trials [85-87] have found an increased risk of EC in tamoxifen treated women versus non-treated. The estimated relative risks were 6.4 [87] (daily dose 40 mg, treatment duration 2 years) and, 2.5 [86] and 7.5 [85] (daily dose 20 mg, treatment duration 5 years) for women treated with tamoxifen versus non-treated.

Therapy for Infertility

Use of fertility drugs has been suggested to increase EC risk [47,88]. In two recent Italian case-control studies, women with a history of treated infertility had a three-fold higher risk of EC [47,88]. The risk was higher for 12 or more months of treatment (OR=6.1) [88]. Moreover, the risk was inversely associated with time since last use (OR=5.3; 25 years or less before the interview versus more than 25 years) and with age at first use (OR=5.1; first use before 30 years) [88].

Dietary Factors

Diet has been suggested to influence EC risk independently from obesity but the relation between EC risk and specific foods or food groups is still limited and controversial [3].

Some studies reported an inverse association with vegetables [89-96] whereas other did not confirm this association [97-102]. Similar inconsistent findings were reported for fruit consumption [90-103]. Several studies investigated the role of cereals [90-95,97-99,101,104], meat [91-95,97-99,101,103-105], fish [91,93,95,97,100,103,105], milk and dairy products [89,91,93-95,97-99,101,103,105], legumes [90-92,97,99-101,103]. They did not report consistent associations with EC.

The identification of low-risk dietary patterns is still under debate. However, considering the well-known relation between estrogen levels and EC risk, it is important to take into account that postmenopausal vegetarian women have lower levels of estriol, total estrogens and prolactin, and higher levels of SHBG than non-vegetarian women, differences not explainable in term of different body weight [93,106].

Some studies have investigated the effect of isoflavone (phytestrogen)-containing food consumption on EC risk [107-109]. The Multiethnic Cohort (MEC) Study including 46,027 non-hysterectomised post-menopausal women (30% were Japanese American), showed a significant reduction in EC risk among women with a total isoflavone intake $\geq$ 7.8 versus $<$ 1.59 mg per 1000 kcal/d (RR=0.66, adjusted for ethnicity) [109]. Consistently, in a population-based case-control study on non-Asian women, the EC risk was 0.59 among women with the highest versus the lowest quartile of total isoflavone intake; the association was stronger in post-menopausal women (OR=0.44) [106].

In another population-based case-control study (EDGE study), the inverse association with total isoflavone intake was limited to women with BMI $<$ 25 (OR=0.5) or with a waist-to-hip ratio $\leq$ 0.85 (OR=0.59) with no evidence of effect modification by HRT use [108].

Coffee and Tea

Coffee has been suggested to reduce the risk of EC through a reduction in the levels of estrogen and insulin, two hormones implicated in endometrial carcinogenesis [110]. A recent meta-analysis [111] and two large prospective studies [110,112] have contributed to define this association.

The meta-analysis, including 2 cohort studies and 7 case-control studies, found a significant reduction in cancer risk of coffee drinkers versus non-drinkers and a reduction in risk of 7% for an increase of 1 cup/die, thus suggesting an inverse relation between coffee and EC [111].

The results of the Nurses' Health Study (NHS), that included women aged 34 to 59, suggested that a coffee intake less than 4 cups of coffee per day was not associated with EC risk but women that consumed 4 cups of coffee or more had a 25% reduction of EC risk as compared to those who consumed 1 cup or less [110]. Consistently, another large prospective study, including women aged 50-71, suggested an inverse relation between coffee intake and EC risk (> 3 cups/day vs. no cups: HR=0.64) and the association was consistent in regular and decaffeinated coffee [112].

No association between tea consumption and EC risk was detected [110,113].

Conclusion

The epidemiological studies have well defined the etiologic role of endogenous and/or exogenous estrogen levels in endometrial carcinogenesis; well recognised risk factors are related to high and prolonged estrogen levels during women life: early age at menarche, nulliparity, late age at menopause, unopposed estrogen HRT use, never OC use, history of diabetes. Other risk factors have a more limited and/or controversial role, and do not help to identify a high risk population.

References

[1] Boyle, P; Levin, B. World Cancer Report 2008. *World Health Organization*. Lyon: International Agency for Research on Cancer; 2008.

[2] Ferlay, J; et al. GLOBOCAN 2008 v1.2, Cancer Incidence and Mortality Worldwide. *IARC CancerBase No. 10*. Lyon: International Agency for Research on Cancer; 2010. http://globocan.iarc.fr

[3] Bravi, F; et al. Food groups and endometrial cancer risk: a case-control study from Italy. *Am. J. Obstet Gynecol* 2009;200:293 e1-7.

[4] Purdie, DM; Green, AC. Epidemiology of endometrial cancer. *Best Prac. Res. Clin. Obstet Gynaecol* 2001;15:341-54.

[5] Friedenreich, C; et al. Anthropometric factors and risk of endometrial cancer: the European prospective investigation into cancer and nutrition. *Cancer Causes Control* 2007;18:399-413.

[6] Devivo, I; et al. Endometrial cancer. In: *Textbook of cancer epidemiology 2nd ed.* New York: Oxford University Press; 2008.

[7] Cook, LS; et al. Endometrial cancer. In: *Cancer epidemiology and prevention. 3rd ed.* New York: Oxford University Press; 2006.

[8] Parazzini, F; et al. The epidemiology of endometrial cancer. *Gynecol Oncol* 1991;41: 1-16.

[9] Ries, LAG; et al. *SEER Cancer Statistics Review 1973-1998.* Bethesda: National Cancer Institute; 2001.

[10] Bray, F; et al. Endometrial cancer incidence trends in Europe: underlying determinants and prospects for prevention. *Cancer Epidemiol Biomarkers Prev.* 2005;14:1132-42.

[11] Murthy, NS; et al. Increase in incidence of cancer of corpus uteri: estimation of time trends - an Indian scenario. *Eur. J. Cancer Prev.* 2011;20:25-32.

[12] Dong, C; Hemminki, K. Modification of cancer risks in offspring by sibling and parental cancers from 2,112,616 nuclear families. *Int. J. Cancer* 2001;92:144-50.

[13] Parazzini, F; et al. Family history and the risk of endometrial cancer. *Int J. Cancer* 1994;59:460-2.

[14] Parslov, M; et al. Risk factors among young women with endometrial cancer: a Danish case-control study. *Am. J. Obstet Gynecol* 2000;182(Pt1):23-9.

[15] Gruber, SB; Thompson, WD. A population-based study of endometrial cancer and familial risk in younger women. Cancer and Steroid Hormone Study Group. *Cancer Epidemiol Biomarkers Prev.* 1996;5:411-7.

[16] Lucenteforte, E; et al. Family history of cancer and the risk of endometrial cancer. *Eur. J. Cancer Prev* 2009;18:95-9.

[17] Kazerouni, N; et al. Family history of breast cancer as a determinant of the risk of developing endometrial cancer: a nationwide cohort study. *J. Med. Genet* 2002;39:826-32.

[18] Olson, JE; et al. Does a family history of cancer increase the risk for postmenopausal endometrial carcinoma? A prospective cohort study and a nested case-control family study of older women. *Cancer* 1999;85:2444-9.

[19] La Vecchia, C; et al. Risk factors for endometrial cancer at different ages. *J Natl Cancer Inst* 1984;73:667-71.

[20] La Vecchia, C; et al. Education and cancer risk. *Cancer* 1992;70:2935-41.

[21] Kelsey, JL; et al. A case-control study of cancer of the endometrium. *Am J. Epidemiol.* 1982;116:333-42.

[22] Renehan, AG; et al. Body-mass index and incidence of cancer: a systematic review and meta-analysis of prospective observational studies. *Lancet* 2008;371:569-78.

[23] Fader, AN; et al. Endometrial cancer and obesity: epidemiology, biomarkers, prevention and survivorship. *Gynecol Oncol* 2009;114:121-7.

[24] Key, TJ; Pike, MC. The dose-effect relationship between 'unopposed' estrogens and endometrial mitotic rate: its central role in explaining and predicting endometrial cancer risk. *Br. J. Cancer* 1988;57:205-12.

[25] Enriori, CL; Reforzo-Membrives, J. Peripheral aromatization as a risk factor for breast and endometrial cancer in postmenopausal women: a review. *Gynecol. Oncol* 1984;17:1-21.

[26] von Gruenigen, VE; et al. Treatment effects, disease recurrence, and survival in obese women with early endometrial carcinoma: a Gynecologic Oncology Group study. *Cancer* 2006;107:2786-91.

[27] Tansavatdi, K; et al. The effects of smoking on estradiol metabolism. *Minerva Ginecol* 2004;56:105-14.

[28] Kaufman, DW; et al. Cigarette smoking and age at natural menopause. *Am. J. Public Health* 1980;70:420-2.

[29] Baron, JA. Smoking and estrogen-related disease. *Am. J. Epidemiol.* 1984;119:9-22.

[30] Conney, AH. Pharmacological implications of microsomal enzyme induction. *Pharmacol. Rev.* 1967;19:317-66.

[31] Key, TJ; et al. Cigarette smoking and urinary estrogen excretion in premenopausal and post-menopausal women. *Br. J. Cancer* 1996;74:1313-6.

[32] Spangler, JG. Smoking and hormone-related disorders. *Prim Care* 1999;26:499-511.

[33] Willett, W; et al. Cigarette smoking, relative weight, and menopause. *Am. J. Epidemiol.* 1983;117:651-8.

[34] MacMahon, B; et al. Cigarette smoking and urinary estrogens. *N Engl. J. Med.* 1982;307:1062-5.

[35] IARC - WHO. Cancer Incidence in Five Continents Vol. IX. *International Association of Cancer Registries*; 2007.

[36] Moore, SC; et al. Physical activity, sedentary behaviours, and the prevention of endometrial cancer. *Br J Cancer* 2010;103:933-8.

[37] Haskell, WL. The influence of exercise training on plasma lipids and lipoproteins in health and disease. *Acta Med Scand* 1986;711(Suppl):25-37.

[38] Hardman, AE; et al. Brisk walking and plasma high density lipoprotein cholesterol concentration in previously sedentary women. *BMJ* 1989;299:1204-5.

[39] Ewertz, M; et al. The joint effect of risk factors on endometrial cancer. *Eur. J. Cancer Clin. Oncol.* 1988;24:189-94.

[40] Kalandidi, A; et al. A case-control study of endometrial cancer in relation to reproductive, somatometric, and life-style variables. *Oncology* 1996;53:354-9.

[41] Dossus, L; et al. Reproductive risk factors and endometrial cancer: the European Prospective Investigation into Cancer and Nutrition. *Int. J. Cancer* 2010;127:442-51.

[42] Peterson, EP. Endometrial carcinoma in young women. A clinical profile. *Obstet Gynecol* 1968;31:702-7.

[43] Tyler, CW Jr; et al. Endometrial cancer: how does cigarette smoking influence the risk of women under age 55 years having this tumor? Am J *Obstet Gynecol* 1985;151:899-905.

[44] Koumantaki, Y; et al. A case-control study of cancer of endometrium in Athens. *Int. J. Cancer* 1989;43:795-9.

[45] The Cancer and Steroid Hormone Study of the Centers for Disease Control and the National Institute of Child Health and Human Development. Combination oral contraceptive use and the risk of endometrial cancer. *JAMA* 1987;257:796-800.

[46] Brinton, LA; et al. Reproductive risk factors for endometrial cancer among Polish women. *Br. J. Cancer* 2007;96:1450-6.

[47] Zucchetto, A; et al. Hormone-related factors and gynecological conditions in relation to endometrial cancer risk. *Eur. J. Cancer Prev* 2009;18:316-21.

[48] Elwood, JM; et al. Epidemiology of endometrial cancer. *J. Natl Cancer Inst.* 1977;59:1055-60.

[49] Parazzini, F; et al. Role of reproductive factors on the risk of endometrial cancer. *Int. J. Cancer* 1998;76:784-6.

[50] Henderson, BE; et al. Re-evaluating the role of progestogen therapy after the menopause. *Fertil Steril* 1988;49(Suppl2):S9-15.

[51] Pocobelli, G; et al. Pregnancy history and risk of endometrial cancer. *Epidemiology* 2011;22:638-45.

[52] Cetin, I; et al. Infertility as a cancer risk factor - a review. *Placenta* 2008;29(SupplB):169-77.

[53] Jensen, A; et al. Risk of breast cancer and gynecologic cancers in a large population of nearly 50,000 infertile Danish women. *Am. J. Epidemiol.* 2008;168:49-57.

[54] Brinton, LA; et al. Reproductive, menstrual, and medical risk factors for endometrial cancer: results from a case-control study. *Am. J. Obstet Gynecol* 1992;167:1317-25.

[55] La Vecchia, C; et al. A case-control study of diabetes mellitus and cancer risk. *Br J Cancer* 1994. 70:950-3.

[56] Shoff, SM; Newcomb, PA. Diabetes, body size, and risk of endometrial cancer. *Am. J. Epidemiol.* 1998;148:234-40.

[57] Parazzini, F; et al. Diabetes and endometrial cancer: an Italian case-control study. *Int. J. Cancer* 1999;81:539-42.

[58] Salazar-Martinez, E; et al. Case-control study of diabetes, obesity, physical activity and risk of endometrial cancer among Mexican women. *Cancer Causes Control* 2000;11:707-11.

[59] Weiderpass, E; et al. Body size in different periods of life, diabetes mellitus, hypertension, and risk of postmenopausal endometrial cancer (Sweden). *Cancer Causes Control* 2000;11:185-92.

[60] Sharma, DN; et al. Medical disorders associated with endometrial carcinoma. *J. Assoc Physicians India* 2001;49:630-3.

[61] Anderson, KE; et al. Diabetes and endometrial cancer in the Iowa women's health study. *Cancer Epidemiol Biomarkers Prev.* 2001;10:611-6.

[62] Friberg, E; et al. Diabetes and risk of endometrial cancer: a population-based prospective cohort study. *Cancer Epidemiol Biomarkers Prev* 2007;16:276-80.

[63] Friberg, E; et al. Diabetes mellitus and risk of endometrial cancer: a meta-analysis. *Diabetologia* 2007;50:1365-74.

[64] Augustin, LS; et al. Glycemic index in chronic disease: a review. *Eur J Clin Nutr 2002;56,1049-1071.*

[65] Mathur, SP; et al. Cervical epidermal growth factor-receptor (EGF-R) and serum insulin-like growth factor II (IGF-II) levels are potential markers for cervical cancer. *Am. J. Reprod Immunol* 2000;44:222-30.

[66] Yu, H; et al. Insulin-like growth factors (IGF-I, free IGF-I and IGF-II) and insulin-like growth factor binding proteins (IGFBP-2, IGFBP-3, IGFBP-6, and ALS) in blood circulation. *J. Clin. Lab Anal.* 1999;13:166-72.

[67] Cohen, P. Serum insulin-like growth factor-I levels and prostate cancer risk--interpreting the evidence. *J. Natl. Cancer Inst* 1998;90:876-9.

[68] Cohen, P; et al. Insulin-like growth factor 1 in relation to prostate cancer and benign prostatic hyperplasia. *Br. J. Cancer* 1998;78:554-6.

[69] Pollak, M. IGF-I physiology and breast cancer. *Recent Results Cancer Res.* 1998;152:63-70.
[70] Galeone, C; et al. Dietary glycemic index, glycemic load, and the risk of endometrial cancer: a case-control study and meta-analysis. *Eur J Cancer Prev* 2012. [Epub ahead of print]. DOI: 10.1097/CEJ.0b013e328354d378
[71] Petridou, E; et al. Endometrial cancer and the IGF system: a case-control study in Greece. *Oncology* 2003;64:341-5.
[72] Friedenreich, CM; et al. Case-control study of the metabolic syndrome and metabolic risk factors for endometrial cancer. *Cancer Epidemiol Biomarkers Prev* 2011;20(11):2384-95.
[73] Rosato, V; et al. Metabolic syndrome and endometrial cancer risk. *Ann. Oncol.* 2011;22:884-9.
[74] Wynder, EL; et al. An epidemiological investigation of cancer of the endometrium. *Cancer* 1966;19:489-520.
[75] Hertig, AT; et al. Genesis of endometrial carcinoma; carcinoma in situ. *Cancer* 1949;2:964-71, illust.
[76] WHO - IARC. Hormonal contraception and post-menopausal hormonal therapy. *IARC Monographs on the Evaluation of Carcinogenic Risks to Humans Vol. 72*; 1999.
[77] Voigt, LF; et al. Recency, duration, and progestin content of oral contraceptives in relation to the incidence of endometrial cancer (Washington, USA). *Cancer Causes Control* 1994;5:227-33.
[78] Prentice, RL; Thomas, DB. On the epidemiology of oral contraceptives and disease. *Adv. Cancer Res.* 1987;49:285-401.
[79] Levi, F; et al. Oral contraceptives and the risk of endometrial cancer. *Cancer Causes Control* 1991;2:99-103.
[80] Nelson, HD; et al. Postmenopausal hormone replacement therapy: scientific review. *JAMA* 2002;288:872-81.
[81] Grady, D; et al. Hormone replacement therapy and endometrial cancer risk: a meta-analysis. *Obstet Gynecol.* 1995;85:304-13.
[82] Doherty, JA; et al. Long-term use of postmenopausal estrogen and progestin hormone therapies and the risk of endometrial cancer. *Am. J. Obstet Gynecol* 2007;197:139 e1-7.
[83] Brown, K. Is tamoxifen a genotoxic carcinogen in women? *Mutagenesis* 2009;24:391-404.
[84] Gottardis, M.M., et al. Contrasting actions of tamoxifen on endometrial and breast tumor growth in the athymic mouse. *Cancer Res* 1988;48:812-5.
[85] Fisher, B; et al. Endometrial cancer in tamoxifen-treated breast cancer patients: findings from the National Surgical Adjuvant Breast and Bowel Project (NSABP) B-14. *J. Natl. Cancer Inst* 1994;86:527-37.
[86] Fisher, B; et al. Tamoxifen for prevention of breast cancer: report of the National Surgical Adjuvant Breast and Bowel Project P-1 Study. *J Natl Cancer Inst* 1998;90:1371-88.
[87] Fornander, T; et al. Adjuvant tamoxifen in early breast cancer: occurrence of new primary cancers. *Lancet* 1989;1:117-20.
[88] Parazzini, F; et al. Use of fertility drugs and risk of endometrial cancer in an Italian case-control study. *Eur. J. Cancer Prev.* 2010;19:428-30.

[89] Barbone, F; et al. Diet and endometrial cancer: a case-control study. *Am. J. Epidemiol.* 1993;137:393-403.
[90] Goodman, MT; et al. Diet, body size, physical activity, and the risk of endometrial cancer. *Cancer Res* 1997;57:5077-85.
[91] Jain, MG; et al. Nutritional factors and endometrial cancer in Ontario, Canada. *Cancer Control* 2000;7:288-96.
[92] Levi, F; et al., Dietary factors and breast cancer risk in Vaud, Switzerland. *Nutr Cancer* 1993;19:327-35.
[93] La Vecchia, C; et al. Nutrition and diet in the etiology of endometrial cancer. *Cancer* 1986;57:1248-53.
[94] Littman, AJ; et al. The association of dietary fat and plant foods with endometrial cancer (United States). *Cancer Causes Control* 2001;12:691-702.
[95] McCann, SE; et al. Diet in the epidemiology of endometrial cancer in western New York (United States). *Cancer Causes Control* 2000;11:965-74.
[96] Tao, MH; et al. A case-control study in Shanghai of fruit and vegetable intake and endometrial cancer. *Br. J. Cancer* 2005;92:2059-64.
[97] Petridou, E; et al. Diet in relation to endometrial cancer risk: a case-control study in Greece. *Nutr. Cancer* 2002;44:16-22.
[98] Potischman, N; et al. Dietary associations in a case-control study of endometrial cancer. *Cancer Causes Control* 1993;4:239-50.
[99] Salazar-Martinez, E; et al. Dietary factors and endometrial cancer risk. Results of a case-control study in Mexico. *Int. J. Gynecol Cancer* 2005;15:938-45.
[100] Shu, X.O; et al. A population-based case-control study of dietary factors and endometrial cancer in Shanghai, People's Republic of China. *Am. J. Epidemiol.* 1993;137:155-65.
[101] Terry, P; et al. Dietary factors in relation to endometrial cancer: a nationwide case-control study in Sweden. *Nutr. Cancer* 2002;42:25-32.
[102] McCullough, ML; et al. A prospective study of fruits, vegetables, and risk of endometrial cancer. *Am. J. Epidemiol* 2007;166:902-11.
[103] Tzonou, A; et al. Dietary factors and the risk of endometrial cancer: a case--control study in Greece. *Br. J. Cancer* 1996;73:1284-90.
[104] Kasum, CM; et al. Whole grain intake and incident endometrial cancer: the Iowa Women's Health Study. *Nutr. Cancer* 2001;39:180-6.
[105] Xu, WH; et al. Animal food intake and cooking methods in relation to endometrial cancer risk in Shanghai. *Br. J. Cancer* 2006;95:1586-92.
[106] Armstrong, BK; et al. Diet and reproductive hormones: a study of vegetarian and nonvegetarian postmenopausal women. *J. Natl. Cancer Inst.* 1981;67:761-7.
[107] Horn-Ross, PL; et al. Phytestrogen intake and endometrial cancer risk. *J. Natl. Cancer Inst* 2003;95:1158-64.
[108] Bandera, EV; et al. Phytestrogen consumption and endometrial cancer risk: a population-based case-control study in New Jersey. *Cancer Causes Control* 2009;20:1117-27.
[109] Ollberding, NJ; et al. Legume, soy, tofu, and isoflavone intake and endometrial cancer risk in postmenopausal women in the multiethnic cohort study. *J. Natl. Cancer Inst* 2012;104:67-76.

[110] Je, Y; et al. A Prospective Cohort Study of Coffee Consumption and Risk of Endometrial Cancer over a 26-Year Follow-Up. *Cancer Epidemiol. Biomarkers Prev.* 2011;20:2487-95.

[111] Bravi, F; et al. Coffee drinking and endometrial cancer risk: a metaanalysis of observational studies. *Am. J. Obstet Gynecol* 2009;200:130-5.

[112] Gunter, MJ; et al. A prospective investigation of coffee drinking and endometrial cancer incidence. *Int. J. Cancer* 2011 Oct 23. [Epub ahead of print]

[113] Bandera, EV; et al. Coffee and tea consumption and endometrial cancer risk in a population-based study in New Jersey. *Cancer Causes Control* 2010;21:1467-73.

In: Endometrial Cancer: Prevention, Diagnosis and Treatment ISBN: 978-1-62257-740-8
Editor: Stefano Greggi

Chapter II

Pathology and Molecular Pathogenesis: A New Way to Read It

Nunzia Simona Losito *

Surgical Pathology, National Cancer Institute "G. Pascale,"
Naples, Italy

Abstract

Endometrial adenocarcinoma is a complex disease whose morphologic heterogeneity, with its biologic and clinical implications, has been well shown by Bokhman's dualistic model until recent years. The classification of endometrial carcinomas in two broad categories, morphologically distinguishable and based on different molecular events during oncogenesis, had relevant clinical consequences identifying groups of tumors with different clinical behavior. In this chapter, we will examine the main histologic variants of endometrial carcinoma, according to World Health Organization (WHO) classification and to Bokhman's dualistic model, focusing on their prognostic value. Other prognostic factors will be considered in order to underline the pathologist's role in taking therapeutic decisions. However, recently Bokhman's model has been questioned, because of the low diagnostic agreement on high grade and mixed carcinomas among expert gynecologic pathologists, because of the identification of ambiguous carcinomas with uninformative morphologic features and because of the presence of a certain grade of overlapping altered molecular pathways in tumors belonging to different categories.

Bokhman's Model

Endometrial cancer is not a single disease: it's a heterogeneous tumor including distinct clinicopathologic entities with different epidemiology, precursors, molecular events during

* E-mail address: n.losito@istitutotumori.na.it.

oncogenesis, clinical behavior and outcome. In 1983, Bokhman [1] proposed a dualistic model of endometrial carcinogenesis classifying endometrial carcinomas into two broad categories. The type I endometrial adenocarcinoma (endometrioid type), represents the vast majority of sporadic endometrial carcinomas (70-80%), arises in pre and perimenopausal women, is estrogen-related, well differentiated, frequently associated to endometrial hyperplasia and endometrial intraepithelial neoplasia (EIN), has diploid DNA content, shows low propensity to myometrial invasion and lymphatic spread, and has a favorable prognosis. The type II endometrial adenocarcinoma (non-endometrioid type), is less frequent (10-20%), occurs in older, postmenopausal women, has aneuploid DNA content, is estrogen-independent and typically arises from atrophic endometrium, which is often in endometrial polyps. Different histotypes, like serous, clear cell, squamous cell and undifferentiated carcinoma belong to type II; clinical behavior is very aggressive, with a tendency to deepen myometrial infiltration, lymphatic spread and cause a fatal outcome (Table 1).

Molecular Alterations

Besides morphologic and clinical differences between the two types of endometrial adenocarcinoma, different molecular pathways have been discovered [2,3].

The most frequent somatic mutations in type I cancers are: 1) alterations of PTEN; 2) alterations in CTNNB-1; 3) K-RAS mutation; 4) microsatellite instability (MI); 5) PIK3CA alterations; 6) ARID1A mutation. The most frequently altered gene in endometrioid adenocarcinoma is PTEN phosphatase and tensin homolog mutated in 35-80% of the cases; a tumor suppressor gene located at chromosome 10p23 [4,5]. PTEN plays a key role in the PTEN-PI3K-AKT pathway [6], activating AKT by phosphorylation. Moreover, loss of PTEN is correlated with the activation of AKT in vivo [7,8].

As a consequence of AKT activation, activation of its downstream target mTOR inhibits apoptosis and cell cycle arrest, and stimulates cell proliferation. PTEN mutation is an early event in endometrial carcinogenesis because it occurs frequently in complex atypical hyperplasia [9]. These types of PTEN mutation are highly variable, including frameshifts, splice-site mutations and point mutations [10,11,12]; are typically hemizygous, involving only one allele; are detectable by immunohistochemistry [9].

Table 1. Bokhman's model for endometrial carcinoma

	Type I (80%)	Type II (20%)
Estrogen-related	Yes	Not
Age	Pre-perimenopausal	Post-menopausal
Precursors	Atypical hyperplasia / EIN	EIC
Grade	Low	High
Myometrial infiltration	Variable / Minimal	Deep
Lymphatic invasion	Not	Yes
Behavior	Indolent	Aggressive
Histotype	Endometrioid	Serous, clear cell, others
DNA content	Diploid	Aneuploid

Legend. EIC: endometrial intraepithelial carcinoma; EIN: endometrial intraepithelial neoplasia.

The prognostic significance of PTEN loss is still uncertain and controversy exists in literature, but many papers, old ones [13] and more recent ones [14,15], have shown its value as an indicator of favorable prognosis.

Mutation in the beta-catenin gene (CTNNB-1) occurs 25-40% of endometrioid adenocarcinomas [16]. Beta-catenin is normally involved in cell adhesion mechanisms; when the gene is mutated, the protein accumulates in the nucleus, activating genes involved in cell cycle regulation. It seems to be associated to indolent behavior, but also to recurrence.

K-RAS is mutated in 14-36% of endometrioid adenocarcinomas and its precursors, suggesting it is an early event in endometrial carcinogenesis [17]. The prognostic significance of this mutation is still controversial; some authors claim it is associated to favorable prognosis [18], while others say the contrary [19]. K-RAS mutation activates MAP-K pathway and up-regulates PIK3CA, promoting transcription of genes involved in cell proliferation [20,21]. Moreover it confers resistance to targeting of the PTEN-PI3K-AKT pathway [22,23]. Microsatellite instability (MI) occurs in endometrial cancers arising in the setting of the hereditary non-polyposis colorectal cancer (HNPCC) syndrome due to the presence of inherited mutations in mismatch repair genes (MSH-2, MLH-1, MSH-6) [24] and in 20-40% of sporadic endometrioid carcinoma, by mismatch repair deficiency due to inactivation of MLH-1 by promoter methylation [25].

PIK3CA mutation occurs in 36-39% of endometrioid adenocarcinomas [26,27] and coexists with PTEN mutation in 27% of endometrial adenocarcinomas. Some authors have claimed it is associated to elevated risk of myometrial invasion and to higher histologic grade [28,29]. Mutation of ARID1A gene, a tumor suppressor gene involved in chromatin remodeling processes, with loss of the corresponding protein BAF 250, has recently been identified in 50% of ovarian clear cell and in 30% of ovarian endometrioid carcinomas [30]. More recently, loss of protein BAF 250 has been demonstrated to be a frequent event in uterine low grade endometrioid carcinomas [31] and, also, in high grade endometrial carcinomas, precisely in 39% of grade 3 endometrioid carcinomas in the uterus [32].

On the other hand, type II non-endometrioid carcinomas are characterized by chromosomal instability, showing loss of heterozygosis (LOH) at multiple foci and by alteration of p53 [33]. P53 is a tumor suppressor gene located on chromosome 17p13.1 that regulates many cellular processes like DNA repair and cell cycle arrest; its mutation occurs in about 90% [34,35,36] of uterine serous carcinomas and its putative precursor endometrial intraepithelial carcinoma (EIC) and in grade 3 endometrial adenocarcinomas and clear cell carcinomas, but less frequently [36,37]. It seems to be associated to poor prognosis [29] (Table 2).

Table 2. More frequent molecular alterations in endometrial adenocarcinomas

Mutation	Incidence
PTEN	35-80% endometrioid adenocarcinomas
CTNNB-1	25-40% endometrioid adenocarcinomas
MI	20-40% endometrioid adenocarcinomas
K-RAS	14-36% endometrioid adenocarcinomas
ARID1-A	30-39% endometrioid adenocarcinomas
p53	90% non-endometrioid adenocarcinomas

Somatic mutation in PPP2R1A, a subunit of protein phosphatase 2A, was observed in 19,2% of type II uterine carcinomas and in only 6,7% of type I uterine endometrioid adenocarcinomas [38]. Recently, genomic studies employing cDNA microarray technology have identified other genes that can help to discriminate between the two types of endometrial adenocarcinomas [6,39,40], like, for instance, EST KIAA1324, identified as one of the best distinguishing molecular signatures [40].

Diagnosis of Malignancy

The pathologist is required making diagnosis of endometrial cancer on endometrial biopsy, before any surgical decision, or on surgical specimen of hysterectomy, to stage the carcinoma. In endometrial biopsy or curettage specimen, one of the three following criteria are required to make diagnosis of cancer [41]:

- a *back-to-back* proliferation of endometrial glands occupying an area measuring at least 2x2 mm;
- an extensive papillary pattern;
- a desmoplastic or fibroblastic stroma infiltrated by irregular glands.

Moreover, in order to ensure proper management of the patient, the pathologist should establish if the tumor represents an endometrial primary or derives from another site (i.e., cervix or extrauterine primary). To this purpose, morphologic and, overall, immunohistochemical features are useful. Papillae in endometrial cancers are thin, sometimes filled with foamy cells and squamous metaplastic morules are not rare; on the contrary, papillae in endocervical cancers are thick and lack foamy cells. Adjacent to invasive component is often found atypical glandular hyperplasia (AH) in endometrial cancer and in situ adenocarcinoma (AIS) in endocervical cancer. Endometrial cancers express vimentin (VIM), estrogen and progesterone receptors (ER, PR) and are carcinoembryonic antigen (CEA) negative.

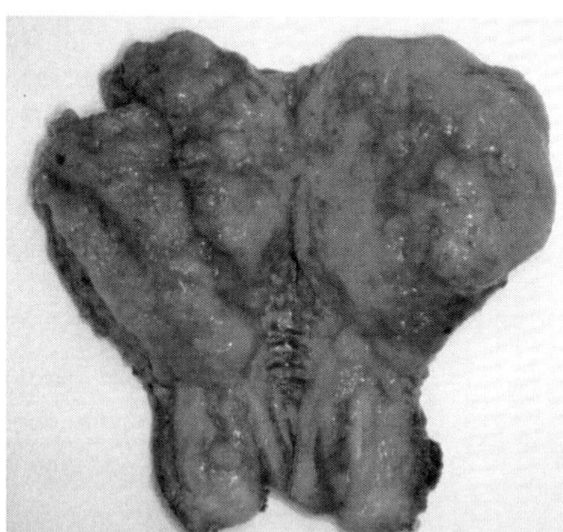

Figure 1. Gross appearance of endometrial carcinoma as vegetant, endoluminal mass.

Endocervical adenocarcinomas are usually CEA and p16 positive, while don't express VIM and hormonal receptors [42]. However, it is necessary to remember that some high-grade endometrial carcinomas, like serous, clear cell and grade 3 endometrioid, can diffusely express p16 [41]. On the surgical specimen, gross appearance is variable, ranging from a diffuse thickening of endometrium to huge, vegetant, polypoid masses (Figure 1) to deeply infiltrating whitish lesions. Tumoral masses can be single or multiple, usually originate from posterior wall of uterine corpus [33] and can also involve endocervix.

Diagnosis of Histotype

The current World Health Organization (WHO) histologic classification of endometrial carcinoma is shown in table 3-1 [43]. We will examine every histologic subtype in this classification as well as other variants not listed by WHO (Table 3).

Table 3. WHO classification of endometrial carcinoma

Endometrioid adenocarcinoma	Serous carcinoma
- Variants	Clear cell carcinoma
with squamous differentiation	Mixed carcinoma
villoglandular	Squamous carcinoma
secretory	Transitional carcinoma
ciliated cells	Undifferentiated carcinoma
Mucinous adenocarcinoma	Others

Legend. WHO: World Health Organization.

Endometrioid Adenocarcinoma (Type I)

Endometrioid adenocarcinoma is the most common histotype arising in the endometrium; it is characterized by glandular growth pattern, resembling normal proliferative endometrium. The typical growth pattern is represented by proliferation of *back-to-back* oval or rounded glands, lined by cylindric epithelial cells with eosinophilic or amphophilic cytoplasm and mild to moderate nuclear atypia. Endometrioid adenocarcinoma can also show more complex pattern of growth like papillary, villoglandular, cribriform and solid areas. Individual tumors can show patchy, focal changes in ciliated, mucinous, squamous cytology.

One of main problems for the pathologist in reporting endometrial adenocarcinoma is to establish the presence of myoinvasion. Endometrial adenocarcinoma can be limited to endometrial mucosa (intraendometrial adenocarcinoma) or can invade myometrium; the endometrial-myometrial boundary is irregular and, therefore, difficult to be assessed; moreover, endometrioid adenocarcinoma can involve adenomyosis foci. While CD10 staining is useful to find adenomyosis foci, highlighting glands-associated stromal cells, is not helpful in the differential diagnosis between invasive carcinoma and adenomyosis involved by carcinoma, because spindled cells surrounding malignant glands may express this marker [44]. Disorganized glandular arrangement and desmoplastic stromal reaction are the clues to diagnose invasion.

The other main difficulty that the pathologist meets is the assessment of lymphatic vessel invasion (LVI). Since the presence of LVI can increase the possibility of lymph node metastasis, it should be reported by the pathologist. Usually, neoplastic cells inside vessels assume an "histiocytoid" appearance and can be highlighted by dense perivascular lymphoid infiltrate. Immunohistochemical staining for D2-40 can be helpful to evidence lymphatic endothelium and to differentiate true LVI from pseudo-invasion due to artifactual displacement during sectioning of the hysterectomy specimen.

Variants of Endometrioid Adenocarcinoma

Four histologic variants of endometrioid adenocarcinoma are recognized [43]. *Endometrioid adenocarcinoma, with squamous differentiation.* Squamous differentiation can be found in different forms: morular (rounded intraluminal masses), islands of clear squamous cells (due to intracytoplasmic glycogen accumulation), sheets of spindled cells, as expression of immature, abortive, squamous differentiation and nests with the appearance of squamous carcinoma [41].

The use of old terms like "adenoacanthoma" and "adenosquamous carcinoma" to indicate well or poorly differentiated squamous component is discouraged today and the WHO recommends the term "adenocarcinoma with squamous differentiation". In many studies, differentiation of the squamous component was shown to parallel that of the glandular component and the prognosis can be predicted by the glandular grade alone [33].

Endometrioid adenocarcinoma, villoglandular variant. The villoglandular variant is characterized by finger-like, slender, long papillae lined by slightly atypical columnar cells, with preservation of polarity of the nuclei. Since these tumors are well differentiated, they are associated to a favorable outcome [45], but tumors with this growth pattern in the invasive component have been found associated to poorer prognosis [46].

Endometrioid adenocarcinoma, secretory variant. It is so called because it resembles early or mid-secretory endometrium. This very rare variant is morphologically characterized by subnuclear or supranuclear glycogen vacuoles (Figure 2). Secretory differentiation can be related to circulating progestins or can be independent from hormonal state. This histotype has, generally, good prognosis [47,48,49].

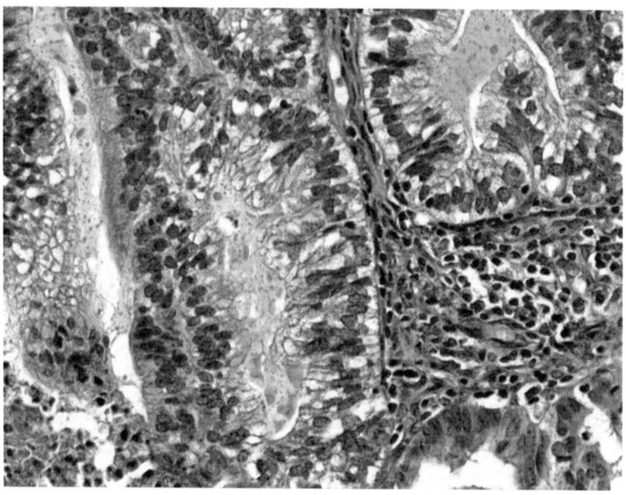

Figure 2. Subnuclear vacuoles are evident in secretory variant of endometrioidadenocarcinoma.

Endometrioid adenocarcinoma, ciliated-cell variant. While focal ciliated cells can be occasionally found in conventional endometrioid carcinoma, extensive ciliated change, in at least 75% of the tumors cells, is rarely found. This variant seems to be associated to good prognosis [50].

Other Variants (not Listed by WHO)

Endometrioid adenocarcinoma, with microglandular pattern. This variant has a typical micropapillary growth pattern with luminal eosinophilic secretions and neutrophils, simulating microglandular hyperplasia of the cervix.

Endometrioid adenocarcinoma, with small non villous papillae. The hallmark of this variant is the presence of small intraluminal papillae without fibrous cores, considered expression of abortive squamous differentiation. In both these variants, morphologic features have no influence on the prognosis.

Endometrioid adenocarcinoma, with mucinous differentiation. Mucinous differentiation is frequently present in endometrioid adenocarcinoma, being characterized by extracellular-intraglandular mucin; on the opposite site, intracytoplasmic mucin is typically found in mucinous adenocarcinoma.

Endometrioid adenocarcinoma, oxyphilic (oncocytic) variant. Rarely, endometrioid adenocarcinomas can be composed of predominant oxyphilic cells, with abundant eosinophilic cytoplasm, rich in mitochondria [51] (Figure 3).

Endometrioid adenocarcinoma, with Sertoliform differentiation. Rare cases of endometrioid adenocarcinoma with closely packed tubules or cords of columnar cells with apical clear cytoplasm, resembling sex cord-stromal tumors have been reported (Figure 4). The clinical behavior of these carcinomas seems to be similar to that of typical endometrioid adenocarcinoma [52,53].

Rarely, endometrioid adenocarcinomas contain signet ring cells, trophoblastic and giant cell, representing a poorly differentiated component [44].

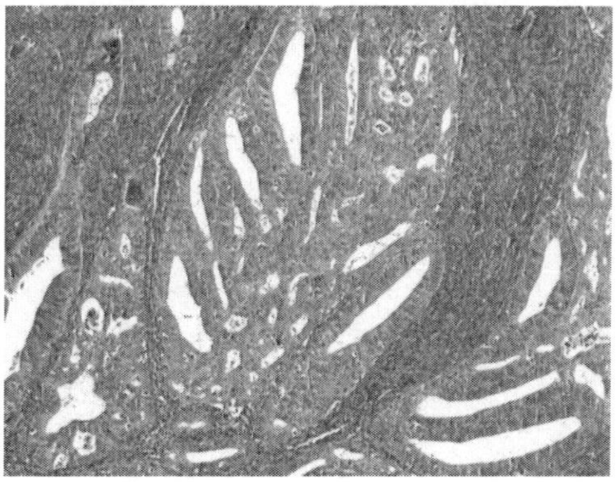

Figure 3. Abundant eosinophilic cytoplasm in oxyphilic variant of endometrioid adenocarcinoma.

Mucinous Adenocarcinoma (Type I)

WHO defines mucinous adenocarcinoma a primary endometrial adenocarcinoma in which most of the tumoral cells contain intracytoplasmic mucin, without specifying the percentage of these cells [43].

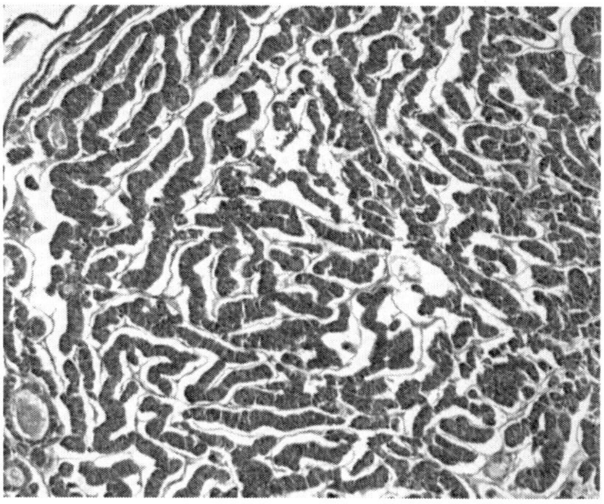

Figure 4. Cords-like growth pattern in sertoliform variant of endometrioid adenocarcinoma.

Some authors have proposed the criterium of > 50% of the tumor cells to have mucinous differentiation to make this diagnosis [54], others the criterium of > 70% [55]; in practice, it is widely accepted the first one [41]. These tumors may have a great architectural complexity, with patterns ranging from glandular, papillary to solid areas. They are usually low grade and the clinical behavior is not different from that of conventional endometrial adenocarcinoma.

Serous Carcinoma (Type II)

Serous carcinoma represents the most frequent histotype of type II endometrial adenocarcinomas, accounting for 10% of all endometrial cancers [56]. It is a typical high grade neoplasia, with papillary or solid growth pattern and marked nuclear atypia. It can arise as small intraepithelial foci in endometrial polyps (EIC) and be associated to diffuse peritoneal disease [57,58], notwithstanding absence of invasion; in this case it is defined as *endometrial intraepithelial carcinoma, minimal uterine serous carcinoma, endometrial carcinoma in situ*. Extensive peritoneal involvement has been explained in different ways: tubal reflux [59], multifocal disease process, spread of carcinomatous cells from fallopian mucosa into the uterine cavity and peritoneal cavity at the meantime [60]. On the other side, serous carcinoma can be deeply infiltrating and associated with extensive lymphatic invasion.

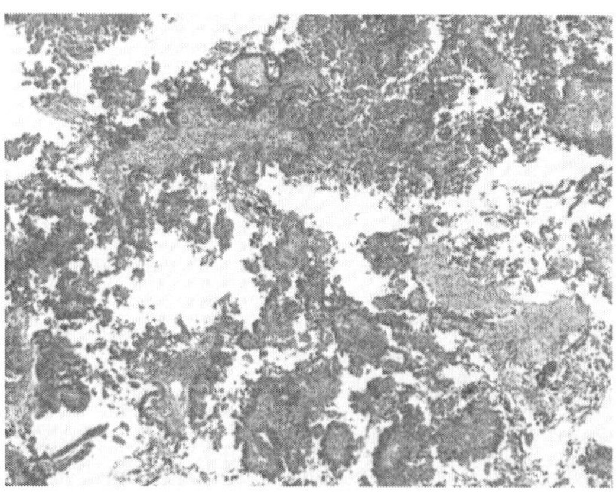

Figure 5. Broad, thick papillae are typical of serous carcinoma adenocarcinoma.

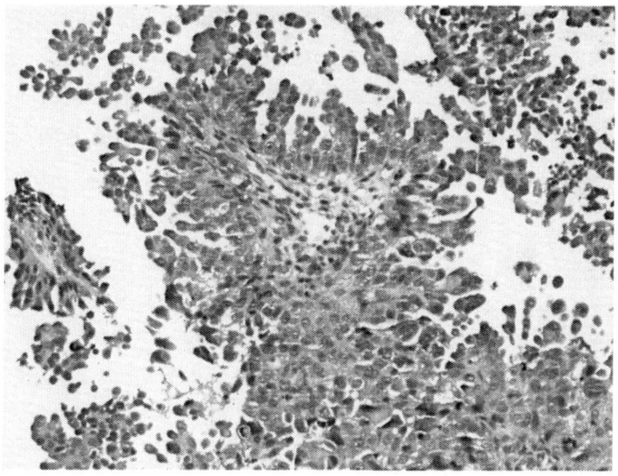

Figure 6. Clusters of highly atypical cells tend to detach from fibrous cores.

Morphologically, papillae are typically thick, with wide fibrous cores, covered by pluristratified, non cohesive, budding and tufting atypical cells (Figures 5,6); nuclei are hyperchromatic, sometimes bizarre, with evident eosinophilic nucleoli and atypical, numerous mitotic figures are easily found. Psammoma bodies are observed in 30% of the cases [44].

Immunohistochemically, serous carcinoma diffusely and strongly express p53 (Figure 7) and p16 stainings, are ER and PR negative and have high levels of Ki67 expression (> 40%). WT_1 expression is rarely (< 10%) seen in serous carcinoma of endometrial origin in contrast to over 90% of extrauterine carcinomas [33].

Clinically, it is a very aggressive neoplasm, presenting at advanced stage and being associated to poor prognosis (14% of 10-year survival).

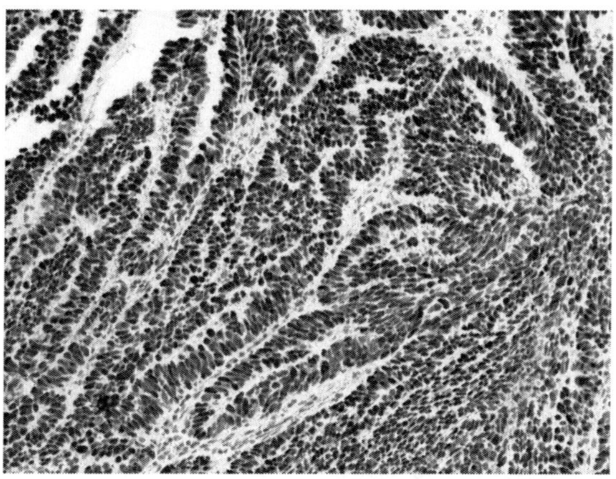

Figure 7. Diffuse and strong immunostaining for p53 in serous carcinoma.

Clear Cell Adenocarcinoma (Type II)

Clear cell adenocarcinoma represents 1-6% of all endometrial carcinomas. It occurs in the old age and is morphologically similar to its equivalent in other female genital organs, like ovary, cervix and vagina. It has a papillary, glandular and solid growth pattern (Figure 8); its cells are characterized by abundant, clear, glycogen-rich cytoplasm, *hobnail* appearance (Figure 9) and marked nuclear atypia. Papillae have typically hyalinized cores;

intracytoplasmic hyalin bodies and eosinophilic intraluminal material can be found [61,62]. Mitotic figures are sparse. It is by definition considered an high grade tumor by WHO classification similarly to serous carcinoma. Immunohistochemically, clear cell adenocarcinoma is negative for progesterone receptor, has a high Ki67 proliferation index and variable expression of p53 and ER [63,64]. It has, like serous carcinoma, poor prognosis.

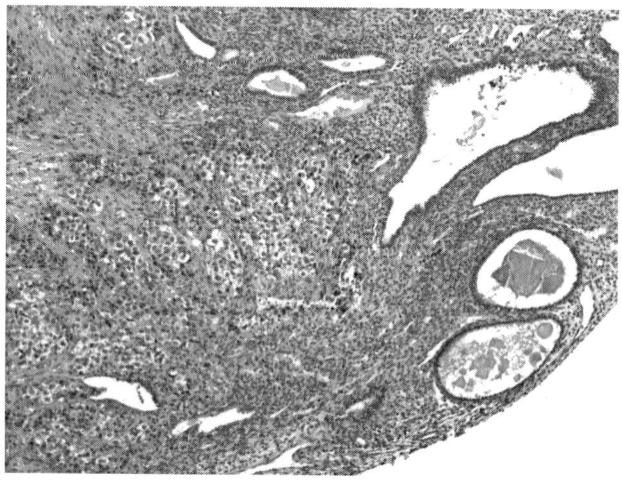

Figure 8. Solid growth pattern clear cell carcinoma in endometrial polyp.

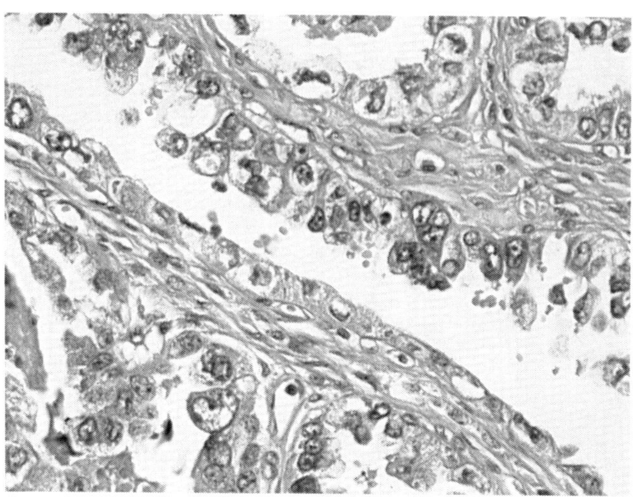

Figure 9. Clear cytoplasm and hobnail, atypical nuclei.

Mixed Adenocarcinomas

Sometimes, different histotypes and, especially, type I endometrial adenocarcinomas and type II carcinomas can coexist; the minor component should comprise at least 10% of the neoplasm. In these cases, the prognosis depends on the amount of the most aggressive component [44].

Squamous Cell Carcinoma (Type II)

It is a very rare histotype in endometrium, accounting for < 1% of all endometrial cancers [65]. It is necessary to exclude the presence of coexisting endometrial adenocarcinoma (endometrioid adenocarcinoma with extensive squamous differentiation) and of synchronous or pre-existing invasive squamous carcinoma of the uterine cervix.

Transitional Cell Carcinoma

The transitional features, similar to those seen in transitional cell carcinoma of the urinary tract, should comprise > 90% of the tumor to formulate this diagnosis. More commonly, these features present admixed with other carcinoma subtypes, such as endometrioid, serous or clear cell carcinomas.

Small Cell Carcinoma

Small cell carcinoma, similar to small cell carcinoma arising in the lung, is much more less common in endometrium than is counterpart in the cervix. In literature, there are single case reports, sometimes associated to paraneoplastic syndrome [66,67]; the larger series are a collection of 16 cases reported by Huntsman et al. [68] and three cases reported by Katahira et al. [69]. The cells are little or medium sized and are arranged in diffuse sheets, cords or nests (Figure 10).

Nuclei are monomorphous, with coarse or granular chromatin and inconspicuous nucleoli and, frequently, present *crushing* artefacts. Mitotic figures as well as apoptotic bodies are numerous and necrosis is easily found.

Immunohistochemically, epithelial markers like cytokeratin (CK), epithelial membrane antigen (EMA) or Cam 5,2 are usually positive, although they can be focal [41]; in particular, we have found CK7 negativity and CK20 dot-like positivity in one case (unpublished data, Figure 11).

Moreover, the tumor cells show positivity for one or more neuroendocrine markers like neuron-specific enolase (NSE), CD56, CD57, synaptophysin, chromogranin, glucagon and calcitonin [68,70]. Intense staining for p16 and p53 has also been described [71,72]. These tumors usually have ominous prognosis, except when polypoid or arising in polyps [72].

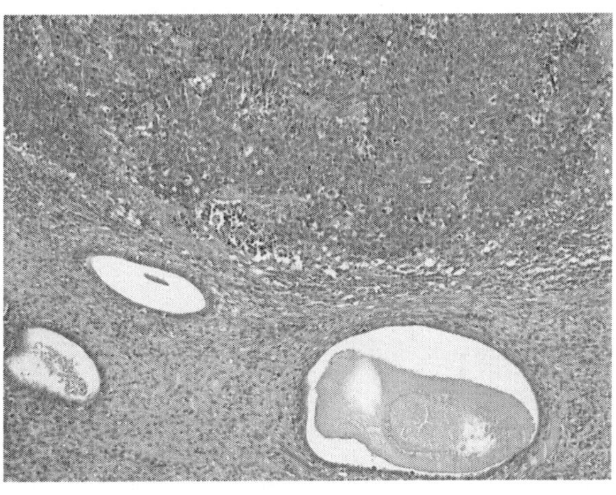

Figure 10. Insular growth pattern in small cell carcinoma.

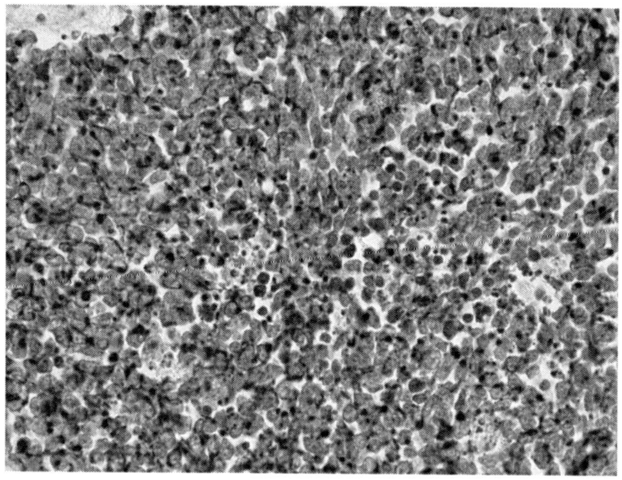

Figure 11. Strong, dot-like CK20 staining in small cell carcinoma.

Large Cell Carcinoma

Less commonly reported is large cell carcinoma. This tumor is characterized by predominant insular growth pattern, but also rosettes can be found [73], geographic (infart-like) necrosis, vascular involvement, abundant, granular eosinophilic cytoplasm, vescicular nuclei with prominent eosinophilic nucleoli and variable expression of neuroendocrine markers. Like in small cell carcinoma, p16 and p53 are often overexpressed [72].

Rarely these neuroendocrine carcinomas present purely; they are usually mixed with conventional endometrial adenocarcinomas [73], but their recognition is very important to clinical purposes because they require different therapeutic regimens.

Undifferentiated Carcinoma

Until a few years ago, there was no standardized definition for this type of tumor. WHO defined undifferential carcinoma of the endometrium in a vague manner, like a "malignant tumor of epithelial structure that is too poorly differentiated to be placed in any other category of carcinomas" [43].

Other authors enclosed in this category carcinomas with minor foci of endometrioid glands, carcinomas with serous type, slit-like glands or papillae and neoplasms traditionally included in the neuroendocrine carcinoma group [74,75]. Only recently, this entity has been recognized like a distinct histopathologic type characterized by "medium-size, monotonous cells in a patternless fashion, with a complete absence of glandular differentiation and with absent or minimal expression of neuroendocrine markers" [76]. This type of tumor has a diffuse, non cohesive, non nested, non trabecular, non glandular pattern of growth (Figure 12); sometimes, cells can assume rabdoid features, resembling lymphoma or plasmocytoma [76,75].

Immunohistochemically, ER, PR and E-cadherin are negative, EMA is positive in 10-20% of cells, CK is positive in 5-10% of cells; in particular, CK18 is expressed, but very strongly, in only rare, scattered cells [6]; neuroendocrine markers like synaptophysin and chromogranin can be expressed, but in less than 10% of cells [78].

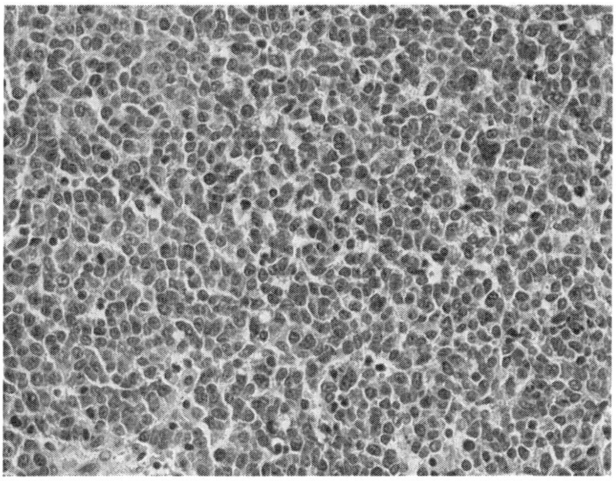

Figure 12. Monotonous, medium-sized, non-cohesive cells with diffuse growth pattern in undifferentiated carcinoma.

When the undifferentiated tumor is associated to a well differentiated endometrioid carcinoma, it can be defined as *dedifferentiated endometrial carcinoma* [6]. Since this pathologic entity is often under-recognized, an extensive sampling is recommended. Its treatment requires an aggressive therapeutic approach.

Finally, a special subgroup of endometrial carcinomas is represented by tumors occurring in Lynch Syndrome (LS), an autosomal dominant cancer susceptibility syndrome characterized by high rate of colorectal, endometrial, ovarian, gastric and urinary cancers and by germ line mutations in one of DNA mismatch repair genes, like hMSH6, hMSH2, hMLH1, hPMS2 [79].

LS-related endometrial cancers have peculiar epidemiologic, clinical and morphologic features: they typically arise in young age women (45-55 years) [80], are not obesity-related, have a more unfavorable course than sporadic cancers, because are more frequently non-endometrioid, high grade, high stage cancers, prone to deep myometrial infiltration and lymph vascular invasion [81,82]. Moreover, unusual morphologic features like high grade, bizarre nuclei, clear cytoplasm, small hyalinized papillae and unusual variants like dedifferentiated/undifferentiated carcinomas are frequently found in LS-related cancers [83,84].

Prognostic Factors in Endometrial Carcinoma

Tumor Type

Histotype has great influence on prognosis. Endometrioid adenocarcinoma, including its variants like villoglandular adenocarcinoma, secretory carcinoma, endometrioid carcinoma with squamous differentiation and mucinous adenocarcinoma have a relatively good prognosis. On the other hand, non-endometrioid carcinomas, like serous carcinoma, clear cell carcinoma, undifferentiated carcinoma and neuroendocrine carcinomas have unfavorable prognosis.

Grading

Histologic grading is clinically prognostic. The grading standard of endometrial endometrioid adenocarcinoma, the International Federation of Gynecology and Obstetrics (FIGO) system [85,86] is based on both architectural and cytologic features:

- Grade 1: ≤5% of a solid, non-morular component;
- Grade 2: 6% - 50% of a solid, non-morular component;
- Grade 3: ≥50% of a solid, non-morular component.

Nuclear grading relies on variation in size and shape of nuclei, variation of staining intensity and distribution of chromatin, presence of prominent nucleoli and of abnormal mitotic figures. The histologic grade should be raised by one level when significant cytologic atypia is observed [33].

This three-tiered grading system is applied to endometrioid and mucinous histotypes and classifies adenocarcinomas as well differentiated (Grade 1), moderately differentiated (Grade 2) and poorly differentiated (Grade 3). Serous, clear cell and undifferentiated tumors are not graded; by definition, they are considered high grade.

The prognostic value of the FIGO grading system has been demonstrated in one univariate study of more than 600 patients with clinical Stage I and/or occult Stage II endometrioid adenocarcinoma. The 5-year relative survival for the patients with Grade 1 tumors was 94%, while it decreased to 84% and 72% for patients with Grade 2 and 3 tumors respectively [44].

More recently several attempts to move to a two-tiered grading system have been proposed [87,88,89] overall in order to improve the reproducibility of diagnosis, but they have not been universally accepted and adopted [90].

Stage and Depth of Myometrial Invasion

The 1988 International Federation of Gynecology and Obstetrics (FIGO) staging system has been found to be the single most important prognostic factor for patients with endometrial carcinoma [44,85]. The 5-year disease free survival is 90% for Stage I, 83% for Stage II and 43% for Stage III tumors. Recently, in 2009, changes in staging carcinoma of uterine corpus have been defined: endocervical glandular involvement only should be considered as stage I and no longer as stage, positive cytology has to be reported separately without changing the stage (Table 4). Tumors with more than 50% myometrial thickness invasion have increased risk of extrauterine metastases, including pelvic and aortic lymph nodes metastases, requiring more aggressive surgical staging [91].

Measurement of depth of invasion, expressed as a percentage of the total myometrial thickness requires a combination of gross and microscopic evaluation and can be problematic because of the difficulty to exactly identify the endometrial-myometrial junction.

Vascular Invasion

Presence of vascular invasion is an independent predictor of recurrence [92] and outcome, being correlated to risk of lymph node metastases. To highlight true neoplastic emboli, immunohistochemical staining for Ulex VIII and DB40 can be useful.

Table 4. FIGO staging of endometrial carcinoma (2009)

I	Tumor confined to the corpus uteri
IA	No or less than half myometrial invasion
IB	Invasion equal to or more than half of the myometrium
II	Tumor invades cervical stroma but does not extend beyond the uterus
III	Local and/or regional spread of the tumor
III	A Tumor invades the serosa of the corpus uteri and/or adnexae
IIIB	Vaginal and/or parametrial involvement
IIIC	Metastases to pelvic and/or para-aortic lymph nodes
IIIC1	Positive pelvic nodes
IIIC2	Positive para-aortic lymph nodes with or without positive pelvic lymph nodes
IV	Tumor invades bladder and/or bowel mucosa, and/or distant metastases
IVA	Tumor invasion of bladder and/or bowel mucosa
IVB	Distant metastases, including intra-abdominal metastases and/or inguinal lymph nodes

Legend. FIGO: International Federation of Gynecology and Obstetrics.

Age

Younger women have better prognosis then old ones. In one study, 5-year survival was 96% for women aged 40-49 years compared with 53% for women of 70-79 years [93]; this is because of the prevalence of high grade non-endometrioid type tumors in older patients.

Steroid Hormone Receptors

Hormones play an important role in the etiopathogenesis of endometrioid (type I) carcinomas. Generally, all endometrioid carcinomas express ER, while PR expression depends on the differentiation of the tumor [94]. Some authors have claimed that immunohistochemical detection of PR can be an independent predictor of clinical course [95,96].

Other Factors

DNA ploidy has been shown to be a useful prognostic factor; about 67% of endometrioid carcinomas are diploid, whereas diploid DNA is found in only 45% of non-endometrioid carcinomas [44].

The expression of some immunohistochemical markers like ER, C-erb B2, p53 and Ki67 has been suggested as of prognostic value, but their significance needs more evaluation, just like molecular alterations like assessment of microsatellite instability and alterations of PTEN and CTNB-1 (beta-catenin) [44].

Beyond Bokhman's Model

Although the Bokhman's dualistic model, relying on molecular data, is appealing to pathologists and clinicians because it provides relevant behavioral information, it seems to be too simplistic [6].

Not all low grade endometrioid adenocarcinomas have indolent behavior, showing deep myometrial infiltration and recurrence and, on the other side, some grade 3 endometrioid adenocarcinomas are superficially invasive and show low risk of recurrence after surgery [6]. Moreover, it is widely accepted that a non endometrioid component can originate from a pre-existing endometrioid adenocarcinoma [33], for probable expansion of an aggressive subclone [3] and that some special histotypes don't exactly fit in any one of the two groups [44]. Overall, it is not always easy for the pathologist to exactly classify an endometrial cancer according to Bockman's categories. So, the term *endometrial carcinoma with ambiguous features* was introduced by R. Soslow to indicate tumors with uninformative morphologic features [97]. In these challenging cases, the introduction of immunohistochemistry or other ancillary techniques could help to elucidate the identity of these tumors.

Some authors suggested to separate endometrial cancers in three categories, according to immunophenotype and to mRNA expression patterns in PI3K/Akt [98,99,29]: the first one, clinically favorable, mostly composed of low grade endometrioid carcinomas, with a small number of high grade carcinomas; the third one, unfavorable, represented by high grade carcinomas; the middle one containing a broad range of types and grades with intermediate prognosis. The low grade endometrioid carcinomas showed ER expression, frequent PTEN mutations and MI, but lacked p53, p16 and HER2 expression; high grade carcinomas, including FIGO 3 endometrioid, non-endometrioid and mixed epithelial carcinomas showed ubiquitous p53 mutations, p16 overexpression and frequent PIK3CA mutations, without PTEN mutation or MI; a third group, represented by a heterogeneous collection of high grade carcinomas, showed not infrequent PTEN, p53, PIK3CA mutations, p16 overexpression and low rates of MI.

Focusing on the issue of endometrioid carcinoma with ambiguous features, an example of ambiguous endometrial carcinoma could be a tumor with a low grade architecture associated to diffuse high nuclear atypia; immunohistochemical stainings for p53, p16, PTEN and hormone receptors could help to distinguish serous carcinomas from endometrioid carcinomas. In particular, loss of PTEN expression together with non overexpression of p16 predicts FIGO grade 3 endometrioid carcinoma with a sensitivity of 90% and specificity of 96,8%, in one study [100]. Other authors have found loss of PTEN expression in 60% of endometrioid carcinomas, but also in 10% of non endometrioid tumors [97].

Sometimes, diagnosis of serous carcinomas with p53 mutations that results in truncated proteins not detectable with commercially available p53 antibodies, can rely on high Ki67 or p16 overexpression, in presence of negative p53 [97].

Other examples of morphologically ambiguous endometrial carcinomas are tumors resembling clear cell carcinoma, but with cylindric or highly pleomorphic cells, tumors resembling serous carcinomas, but with clear cell and tumors thought to be mixed. [97]. Again, immunohistochemistry can be useful, since clear cell carcinomas less frequently than endometrioid carcinomas express hormone receptors, don't show PTEN mutations and have higher proliferative indexes with Ki67; compared to serous carcinomas, Ki67, p16 and p53 overexpression rates are lower, while, on the other hand, diffuse and strong staining for hepatocyte nuclear factor-1beta has been reported [101,102,103].

In conclusion, serous carcinomas can be diagnosed with certainty in the presence of the least focal papillary growth pattern and marked nuclear atypia and endometrioid carcinomas can confidently be diagnosed when glandular and papillary areas are associated to low nuclear grade and when solid growth pattern is accompanied by squamous, mucinous, secretory changes. When a morphologically ambiguous tumor is found in an endometrial biopsy or curettage, a attempt to assess grade and tumor type should be made [97]. FIGO grading system should not be applied when tumor type is uncertain; in these cases, the binary grading system proposed by Gilks [88] should be used. Cancers showing papillary or solid architecture, high nuclear grade and > 5 mitoses x 10HPF should be diagnosed as high grade tumors [97]; staining for p53 could be useful to separate low from high grade tumors and to individuate tumors prone to peritoneal dissemination [104]; afterword, immunohistochemical markers can be applied as previously shown.

If, notwithstanding immunohistochemistry, the tumor is still ambiguous, the best thing to do should be assign a grade, with an accurate description of morphologic features and of differential diagnoses [97].

References

[1] Bokhman, JV. To pathogenetic types of endometrial carcinoma. *Gynecol. Oncol.* 1983;15:10-7.

[2] Lax, SF. Molecular genetic pathways in various types of endometrial carcinoma: from a phenotypical to a molecular-based classification. *Virchows Arch.* 2004;444:213-23.

[3] Matias-Guiu, X; Catasus, L; Bussaglia, E; et al. Molecular pathology of endometrial hyperplasia and carcinoma. *Hum. Pathol.* 2001;32:569-77.

[4] Steck, PA; Pershouse, MA; Jasser, SA; et al. Identification of a candidate tumor suppressor gene, MMAC1, et chromosome 10q23.3 that is mutated in multiple advanced cancers. *Nat. Genet.* 1997;15:356-62.

[5] Li, J; Yen, C; Liaw, D; et al. PTEN, a putative protein tyrosine phosphatase gene mutated in human brain, breast, and prostate cancer. *Science* 1997;275:2742-6.

[6] Soslow, RA; Goldblum, JR. *Current Concepts in Gynecologic Pathology: Epithelial Tumors of Gynecologic Tract. Surgical Pathology Clinics.* Philadelphia: Saunders; 2011.

[7] Choe, G; Horvath, S; Cloughesy, TF; et al. Analysis of the phosphatidylinositol 3-kinase signaling pathway in glioblastoma patients in vivo. *Cancer Research* 2003;63:2742-6.

[8] Terakawa, N; Kanamori, Y; Yoshida, S. Loss of PTEN expression followed by Akt phosphorylation is a poor prognostic factor for patients with endometrial cancer. *Endocr. Relat. Cancer* 2003;10:203-8.

[9] Mutter, GL; Lin, MC; Fitzgerald, JT; et al. Altered PTEN expression as a diagnostic marker for the earliest endometrial precancers. *J. Natl. Cancer Inst.* 2000;92:924-30.

[10] Kong, D; Suzuki, A; Zou, TT; et al. PTEN1 is frequently mutated in primary endometrial carcinomas. *Nat. Genet.* 1997;17:143-4.

[11] Bussaglia, E; del Rio, E; Matias Guiu, X; et al. PTEN mutations in endometrial carcinomas: a molecular and clinicopathologic analysis of 38 cases. *Hum. Pathol.* 2000;31:312-7.

[12] Minaguchi, T; Yoshikawa, H; Oda, K; et al. PTEN mutation located only outside exons 5,6 and 7 is an independent predictor of favorable survival in endometrial carcinomas. *Clin. Cancer Res.* 2001;7:2636-42.

[13] Risinger, JI; Hayes, K; Maxwell, GL; et al. PTEN mutation in endometrial cancer is associated with favorable clinical and pathologic characteristics. *Clin. Cancer Res.* 1998;4:3005-10.

[14] Kanamori, Y; Kigawa, J; Itamochi, H; et al. PTEN expression is associated with prognosis for patients with advanced endometrial carcinoma undergoing postoperative chemotherapy. *Int. J. Cancer* 2002;100:686-9.

[15] Uegaki, K; Kanamori, Y; Kigawa, J; et al. PYEN-positive and phosphorylated-Akt-negative expression is a predictor of survival for patients with advanced endometrial carcinoma. *Oncol. Rep.* 2005;14:389-92.

[16] Fukuchi, T; Sakamoto, M; Tsuda, H; et al. Beta-catenin mutation in carcinoma of the uterine endometrium. *Cancer Res.* 1998;58:3526-8.

[17] Lagarda, H; Catasus, L; Arguelles, R; et al. K-ras mutations in endometrial carcinoma with microsatellite instability. *J. Pathol.* 2001;193:193-9.

[18] Sasaki, H; Nishii, H; Takahashi, H; et al. Mutation of the Ki-ras proto-oncogene in human endometrial hyperplasia and carcinoma. *Cancer Res.* 1993;53(8):1906-10.

[19] Fujimoto, I; Shimizu, Y; Hirai, Y; e al. Studies on ras oncogene activation in endometrial carcinoma. *Gynecol. Oncol.* 1993;48:196-202.

[20] Chon, HS; Hu, W; Kavanagh, JJ. Targeted therapies in gynecologic cancers. *Cur. Cancer Drug Targets* 2006;6:333-63.

[21] Catasus, L; Gallardo, A; Prat, J. Molecular genetics of endometrial carcinoma. *Diagn. Histopathol.* 2009;15:554-63.

[22] Engelman, JA; Chen, L; Than, X; et al. Effecive use of PI3K and MAK inhibitors to treat mutant Kras G12D and PIK3CA H1047R murine lung cancers. *Nat. Med.* 2008;14:1351-6.

[23] Ihle, NT; Lemos, R Jr; Wipf, P; et al. Mutations in the phosphatidylinositol 3-kinase pathway predict for antitumor activity of the inhibitor PX-866 whereas oncogenic Ras is a dominant predictor for resistence. *Cancer Res.* 2009;69:143-50.

[24] Parc, YR; Halling, KC; Burgart, LG; et al. Microsatellite instability and hMLH1/hMSH2 expression in young endometrial carcinoma patients: association with family history and histopathology. *Int. J. Cancer* 2000; 86:60-6.

[25] Esteller, M; Levine, R; Bylin, SB; et al. MLH1 promoter hypermethylation is associated with the microsatellite instability phenotype in sporadic endometrial carcinomas. *Oncogene* 1998;17:2413-17.

[26] Oda, K; Stokoe, D; Taketani, Y; et al. High frequency of coexistent mutations of PIK3CA and PTEN genes in endometrial carcinoma. *Cancer Res.* 2005;65:10669-73.

[27] Hayes, MP; Wang, H; Espinal-Witter, R; et al. PIK3CA and PTEN mutations in uterine endometrioid carcinoma and complex atypical hyperplasia. *Clin. Cancer Res.* 2006;12:5932-5.

[28] Catasus, L; Gallardo, A; Cuatrecasas, M; et al. PIK3-CA mutations in the kinase domain (exon 20) of uterine endometrial adenocarcinomas are associated with adverse prognostic parameters. *Mod. Pathol.* 2008;21:131-9.

[29] Catasus, L; Gallardo, A; Cuatrecasas, M; et al. Concomitant PI3K-AKT and p53 alterations in endometrial carcinomas are associated with poor prognosis. *Mod. Pathol.* 2009;22:522-9.
[30] Wiegand, KC; Shah, SP; Al-Agha, OM; et al. ARID1A mutations in endometriosis associated ovarian carcinomas. *N. Engl. J. Med.* 2010;363:1532-43.
[31] Guan, B; Mao, TL; Panuganti, PK; et al. Mutation and loss expression of ARID1A in uterine low-grade endometrioid carcinoma. *Am. J. Surg. Pathol.* 2011;35:625-32.
[32] Wiegand, KC; Lee, AF; Al-Agha, OM; et al. Loss of BAF250a (ARID1A) is frequent in high-grade endometrial carcinomas. *J. Pathol.* 2011;224:328-33.
[33] Robboy, SJ; Mutter, GL; Prat, J; et al. *Pathology of the Female Reproductive Tract.* II Ed. Philadelphia: Churchill Livingstone; 2009.
[34] Sherman, ME; Bur, ME; Kurman, RJ. P53 in endometrial cancer and its putative precursors: evidence for diverse pathways of tumorigenesis. *Hum. Pathol.* 1995;26:1268-74.
[35] Trahan, S; Tetu, B; Raymond, PE. Serous papillary carcinoma of the endometrium arising from endometrial polyps: a clinical, histological, and immunohistochemical study of 13 cases. *Hum. Pathol.* 2005;36:1316-21.
[36] Lax, SF; Kendall, B; Tashiro, H; et al. The frequency of p53, K-ras mutations, and microsatellite instability differs in uterine endometrioid and serous carcinoma: evidence of distinct molecular genetic pathways. *Cancer* 2000;88:814-24.
[37] An, HJ; Logani, S; Isacson, C; et al. Molecular characterization of uterine clear cell carcinoma. *Mod. Pathol.* 2004;17:530-7.
[38] Shih, IeM; Panuganti, PK; Kuo, KT; et al. Somatic mutations of PPP2R1A in ovarian and uterine carcinomas. *Am. J. Pathol.* 2011;178:1442-7.
[39] Risinger, JI; Maxwell, GL; Chandramouli, GV; et al. Microarray analisys reveals distinct gene expression profiles associated with different histologic types of endometrial cancer. *Cancer Res.* 2003;63:6-11.
[40] Maxwell, GL; Chandramouli, GV; Dainty, L; et al. Microarray analisys of endometrial carcinomas and mixed mullerian tumors reveals distinct gene expression profiles associated with different histologic types of uterine cancer. *Clin. Cancer Res.* 2005;11:4056-66.
[41] Malpica, A; Deavers, MT; Eusher, E. *Biopsy Interpretation of the Uterine Cervix and Corpus.* Philadelphia: Lippincot Williams and Wilkins; 2010.
[42] Zaino, RJ. The fruits of our labours: distinguishing endometrial from endocervical adenocarcinoma. *Int. J. Gynecol. Pathol.* 2002;21:1-3.
[43] Tavassoli, FA; Stratton, MR. *WHO Classification of Tumors: Pathology and Genetics of Tumors of the Breast and Female Genital Organs.* Lyon: IARC Press; 2003.
[44] Oliva, E; Malpica, A; Deavers, MT; Eusher, E. *Biopsy Interpretation of the Uterine Cervix and Corpus.* Philadelphia: Lippincot Williams and Wilkins; 2010.
[45] Esteller, M; Garcia, A; Martinez-Palones, JM; et al. Clinicopathologic features and genetic alterations in endometrioid carcinoma of the uterus with villoglandular differentiation. *Am. J. Clin. Pathol.* 1999;111:336-42.
[46] Ambros, RA; Ballouk, F; Malfetano, JH; et al. Significance of papillary (villoglandular) differentiation in endometrioid carcinoma of the uterus. *Am. J. Surg. Pathol.* 1994;18:569-75.

[47] Christopherson, WM; Alberhasky, RC; Connelly, PJ. Carcinoma of the endometrium: I. A clinicopathologic study of clear-cell carcinoma and secretory carcinoma. *Cancer* 1992;49:1511-23.

[48] Tobon, H; Watkins, GJ. Secretory adenocarcinoma of the endometrium. *Int. J. Gynecol. Pathol.* 1985;4:328-335.

[49] Silverberg, SG; Kurman, RJ. *Endometrial Carcinoma. Tumors of the uterine corpus and Gestational Trophoblastic Disease*. Washington, DC: Armed Forces Institute of Pathology; 1991.

[50] Hendrickson, MR; Kempson, RL. Ciliated carcinoma - a variant endometrial adenocarcinoma: a report of 10 cases. *Am. J. Pathol.* 1983;2:1-12.

[51] Silver, SA; Cheung, ANY; Tavassoli, FA. Oncocytic metaplasia and carcinoma of the endometrium: an immunohistochemical and ultrastructural study. *Int. J. Gynecol. Pathol.* 1999;18:12-19.

[52] Usadi, RS; Bentley, RC. Endometrioid carcinoma of the endometrium with sertoliform differentiation. *Int. J. Gynecol. Pathol.* 1995;14:360-64.

[53] Eichhorn, JH; Young, RH; Clement, PB. Sertoliform endometrial adenocarcinoma: a study of four cases. *Int. J. Gynecol .Pathol.* 1996;15:9-26.

[54] Ross, JC; Eifel, PJ; Cox, RS; et al. Primary mucinous adenocarcinoma of the endometrium . A clinicipathologic and histochemical study. *Am. J. Surg. Pathol.* 1983;7:715-29.

[55] Melham, MF; Tobon, H. Mucinous adenocarcinoma of the endometrium: a clinicopathological review of 18 cases. *Int. J. Gynecol. Pathol.* 1987;6:347-55.

[56] Bancher-Todesca, D; Neunteufel, W; Williams, KE; et al. Influence of postoperative treatment on survival in patients with uterine papillary serous carcinoma. *Gynecol. Oncol.* 1998;71:344-7.

[57] Wheeler, DT; Bell, KA; Kurman, RJ; et al. Minimal uterine serous carcinoma. *Ham. J. Surg. Pathol.* 2000;24:797-806.

[58] Soslow, RA; Pirog, E; Isacson, C. Endometrial intraepithelial carcinoma with associated peritoneal carcinomatosis. *Ham. J. Surg. Pathol.* 2000;24:726-32.

[59] Snyder, MJ; Bentley, R; Robboy, SJ. Transtubal spread of serous adenocarcinoma of the endometrium: an uderrecognized mechanism of metastis. *Int. J. Gynecol. Pathol.* 2006;25:155-60.

[60] Crum, CP; Drapkin, R; Miron, A; et al. The distal fallopian tube: a new model for pelvic serous carcinogenesis. *Curr. Opin. Obstet. Gynecol.* 2007;19:3-9.

[61] Kurman, RJ; Scully RE. Clear cell carcinoma of the endometrium: an analysis of 21 cases. *Cancer,* 1976;37:872-82.

[62] Kanbour-Shakir, A; Tobon, H. Primary clear cell carcinoma of the endometrium: a clinicopathologic study of 20 cases. *Int. J. Gynecol. Pathol.* 1991;10:67-78.

[63] Lax, SF; Pizer, ES; Ronnett, BM; et al. Clear cell carcinoma of the endometrium is characterized by a distinctive profile of p53, Ki-67, estrogen and progesterone receptor expression. *Hum. Pathol.* 1998;29:551-8.

[64] Vang, R; Whitaker, BP; Farhood, AI; et al. Immunohistochemical analysis of clear cell carcinoma of gynecologic tract. *Int. J. Gynecol. Pathol* 2001;20:252-9.

[65] Goodman, A; Zukerberg, LR; Rice, LW; et al. Squamous cell carcinoma of the endometrium: a report of eight cases and a review of the literarture. *Gynecol. Oncol.* 1996;61:54-60.

[66] Campo, E; Brunier, MN; Merino, MJ. Small cell carcinoma of the endometrium with associated ovular paraneoplastic syndrome. *Cancer* 1992;69:2283-8.

[67] Sekiguchi, I; Suzuki, M; Sato, I; et al. Rare case of small cell carcinoma arising from endometrium with paraneoplastic retinopathy. *Gynecol. Oncol.* 1998;71:454-7.

[68] Huntsman, DG; Clement, PB; Gilks, CB; et al. A clinicopathological study of sixteen cases. *Am. J. Surg. Pathol.* 1994;18:364-75.

[69] Katahira, A; Akahira, J; Niikura, H; et al. Small cell carcinoma of the endometrium: report of three cases and literature review. *Int. J. Gynecol. Cancer* 2004;145:1018-23.

[70] van Hoeven, KH; Hudock, JA; Woodruff, JM; et al. A small cell neuroendocrine carcinoma of the endometrium. *Int. J. Gynecol. Pathol.* 1995;14:21-9.

[71] Melgoza, F; Brewster, WR; Wilczynski, S; et al. p16 positive small cell neuroendocrine carcinoma of the endometrium. *Int. J. Gynecol. Pathol.* 2006;25:252-6.

[72] Albores-Savedra, J; Martinez-Benitez, B; Luevano, E. Small cell and large cell neuroendocrine carcinomas of the endometrium and cervix: polypoid tumors and those arising in polyps may have a favorable prognosis. *Int. J. Gynecol. Pathol.* 2008;27: 333-9.

[73] Mulvany, NJ; Allen, DG. Combined large cell neuroendocrine and endometrioid carcinoma of the endometrium. *Int. J. Gynecol. Pathol.* 2008;27:49-57.

[74] Abeler, VM; Kjorstad, KE; Nesland JM. Undifferentiated carcinoma of the endometrium. A histopathologic and clinical study of 31 cases. *Cancer* 1991;1;68: 98-105.

[75] Clement, PB; Young, RH. Non endometrioid carcinoma of the uterine corpus: a review of their pathology with emphasis on recent advances and problematic aspects. *Adv. Anat. Pathol.* 2004;11:117-42.

[76] Altrabusi, B; Malpica, A; Deavers, MT; et al. Undifferentiated carcinoma of the endometrium. *Am. J. Surg. Pathol.* 2005;29:1316-21.

[77] Tafe, LJ; Garg, K; Chew, I; et al. Endometrial and ovarian carcinomas with undifferentiated components: clinically aggressive and frequently underrecognized neoplasms. *Mod. Pathology* 2010;23:781-9.

[78] Taraif, SH; Malpica, A; Silva, EG; et al. The significance of neuroendocrine expression in undifferentiated carcinoma of the endometrium. *Int. J. Gynecol. Pathol.* 2009;28:142-7.

[79] Hampel, H; Frankel, W; Panescu, J; et al. Screening for Lynch syndrome (hereditary nonpolyposis colorectal cancer) among endometrial cancer patients. *Cancer Res.* 2006;66:7810-7.

[80] Vasen, HF; Wijnen, JT; Menko, FH; et al. Cancer risk in families with hereditary nonpolyposis colorectal cancer diagnosed by mutation analysis. *Gastroenterology* 1996;110:1020-7.

[81] Carcangiu, ML; Dorji, T; Radice, P; et al. HNPCC-related endometrial carcinomas show a high frequency of non-endometrioid types and of high FIGO grade endometrioid carcinomas. *Mod. Pathol.* 2006;19:173.

[82] Garg, K; Shih, K; Barakat, RR; et al. Endometrial carcinomas in women age 40 years and younger: tumors associated with loss of DNA mismatch repair proteins appear to be a distinct clinicopathologic subset. *Am. J. Surg. Pathol.* 2009;33:1869-77.

[83] Garg, K; Leitao, MM Jr; Kauff, ND; et al. Selection of endometrial carcinomas for DNA mismatch repair protein immunohistochemistry using patient age and tumor

morphology enhances detection of DNA mismatch repair abnormalities. *Am. J. Surg. Pathol.* 2009;33:925-33.

[84] Garg, K; Soslow, RA. Lynch syndrome (hereditary nonpolyposis colorectal cancer) and endometrial carcinoma. *J. Clin. Pathol.* 2009;62:679-84.

[85] Pecorelli, S. Revised FIGO staging for carcinoma of the vulva, cervix, and endometrium. *Int. J. Gynaecol. Obstet.* 2009;105:103-4.

[86] Zaino, RJ; Kurman, RJ; Diana, KL; et al. The utility of the revised International Federation of Gynecology and Obstetrics histologic grading of endometrial adenocarcinoma using a defined nuclear grading system. A Gynecology Oncology Group study. *Cancer* 1995;75:81-6.

[87] Lax, SF; Kurman, RJ; Pizer, ES; et al. A binary architectural grading system for uterine endometrial endometrioid carcinoma has superior reproducibility compared with FIGO grading and identifies subsets of advance-stage tumors with favorable and unfavorable prognosis. *Am. J. Surg. Pathol.* 2000;24:1201-8.

[88] Alkushi, A; Abdul-Rahman, ZH; Lim, P; et al. Description of a novel system for grading of endometrial carcinoma and comparison with existing grading systems . *Am. J. Surg. Pathol.* 2005;29:295-304.

[89] Taylor, RR; Zeller, J; Lieberman, RW; et al. An analysis of two versus three grades for endometrial carcinoma. *Gynecol. Oncol.* 1999;74:3-6.

[90] Gemer, O; Uriev, L; Voldarsky, M; et al. The reproducibility of histological parameters employed in the novel binary grading systems of endometrial cancer. *Eur. J. Surg. Oncol.* 2009;35:247-51.

[91] Larson, DM; Connor, GP; Broste, SK; et al. Prognostic significance of gross myometrial invasion with endometrial cancer. *Obstet. Gynecol.* 1996;88:394-8.

[92] Morrow, CP; Bundy, BN; Kurman, RJ; et al. Relationship between surgical-pathological risk factors and outcome in clinical stage I and II carcinoma of the endometrium: a Gynecology Oncology Group study. *Gynecol. Oncol.* 1991;40:55-65.

[93] Connelly, PJ; Alberhasky, RC; Christopherson, WM. Carcinoma of the endometrium III. Analysis of 865 cases of adenocarcinoma and adenoacanthoma. *Obstet. Gynecol.* 1982;59:569-75.

[94] Satyaswaroop, PG; Mortel, R. Sex steroid receptors in endometrial carcinoma. *Gynecol. Oncol.* 1993;50:278-80.

[95] Fukuda, K; Mori, M; Uchiyama, M; et al. Prognostic significance of progesterone receptor immunohistochemistry in endometrial carcinoma. *Gynecol. Oncol.* 1998;69:220-5.

[96] Kerner, H; Sabo, E; Friedman, M; et al. An immunohistochemical study of estrogen and progesterone receptors in adenocarcinoma of the endometrium and in the adjacent mucosa. *Int. J. Gynecol. Cancer* 1995;5:275-81.

[97] Soslow, RA. Endometrial carcinomas with ambiguous features. *Seminars in Diagnostic Pathology* 2010;27:261-73.

[98] Alkushi, A; Clarke, BA; Akbari, M; et al. Identification of prognostically relevant and reproducible subsets of endometrial adenocarcinoma based on clustering analysis of immunostaining data. *Mod. Pathol.* 2007;20:1156-65.

[99] Catasus, L; D'Angelo, E; Pons, C; et al. Expression profiling of 22 genes involved in the PI3K-AKT pathway identifies to subgroups of high-grade endometrial carcinomas with different molecular alterations. *Mod. Pathol.* 2010;23:694-702.

[100] Alkushi, A; Kobel, M; Kalloger, SE; et al. High-grade endometrial carcinoma: serous and grade 3 endometrioid carcinomas have different immunophenotypes and outcomes. *Int. J. Gynecol. Pathol.* 2010;29:343-350.

[101] Yamamoto, S; Tsuda, H; Aida, S; et al. Immunohistochemical detection of hepatocyte nuclear factor 1beta in ovarian and endometrial clear cell adenocarcinomas and non-neoplastic endometrium. *Hum. Pathol.* 2007;38:1074-80.

[102] Han, G; DeLair, D; Gilks, CB; et al. Endometrial adenocarcinoma with clear cell morphology: interobserver variability and immunohistochemical analysis using hepatocyte nuclear factor-1 beta. *Mod. Pathol.* 2010;23(Suppl 1):245A.

[103] Yemelyanova, A; Vang, R; Ronnett, BM. Immunohistochemical profile of endometrial clear cell carcinoma. *Mod. Pathol.* 2010;23(Suppl.1):269A.

[104] Garg, K; Leitao, MM Jr; Wynveen, CA; et al. p53 overexpression in morphologically ambiguous endometrial carcinomas correlates with adverse clinical outcomes. *Mod. Pathol.* 2010;23:80-92.

In: Endometrial Cancer: Prevention, Diagnosis and Treatment ISBN: 978-1-62257-740-8
Editor: Stefano Greggi

Chapter III

The Role of Ultrasound in Early Diagnosis and Clinical Staging

Antonia Carla Testa*, Floriana Mascilini and Maria Cristina Moruzzi
Obstetrics and Gynecology, Catholic University of the Sacred Heart, Rome, Italy

Abstract

Transvaginal or transrectal ultrasonography is an accurate method in recognizing the endometrial pathology but the diagnosis of specific disease is sometimes very difficult.

In women with postmenopausal bleeding a simple measurement of endometrial thickness can reliably discriminate between women who are at low or high risk of endometrial cancer, with an endometrial thickness of 4 mm or less decreasing the likelihood of endometrial cancer by a factor of ten both in users and non-users of hormone replacement therapy.

In the high-risk group of women, i.e. those with an endometrial thickness of 5 mm or more, an evaluation of endometrial morphology and vascularization using gray-scale and Doppler ultrasound imaging with or without the added use of sonohysterography can be used to further refine the estimation of risk of pathology and, in particular, the risk of endometrial cancer.

The usefulness of an ultrasound examination of the endometrium in premenopausal women with bleeding problems is much less obvious. Most studies reporting on ultrasonography of the uterine cavity are small, and the results are sometimes conflicting.

In patients with already diagnosed endometrial cancer a pretreatment evaluation using modern imaging methods is becoming more common as a result of the benefits of such techniques in tailoring treatment.

As transvaginal examination and Magnetic Resonance Imaging are comparable in assessing the local extent of the disease, transvaginal examination is currently considered the first-line imaging modality in patients with endometrial carcinoma.

* E-mail address: atesta@rm.unicatt.it.

Introduction

Over recent years transvaginal sonography has significantly improved the ability to accurately diagnose and manage intrauterine abnormalities.

It is widely accepted that transvaginal or transrectal ultrasonography (TVUS and TRUS) is an accurate method in recognizing the endometrial pathology, but the diagnosis of specific disease is sometimes very difficult.

In the case of endometrial cancer, the main areas for the application of ultrasonography are the evaluation of the patient with postmenopausal bleeding with an attempt to discriminate between benign and malignant endometrium, and the pretreatment evaluation of the patient with already diagnosed endometrial cancer in order to define the local extent of the disease.

The Role of Ultrasound in Diagnosing Endometrial Cancer in Women with Postmenopausal Bleeding

Postmenopausal bleeding (PMB) defined as blood loss occurring at least 12 months after menopause, signals endometrial carcinoma in around 10% of cases [1], cervical carcinoma in 1% of cases, or less serious conditions, such as benign endometrial polyps, in a further 20-40% [1].

The normal postmenopausal endometrium is thin, uniform and made up of the basalis layer, which is anatomically less than 1 mm thick. There is usually a slight tendency for sonographic endoluminal measurements to overestimate the anatomical endometrial thickness of the endometrium, but a normal unstimulated postmenopausal endometrium should not exceed 4-5 mm in thickness when measured with ultrasound (Figure 1) [2].

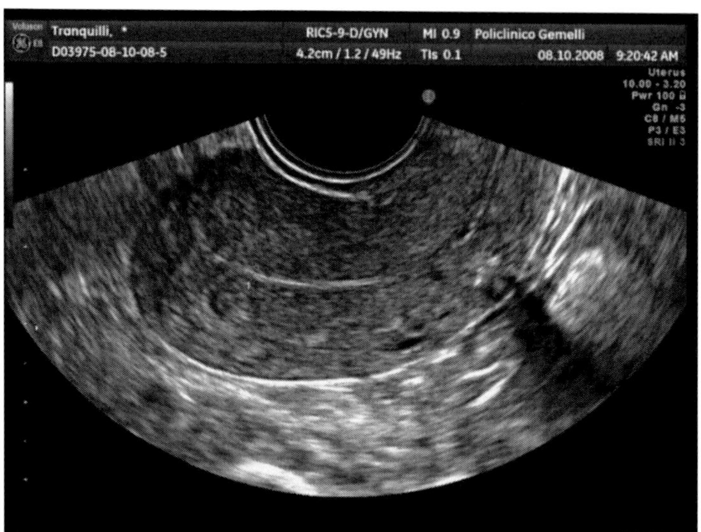

Figure 1. Transvaginal sonographic longitudinal section of the uterus in a postmenopausal patient with a thin and regular endometrium (2 mm).

A thin, 1-2 mm hypoechoic rim (also called the subendometrium) between the echogenic endometrium and the myometrium, usually surrounds the normal postmenopausal endometrium. This halo must not be included in the measurement of endometrial thickness [3].

For women with an endometrium of ≥ 4.5 mm and with postmenopausal bleeding, the sonographic measurement of endometrial thickness is crucial, as the risk of endometrial cancer increases with every additional millimeter [4]. Conversely, an endometrial measurement, which result less than a suggested cut-off, should not indicate the presence of an endometrial cancer. Several large prospective multicenter trials have been carried out to validate the concept that a thin distinct endometrial echo in a postmenopausal woman with bleeding could reliably exclude cancer and thus avoid any further endometrial tests and expense.

Almost every guideline, which uses the cut-off of 5 mm to exclude endometrial cancer, refers to a meta-analysis performed in 1998 by Smith-Bindman et al. [2].

With a cut-off value of 5mm, the sensitivity for detecting endometrial carcinoma was 96%, and the specificity 61%. This combination of sensitivity and specificity reduces a pretest probability of 10% for endometrial cancer to a post-test probability (for a negative test) of 1% [5]. Thus, based on the post-test probability of 1%, the authors recommended a conservative management to women with an endometrial thickness of ≤ 5 mm.

The three other meta-analyses dealing with TVUS in symptomatic postmenopausal patients, reached different conclusions.

A meta-analysis of nine studies conducted by Tabor et al. [6] included only studies where the corresponding author was able to provide original data and obtained a sensitivity of 96% and a specificity of 50% were found. These values give a post-test probability for a negative test of about 1% with a pre test probability of carcinoma of 10% [6]. These results are comparable to those of Smith-Bindman et al., but the authors disagreed on the interpretation of the results. The conclusion of Tabor et al. was that a 4% false-negative rate is not acceptable and concluded that the use of TVUS in the evaluation of PMB is not recommended prior to invasive testing [6].

Gupta et al. performed a systematic quantitative review in which they focused on study quality assessment. Their conclusion was that TVUS could be used to rule out endometrial hyperplasia or carcinoma using an endometrial thickness of ≤ 5 mm [7]. However, the meta-analyses done by Tabor, Gupta and Smith-Bindman are limited because they are based on previously published data, and probably overestimate the accuracy of predictions based on endometrial thickness. The use of individual patient data instead of published summary data gives less optimistic but more accurate conclusions. In diagnostic reviews the same might apply. Timmermans et al. tried to overcome this limitation using a meta-analytic approach in which individual patient data from a series of original studies were combined [8]. This study showed that in previous studies and meta-analyses, the diagnostic accuracy of TVS had been overestimated. Timmermans et al. found a lower diagnostic accuracy for TVS than was reported previously: a sensitivity of 95% and a specificity of 47% at a cut-off of ≤ 4 mm, giving a post-test probability for a negative test of 1.2%. At a cut-off of ≤ 3 mm, they found a sensitivity of 98% and a specificity of 35%, giving a LR for a negative test result of 0.06. Thus, a cut-off level of ≤ 3 mm reduced a pre-test probability of 10% to a 0.7% posttest probability. This article concluded that the use of TVS in the measurement of endometrial thickness remains justified, but with a recommended cut-off level of ≤ 3 mm [5].

Besides the measurement of the thickness, the morphology of the endometrium could be evaluated by means of two-dimensional (2D) grayscale ultrasound. Suspicious sonomorphological signs of endometrial cancer are heterogenous endometrial echogenicity [3] and an irregular endometrial-myometrial border [9]. Its echogenicity is related to the amount of mucin in the endometrium, whilst areas of haemorrhage and necrosis may explain the heterogenous endometrial echogenicity and indicate endometrial cancer [10].

An irregular endometrial-myometrial border reflects the invasion on endometrial cancer into the myometrium [11].

Recently, three-dimensional (3D) volume acquisition was utilized for the assessment of endometrium. However, when the endometrial echo is thin, 3D volumes are generally difficult to produce. It has been demonstrated that the diagnostic performance for the discrimination between benign and malignant endometrium of 3D imaging was not superior to that of endometrial thickness as measured by 2D ultrasonography, and 3D Power Doppler imaging added little to endometrial thickness determinations [12].

Power Doppler may be used to examine small, tortuous vessels and visualize their branching in endometrial tumor. Increased angiogenesis with the formation of new capillaries, and increased microvascular density in the tissue are the signs of tumor [12]. Irregular branching of vessels [13] and an increased number of vessels (a multiple vessel pattern) [14] as assessed by Power Doppler are the usual characteristics of endometrial cancer. The degree of endometrial vascularity can be assessed subjectively or objectively by quantifying the color content of the endometrial scan obtained by using Power Doppler ultrasound. High color content indicates an increased risk of endometrial cancer [11].

3D Power Doppler ultrasound with some specialized computer programs allows calculate the volume of the tissue being investigated enabling the characterization of the vascularity of the entire endometrium. It has been reported that high endometrial volume and high indices of vascularity are associated with endometrial cancer, and can thus be used to predict endometrial malignancy [15].

Saline infusion ultrasonography, also called hydrosonography, is a complement to standard TVUS and facilitates the evaluation of the whole uterine cavity during the ultrasound examination. The method allows accurate discrimination between focal endometrial lesions and global endometrial thickening [9]. Hydrosonographic features indicating endometrial cancer are irregular thickening of the endometrium with variable echogenic texture, irregular myometrial-endometrial border, difficulties with distending the uterine cavity during the procedure and an irregular surface of a focal lesion [13]. Concern has been expressed about performing hydrosonography when TVUS strongly suggests endometrial cancer [16], as there is a small risk of malignant cells finding their way into abdominal cavity via the fallopian tube [17], however this was not confirmed by other studies.

The Role of Ultrasound in Staging Endometrial Cancer

Prognosis of endometrial cancer depends on age of the patient, histological type and grade of tumor, tumor size, depth of myometrial invasion, cervical stromal invasion and lymph node metastases [18].

Tumor size and assessment of the degree of myometrial and cervical invasion cannot be revealed by clinical examination and endometrial biopsy. Preoperative knowledge of all these parameters is advantageous when planning treatment, in order to define the appropriate type of surgery, to properly counsel patients, and avoid the morbidity associated with unnecessary lymphadenectomy or radical hysterectomy.

Several techniques have been studied as tools for preoperative staging of endometrial carcinoma. Magnetic resonance imaging (MRI), computed tomography (CT) and transvaginal sonography (TVS) have all been proven to be accurate in the assessment of depth of myometrial infiltration [19-28].

The diagnostic accuracy of the three imaging modalities has been compared in a large-scale meta-analysis [29], which demonstrated that the summary receiver-operating characteristics (ROC) curves of CT, sonography and MRI were of similar shape, and showed no significant differences in performance, although MRI showed a trend toward better results. In particular, it has been demonstrated that contrast-enhanced MRI performs better than helical CT in the preoperative staging of endometrial cancer [30]. However, MRI is costly, time consuming and has limited availability, and so may not be appropriate for all patients [28].

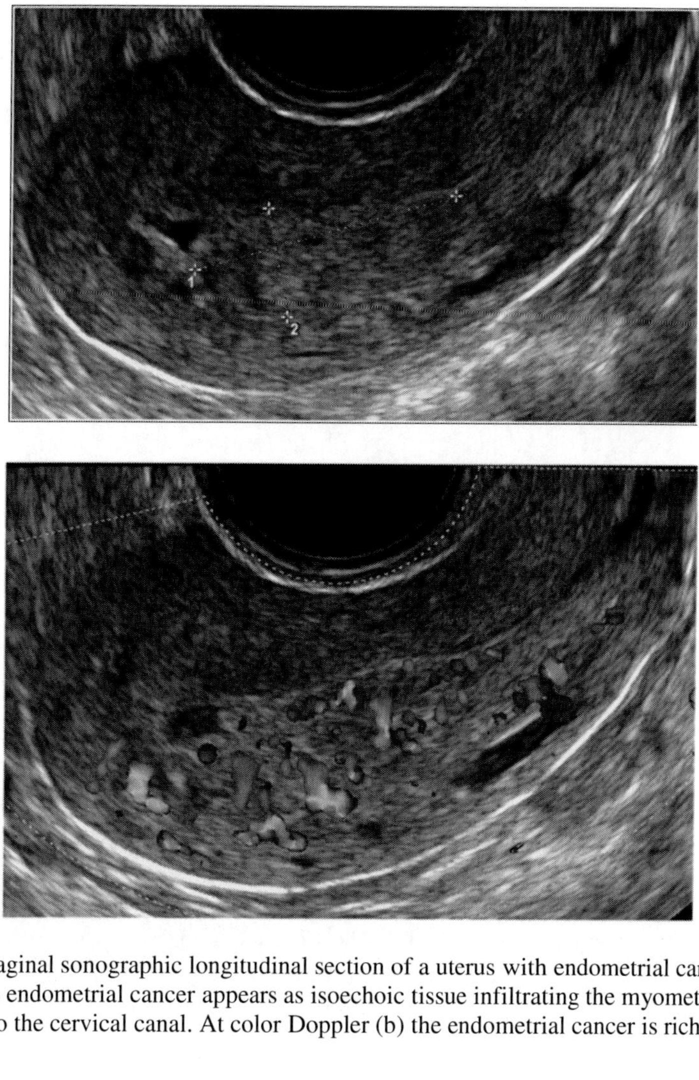

Figure 2. Transvaginal sonographic longitudinal section of a uterus with endometrial carcinoma. At gray scale (a) the endometrial cancer appears as isoechoic tissue infiltrating the myometrial wall with no protrusion into the cervical canal. At color Doppler (b) the endometrial cancer is richly vascularized.

In a prospective multicenter study, we evaluated and compared the accuracy of high-frequency TVS and contrast-enhanced MRI in preoperative staging of endometrial carcinoma [31]. We have shown that contrast-enhanced MRI and TVS perform equally well in the evaluation of myometrial invasion, whereas TVS shows a trend towards better performance in the detection of cervical tumor spread.

Currently, transvaginal ultrasound examination is widely accepted as the first-line imaging modality for early-stage endometrial cancer [18]. As suggested by Vergote and colleagues, the preoperative assessments of patients with endometrial cancer could also include computed tomography of lungs, liver, and retroperitoneal lymph nodes [32].

MRI, which is more expensive and time consuming, could be employed as a second-line imaging technique in patients in whom TVS gives images of poor quality.

Sonographic examination of a patient with known endometrial cancer should provide the clinician with information regarding the tumor location, size (three diameters), sonomorphology (e.g., echogenicity, homogeneity, endometrial-myometrial junction) and vascular pattern [11]. Moreover, it offers the possibility of evaluating the extent of tumor infiltration into the myometrium and towards the cervix (Figures 2,3).

Ideally, the depth of myometrial tumor invasion should be measured from the endometrial-myometrial interface to the deepest border of the tumor extension into the myometrium and should be related to the width of the normal myometrium [33]. However, in some cases the normal myometrium is not accessible as it is either consumed by the tumor or greatly thinned by pressure from exophytically grown tumor.

Another means of measuring the degree of myometrial infiltration is to determine the relationship between the maximum tumor thickness (d1) and the anteroposterior diameter of the uterus (d2) in the sagittal plane, as proposed by Karlsson and colleagues [20]. Invasion of less than half the myometrium is recorded when the ratio of d1 to d2 is $< 50\%$ (Stage T1a), and invasion equal to or greater than half the myometrium is recorded when the ratio of d1 to d2 equals or exceeds 50% (Stage T1b) [20].

This approach seems less operator-dependent, although the extent of invasion may be overestimated in cases of large polypoid exophytic tumors with thinned myometrium or underestimated in cases of asymmetrical, mainly infiltrating growth pattern. Both methods have over 80% accuracy in assessing the extent of myometrial infiltration [20,31,34]. Another option is to measure instead the minimum thickness of tumor free myometrium (the distance between the deepest tumor margin and the serosa). This parameter is easily assessed and seems also to be a useful prognostic factor for recurrence, using a cut-off of 10 mm (area under the receiver-operating characteristics curve, 0.76) [35].

When the tumor infiltrates the cervical stroma, it usually appears at color Doppler as hypoechoic richly vascularized tissue.

In order to assess cervical stromal involvement, it is important to visualize the level of the uterine artery entries into the uterus. By moving the probe from side to side to assess the whole uterus in the sagittal plane, the level of entry of the left and right uterine arteries can be determined by Doppler.

This level corresponds approximately to the internal cervical os [33]. In cases in which the endometrial tumor only protrudes into the cervical canal and has not infiltrated the cervical stroma, by applying slight pressure with the transvaginal probe the sliding effect of tumor mass against the endocervical mucosa can be observed.

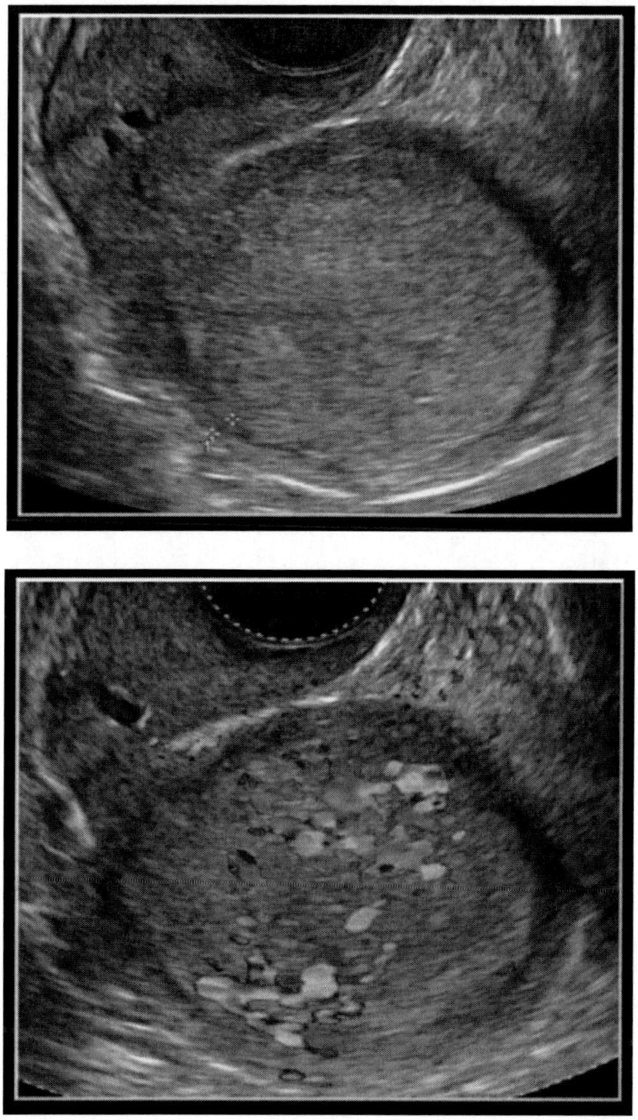

Figure 3. Transvaginal sonographic longitudinal section of a uterus with endometrial carcinoma. At gray scale (a) the endometrial cancer appears as hyperechoic mass of large dimensions, with deep myometrial infiltration and no cervical stroma infiltration. At color Doppler (b) the endometrial cancer appears richly vascularized.

Color and Power Doppler can be useful to assess the vascular pattern of endometrial cancer. In some cases, the presence of abnormal perfusion permits a better recognition of the tumor border in less visible tumors (i.e. those that are isoechogenic with the myometrium).

In cases of mainly polypoid growing tumors, the detection with Doppler of dominant feeding vessels enables more detailed examination of the endometrial–myometrial junction at the insertion of the feeding vessels (entry point of feeding artery) in order to assess more accurately the depth of myometrial invasion [33].

The possibility to predict lymph node metastasis by intratumoral Doppler analysis has been reported [36]. Unfortunately, it has not been confirmed by other studies with only significant difference of color score between early and advanced stages and a slight correlation with myometrial invasion reported [37]. In a collaborative multicenter prospective study we analyzed the gray-scale and vascular characteristics of endometrial cancer in relation to stage, grade and size using 2D / 3D transvaginal ultrasound. We have shown that gray-scale and vascular morphology characteristics of endometrial cancer are significantly related to tumor stage, grade and size. Tumors of Stage IB or greater, of Grade 3 or with a tumor/uterine AP ratio of ≥ 50% are more often hypo- echoic or have a mixed echogenicity, have a higher color score and more often display multiple globally entering vessels, whereas tumors of Stage IA, of Grade 1 or Grade 2, or with a tumor/uterine AP ratio of < 50% are more often hyperechoic, and have more frequently low or no vascularization [38].

Conclusion

Transvaginal sonography represents an accurate method to diagnose and manage intrauterine abnormalities.

In women with postmenopausal bleeding the measurement of endometrial thickness can reliably discriminate between women who are at low or high risk of endometrial cancer, with an endometrial thickness of 4 mm or less decreasing the likelihood of endometrial cancer by a factor of ten both in users and non-users of hormone replacement therapy [2,39-43].

In patients with endometrial cancer transvaginal ultrasound examination is considered the first-line imaging modality for preoperative assessment of local extension of the disease.

References

[1] Dijkhuizen, FP; Brölman, HA; Potters, AE; et al. The accuracy of transvaginal ultrasonography in the diagnosis of endometrial abnormalities. *Obstet. Gynecol.* 1996;87:345-9.

[2] Smith-Bindman, R; Kerlikowske, K; Feldstein, VA; et al. Endovaginal ultrasound to exclude endometrial cancer and other endometrial abnormalities. *JAMA* 1998;280:1510-7.

[3] Epstein, E. Management of postmenopausal bleeding in Sweden: a need for increased use of hydrosonography and hysteroscopy. *Acta. Obstet. Gynecol. Scand.* 2004;83: 89-95.

[4] Epstein, E; Valentin, L. Rebleeding and endometrial growth in women with postmenopausal bleeding and endometrial thickness < 5 mm managed by dilatation and curettage or ultrasound followup: a randomized controlled study. *Ultrasound Obstet. Gynecol.* 2001;18:499-504.

[5] VanHanegem, N; Breijer, MC; Khan, KS; et al. Diagnostic evaluation of the endometrium in postmenopausal bleeding: An evidence-based approach. *Maturitas* 2011;68:155-64.

[6] Tabor, A; Watt, HC; Wald, NJ. Endometrial thickness as a test for endometrial cancer in women with postmenopausal vaginal bleeding. *Obstet. Gynecol.* 2002;99:663-70.

[7] Gupta, JK; Chien, PF; Voit, D; et al. Ultrasonographic endometrial thickness for diagnosing endometrial pathology in women with postmenopausal bleeding: ameta-analysis. *Acta Obstet. Gynecol. Scand.* 2002;81:799-816.

[8] Timmermans, A; Opmeer, BC; Khan, KS; et al. Endometrial thickness measurement for detecting endometrial cancer in women with postmenopausal bleeding: a systematic review and meta-analysis. *Obstet. Gynecol* 2010;116:160-7.

[9] Goldstein, RB; Bree, RL; Benson, CB; et al. Evaluation of the woman with postmenopausal bleeding: society of radiologists in ultrasound-sponsored consensus conference statement. *J. Ultrasound Med.* 2001;20:1025-36.

[10] Sheth, S; Hamper, UM; Kurman, RJ. Thickened endometrium in the postmenopausal woman: sonographic-pathologic correlation. *Radiology* 1993;187:135-9.

[11] Leone, FP; Timmerman, D; Bourne, T; et al. Terms, definitions and measurements to describe the sonographic features of the endometrium and intrauterine lesions: a consensus opinion from the International Endometrial Tumor Analysis (IETA) group. *Ultrasound Obstet. Gynecol.* 2010;35:103-12.

[12] Opolskiene, G; Sladkevicius, P; Jokubkiene, L; et al. Three dimensional ultrasound imaging for discrimination between benign and malignant endometrium in women with postmenopausal bleeding and sonographic endometrial thickness of at least 4.5 mm. *Ultrasound Obstet. Gynecol.* 2010; 35:94-102.

[13] Epstein, E; Valentin, L. Gray-scale ultrasound morphology in the presence or absence of intrauterine fluid and vascularity as assessed by color Doppler for discrimination between benign and malignant endometrium in women with postmenopausal bleeding. *Ultrasound Obstet. Gynecol.* 2006;28:89-95.

[14] Alcázar, JL; Castillo, G; Mínguez, JA; et al. Endometrial blood fl ow mapping using transvaginal power Doppler sonography in women with postmenopausal bleeding and thickened endometrium. *Ultrasound Obstet. Gynecol.* 2003;21:583-8.

[15] Alcázar, JL; Galván, R; Albela, S; et al. Assessing myometrial infi ltration by endometrial cancer: uterine virtual navigation with three-dimensional US. *Radiology* 2009;250:776-83.

[16] Amant, F; Moerman, P; Neven, P; et al. Endometrial cancer. *Lancet* 2005;366:491-505.

[17] Alcázar, JL; Errasti, T; Zornoza, A. Saline infusion sonohysterography in endometrial cancer: assessment of malignant cells dissemination risk. *Acta Obstet. Gynecol. Scand. 2000*;79:321-2.

[18] Benedet, JL; Bender, H; Jones, H3rd; et al. FIGO staging classifications and clinical practice guidelines in the management of gynecologic cancers. FIGO Committee on Gynecologic Oncology. *Int. J. Gynaecol. Obstet.* 2000;70:209-262.

[19] Varpula, MJ; Klemi, PJ. Staging of uterine endometrial carcinoma with ultra-low field (0.02 T) MRI: a comparative study with CT. *J. Comput. Assist. Tomogr.* 1993;17:641-7.

[20] Karlsson, B; Norstrom, A; Granberg, S; et al. The use of endovaginal ultrasound to diagnose invasion of endometrial carcinoma. *Ultrasound Obstet. Gynecol.* 1992;2:35-9.

[21] Kim, SH; Kim, HD; Song, YS; et al. Detection of deep myometrial invasion in endometrial carcinoma: comparison of transvaginal ultrasound, CT, and MRI. *J. Comput. Assist. Tomogr.* 1995;19:766-72.

[22] Hasami, K; Matsuzawa, M; Chen, HF; et al. Computed tomography in the evaluation and treatment of endometrial carcinoma. *Cancer* 1982;50:904-8.

[23] Teefey, SA; Stahl, JA; Middleton, WD; et al. Local staging of endometrial carcinoma: comparison of transvaginal and intraoperative sonography and gross visual inspection. *AJR Am. J. Roentgenol.* 1996;166:547-52.

[24] Joja, I; Asakawa, M; Asakawa, T; et al. Endometrial carcinoma: dynamic MRI with turbo-flash technique. *J .Comput. Assist. Tomogr.* 1996; 20: 878–887.

[25] Seki, H; Kimura, M; Sakai, K. Myometrial invasion of endometrial carcinoma: assessment with plain and gadoliniumenhanced MR imaging. *Radiology* 1992;185: 207-12.

[26] Arko, D; Takac, I. High frequency transvaginal ultrasonography in preoperative assessment of myometrial invasion in endometrial cancer. *J. Ultrasound Med.* 2000;19:639-43.

[27] Manfredi, R; Mirk, P; Maresca, G; et al. Local-regional staging of endometrial carcinoma: role of MR imaging in surgical planning. *Radiology* 2004;231:372-8.

[28] De Smet, F; De Brabanter, J; Van den Bosch, T; et al. New models to predict depth of infiltration in endometrial carcinoma based on transvaginal sonography. *Ultrasound Obstet. Gynecol.* 2006;27:664-71.

[29] Kinkel, K; Kaji, Y; Yu, KK; et al. Radiologic staging in patients with endometrial cancer: a metaanalysis. *Radiology* 1999;212:711-8.

[30] Hardesty, LA; Sumkin, JH; Hakim, C; et al. The ability of helical CT to preoperatively stage endometrial carcinoma. *AJR Am. J. Roentgenol.* 2001;176:603-6.

[31] Savelli, L; Ceccarini, M; Ludovisi, M; et al. Preoperative local staging of endometrial cancer: transvaginal sonography vs. magnetic resonance imaging. *Ultrasound Obstet. Gynecol.* 2008;31:560-6.

[32] Amant, F; Moerman, P; Neven, P; et al. Endometrial cancer. *Lancet* 2005;366:491-505.

[33] Fischerova, D. Ultrasound scanning of the pelvis and abdomen for staging of gynecological tumors: a review. *Ultrasound Obstet. Gynecol.* 2011;38:246-66.

[34] Weber, G; Merz, E; Bahlmann, F; et al. Assessment of myometrial infiltration and preoperative staging by transvaginal ultrasound in patients with endometrial carcinoma. *Ultrasound Obstet. Gynecol.* 1995;6:362-7.

[35] Lindauer, J; Fowler, JM; Manolitsas, TP; et al. Is there a prognostic difference between. depth of myometrial invasion and the tumor-free distance from the uterine serosa in endometrial cancer? *Gynecol. Oncol.* 2003;91:547-51.

[36] Ercoli, A; Delmas, V; Fanfani, F; et al. Terminologia Anatomica versus unofficial descriptions and nomenclature of the fasciae and ligaments of the female pelvis: a dissection-based comparative study. *Am. J. Obstet. Gynecol.* 2005;193:1565-73.

[37] Testa, AC; Scambia, G; Caruso, A. The clinical usefulness of preoperative intratumoral Doppler analysis in predicting lymph node metastasis in patients with endometrial carcinoma. *Gynecol. Oncol.* 2000;79:522-3.

[38] Epstein, E; Van Holsbeke, C; Mascilini, F; et al. Gray-scale and color Doppler ultrasound characteristics of endometrial cancer in relation to stage, grade and tumor size. *Ultrasound Obstet. Gynecol.* 2011;38:586-93.

[39] ACOG Committee. ACOG Committee Opinion No. 426: the role of transvaginal ultrasonography in the evaluation of postmenopausal bleeding. *Obstet. Gynecol.* 2009;113:462-4.

[40] Ferrazzi, E; Torri, V; Trio, D; et al. Sonographic endometrial thickness: a useful test to predict atrophy in patients with postmenopausal bleeding. An Italian multicenter study. *Ultrasound Obstet. Gynecol.* 1996;7:315-21.

[41] Van den Bosch, T; Van Schoubroeck, D; Domali, E; et al. A thin and regular endometrium on ultrasound is very unlikely in patients with endometrial malignancy. *Ultrasound Obstet. Gynecol.* 2007;29:674-9.

[42] Gull, B; Karlsson, B; Milsom, I; et al. Can ultrasound replace dilation and curettage? A longitudinal evaluation of postmenopausal bleeding and transvaginal sonographic measurement of the endometrium as predictors of endometrial cancer. *Am. J. Obstet. Gynecol.* 2003;188:401-8.

[43] Karlsson, B; Granberg, S; Wikland, M; et al. Transvaginal ultrasonography of the endometrium in women with postmenopausal bleeding – a Nordic multicenter study. *Am. J. Obstet. Gynecol.* 1995;172:1488-94.

In: Endometrial Cancer: Prevention, Diagnosis and Treatment ISBN: 978-1-62257-740-8
Editor: Stefano Greggi

Chapter IV

Hysteroscopic Diagnosis: Is There Any Doubt?

Valeria Masciullo[1*] and Ivan Mazzon[2]
[1]Gynecologic Oncology, Catholic University of the Sacred Heart, Rome, Italy
[2]Gynecologic Endoscopy, "Nuova Villa Claudia," Rome, Italy

Abstract

Hysteroscopy (direct endoscopic visualization of the endometrial cavity) has emerged as a useful and safe diagnostic procedure for investigating postmenopausal bleeding with a low incidence of clinically significant complications. An endometrial carcinoma can be detected in 7-11% of postmenopausal patients and 2-3% of premenopausal patients submitted to hysteroscopy. Compared with traditional methods such as curettage, hysteroscopy offers the possibility of visualizing macroscopic or focal abnormalities and taking direct biopsies increasing the accuracy of cancer diagnosis. Moreover with the introduction of smaller diameter hysteroscopic systems and the "vaginoscopic" approach, patient acceptance has improved considerably and hysteroscopy is routinely performed in an outpatient setting without the use of anesthesia. Regarding the risk of peritoneal dissemination of cancer cells, there is no evidence to support an association between preoperative hysteroscopic examination and worse prognosis.

Additional roles for hysteroscopy in endometrial cancer have been recently established in clinical staging and sentinel node mapping. Recent studies demonstrated that in women with endometrial carcinoma the exclusion of cervical canal involvement at hysteroscopy is more reliable than at magnetic resonance and transvaginal ultrasound, whereas magnetic resonance remains the most reliable technique for predicting cervical involvement. Although the role of sentinel node in endometrial cancer is still controversial, intraoperative sentinel node detection is feasible using hysteroscopy for

* E-mail address: valeriamasciullo@yahoo.com.

injection of blue dye and technetium-99m beneath the tumor. This technique may actually enhance the chances to detect metastatic disease, while reducing the extent of surgery.

In conclusion, hysteroscopy seems an accurate and promising technique in the diagnosis and management of endometrial cancer.

Introduction

Endometrial cancer has a high diagnostic rate in the early stage, approximately 80% in stage I and 13% in stage II [1]. This is due to the abnormal uterine bleeding as the presenting symptom in 90% of the cases. The best diagnostic strategy in patients with postmenopausal bleeding (PMB) still remains controversial. In the past, the principal method of investigation was dilatation and curettage (DandC), which has been recently almost completely replaced by endometrial biopsy and hysteroscopy. In fact, in approximately 60% of the DandC procedure less than half of the uterine cavity is curetted, whereas hysteroscopy offers the possibility of visualizing macroscopic or focal abnormalities (Figure 1) and taking direct biopsies [2].

Hysteroscopy: Technique, Limits and Complications

Hysteroscopy is the direct endoscopic visualization of the endometrial cavity, which is used extensively in the evaluation of gynecological problems, such as menorrhagia and PMB. The procedure is considered safe and acceptable and is used extensively in Europe and North America [3]. A hysteroscope consists of an outer sheath, which contains a valve through which the fluid or gas used to distend the uterine cavity is circulated. There is no gold standard concerning the preferential distension medium. The simplest and cheapest methods are represented by carbon dioxide (CO_2) or a solution of 5% dextrose in water or normal saline (NaCl).

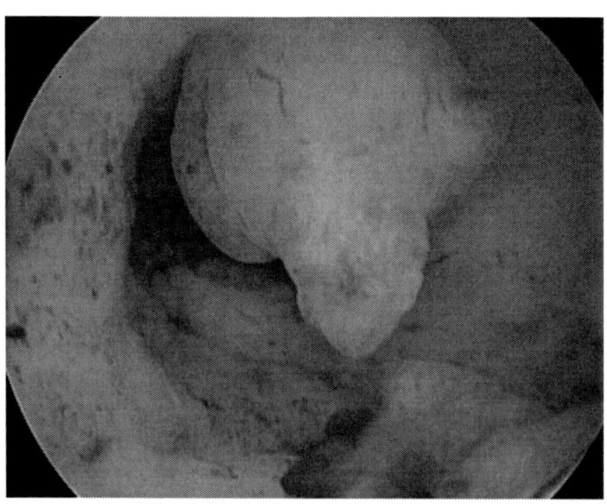

Figure 1. Hysteroscopic view of endometrial adenocarcinoma.

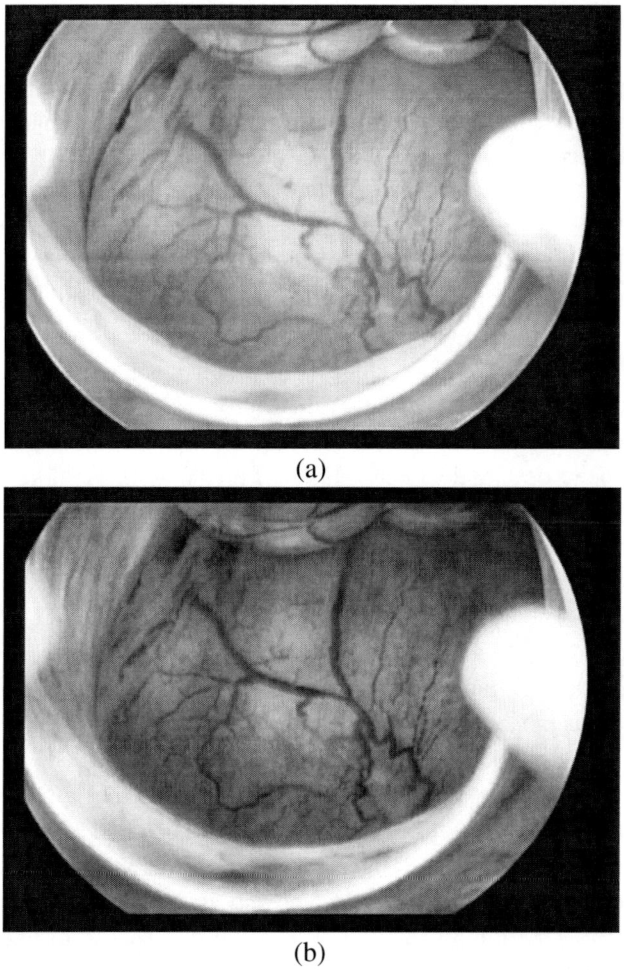

Figure 2. Endometrial adenocarcinoma onset on polyp: (a) hysteroscopic view in white light, and (b) in narrow band imaging technology.

Recent advance in instrumentation have allowed hysteroscopy to be performed in an ambulatory setting without premedication or anesthesia with a given obvious advantage to the patients and the cost effectiveness (Figure 2a). The main complications of hysteroscopy, either the failure to observe the uterine cavity because of bleeding or air bubbles, are hemorrhage, perforation of the uterus, infection and cervical laceration. However, these complications are infrequent and are usually easy to manage [4].

Role of Hysteroscopy in the Diagnosis of Endometrial Carcinoma

The main objective in the diagnostic work up of postmenopausal women presenting with abnormal uterine bleeding is to detect or rule out endometrial cancer. Approximately 90% of women with endometrial carcinoma report vaginal bleeding as their only complaint, thus this symptom should always be carefully investigated.

The best diagnostic strategy in patients with PMB still remains controversial. The probability of endometrial pathology is strongly reduced in the presence of an endometrial ultrasound with an endometrial thickness $\leq$ 4 mm and endometrial sampling is not recommended below this cut off value [5]. However, different authors have come to a different conclusion suggesting systematic sampling from symptomatic patients regardless of endometrial thickness [6]. Guidelines advocate office endometrial sampling to rule out endometrial carcinoma in women with PMB and endometrial thickness as assessed by transvaginal ultrasonography (TVS). Before TVS was introduced in the early 1990s, women with PMB were scheduled for DandC. DandC is now considered an outdated practice and has been replaced by less invasive outpatient evaluation using endometrial biopsy devices and outpatient hysteroscopy guided biopsies [7].

The Pipelle (Pipelle de Cornier, Paris, France) or the Vabra (Berkeley Medevices Inc., Richmond, CA, USA) devices used for endometrial sampling are very sensitive techniques for the detection of endometrial carcinoma (99.6 and 97.1%, respectively) [8]. However, the amount of tissue obtained by office sampling is extremely variable and sometimes insufficient for diagnosis.

In the presence of intracavitary lesion, hysteroscopy offers the possibility of visualizing macroscopic or focal lesions and taking direct biopsies by curettes or forceps, yielding an accurate histological diagnosis [9]. Moreover, the introduction of the microhysteroscope and the vaginoscopic approach have improved significantly patient compliance allowing to perform the procedure in an outpatient setting without anesthesia. However, the role of hysteroscopy in the diagnosis of endometrial cancer is still debated because individual studies are small, leading to imprecise and heterogeneous estimates of accuracy.

A recent quantitative review analysis [2] showed an overall sensitivity of 86.4% and a specificity of 99.2% according to 56 studies of hysteroscopy for endometrial cancer. Diagnostic accuracy was lower for endometrial disease than endometrial cancer. However, its high accuracy relates to diagnosing cancer rather than excluding it. Interestingly, the accuracy tended to be higher among postmenopausal women and in the outpatient setting. Failed hysteroscopy in the outpatient setting is due to technical problems (cervical stenosis or structural abnormalities), inadequate visualization (bleeding, debris) or patient factors (pain, intolerance).

Outpatient hysteroscopy appears to be of reasonable, although more modest, accuracy in endometrial hyperplasia as well [10]. The recent introduction of an optical image enhancement technology such as narrow band imaging - NBI (Olympus, Hamburg, Germany) that enhances the visibility of vessels and other structures on the mucosal surface (Figure 2b) has further improved the accuracy of hysteroscopy in predicting endometrial cancer [11].

Approximately 10-15% of women with PMB have endometrial carcinoma whereas the prevalence of endometrial polyps in these patients is estimated to be around 40%. Nevertheless, histological examination, following total removal of these polyps, proves the presence of an endometrial carcinoma hidden in 20% of cases despite negative biopsy, raising questions whether an endometrial polyp should always be resected [5]. The most important benefit of hysteroscopy is its "see and treat" potential, which not only avoids multiple hospital visits, but also provide higher patient satisfaction [12].

Role of Hysteroscopy in Staging Endometrial Cancer

Stromal invasion to the cervix occurs in 10 to 20% of endometrial cancer cases altering the pattern of spread involving parametrium and reducing the 5-year survival rate to 60-70%. Consequently, in stage II disease radical hysterectomy with bilateral salpingo-oophorectomy and systematic pelvic lymphadenectomy with or without para-aortic lymphadenectomy is performed whenever feasible [13]. In fact, it has to be taken into account that patients affected by endometrial carcinoma, who are often elderly, obese and have cardiovascular comorbidities may benefit of a vaginal approach to total hysterectomy in order to reduce the risks of complications [14].

In this setting, a thorough preoperative clinical and instrumental work-up is critical to minimize the risk of understaging the disease and to tailor the extent and the radicalness of surgery. Several diagnostic techniques have been proposed to assess cervical involvement (endocervical curettage, TVS, computed tomography - CT, magnetic resonance imaging - MRI) although they have not produced very reliable results [15,16]. Endocervical curettage was found to have a 50% false-positive rate and a 13% false-negative rate [15,17]. TVS was the first diagnostic imaging method to be introduced for cervical assessment [18], however, it has since been replaced by MRI due to the high success rate of the last [19].

If hysteroscopy is considered the best technique for investigating uterine cavity, its role in the tumor staging and assessment of cervical involvement, either or not combined with directed biopsies, is still controversial. Lo et al. in a retrospective study conducted in 200 patients with endometrial carcinoma, demonstrated that hysteroscopy using saline has a high accuracy and negative predictive value (NPV: 96.4%) in assessing tumor spread to the cervix [20]. This finding that hysteroscopy is a reliable diagnostic tool for excluding cervical involvement has been further supported [21]. However, in a recent study [22] conducted in 100 patients, hysteroscopy showed a positive predictive value of 0.58 that was about half that previously shown [20], raising questions on the limits of hysteroscopy in diagnosing cervical involvement even when combined with directed biopsies. Technical factors and characteristic of the tumors may account for different results. To date, data from the literature seems to suggest that MRI shows the highest positive predictive value, especially when the stroma is invaded [15].

In conclusion, in women with endometrial carcinoma the exclusion of cervical involvement is more reliable at hysteroscopy than at MRI and TVS, whereas MRI remains the most unfailing technique for predicting cervical involvement.

Does Hysteroscopy Facilitate Tumor Cell Dissemination?

Although hysteroscopy is generally considered a valuable tool in the diagnosis of endometrial cancer, its use is limited in many European and North American cancer centers mostly for the potential risk of cancer cells dissemination throughout the tubes into the peritoneal cavity [23]. During hysteroscopic examination, tissue fragments and malignant cells may disseminate into peritoneal cavity under the pressure of the medium used for distension of the uterine cavity [24,25], worsening the prognosis of the disease. If several studies have confirmed a high association between positive peritoneal cytology and hysteroscopy [24,26], others have failed to show this correlation [27,28]. Nevertheless, most of the studies are not adequately designed, thus no definitive conclusion has been drawn about this issue.

A recent meta-analysis on 2,944 women enrolled in selected studies suggests that hysteroscopy increases significantly the risk for peritoneal dissemination of malignant cells, especially when 0.9% sodium chloride is used as distension medium [29]. The distension pressure does not contribute to the risk as previously reported [30] especially when the tumor is localized at the early stage (stage I or II).

Moreover, although endometrial cancer cells may disseminate into the peritoneal cavity during hysteroscopy, it does not seem to affect the prognosis. Some authors have hypothesized that spread of cancer cells into the peritoneal cavity during hysteroscopy is a passive and transient process and that cytology would return to negative after a period of time [31].

In the past years, the presence of positive peritoneal cytology has not been indicated as an independent prognostic factor for survival of endometrial cancer [32]. Additionally, the current International Federation of Gynecology and Obstetrics (FIGO) staging has recently been revised according to the fact that positive peritoneal cytology does not affect stage of disease and should be reported separately [33].

In conclusion, there is no reason to avoid diagnostic hysteroscopy before to surgery in patients with endometrial cancer, especially in early stages.

Role of Hysteroscopy in Lymphatic Mapping and Sentinel Node Biopsy in Endometrial Cancer

In early stage endometrial cancer, the frequency of lymph node metastases ranges between 0 and 34% [34]. Their identification represents an integral part of surgical staging since the presence of lymph nodes metastasis is an important prognostic factor [35]. Several papers also support the potential therapeutic value of lymphadenectomy [36,37].

The sentinel node (SN) is defined as the first node in the lymphatic system that drains a tumor site. If the SN is not metastatic, then all other nodes should also be disease-free. Few studies have assessed the feasibility of sentinel node biopsy in endometrial cancer by using hysteroscopy [38-42]. The technique consists of an injection of 2 ml of blue dye, followed by 20-50 MBq technetium-99 m-labelled nanocolloids into the subendometrial layer underlying endometrial cancer using an hysteroscope. In a series of 28 patients [38], injections were performed at four sites under the endometrium and sentinel nodes were identified intraoperatively by a gamma probe and removed. Detection rate was reported to be 82%, with 100% sensitivity and 100% specificity. The location of SN was in agreement with the spread pattern in endometrial cancer, with an incidence of metastatic lymph nodes of approximately 50% in the pelvis, 30% in both the pelvis and the para-aortic site and 20% in the para-aortic area alone [34].

Other two studies [39,40] compared a radioactive tracer and a blue dye injected hysteroscopically for the identification of SN. In both cases they performed a lymphoscintigraphy 15 minutes after the hysteroscopy injection and then 5 minutes for up to 1 hour or until few nodes were identified. Surgery was then performed using an intraoperative gamma probe and direct identification of blue-stained nodes. After removal of SN, a pelvic lymphadenectomy was performed in all cases and para-aortic lymphadenectomy only in cases of special hystotypes. Scintigraphy has a 100% success rate in detecting sentinel nodes compare to blue dye (57-83%) whereas the combination of both yields the best results. Other studies failed or showed a low detection rate in the identification of SN [41,42].

Some authors perform intramyometrial [41] and/or intracervical injections, however in this last case the tracer distribution is not reflecting the corpus uterine drainage but the cervical pathway.

The main problem with SN is represented by the false negative rate which understages the patients and influences the need for adjuvant therapy. To date calculation of false negative rates cannot be achieved due to the small number of series, however an acceptably low false-negative rate is crucial before SN can be considered as an alternative to the current standard treatment.

References

[1] Colombo, N; Preti, E; Landoni, F; Carinelli, S; Colombo, A; Marini, C; et al; ESMO Guidelines Working Group. Endometrial cancer: ESMO Clinical Practice Guidelines for diagnosis, treatment and follow-up. *Ann. Oncol.* 2011;22(Suppl 6):vi35-9.

[2] Clark, TJ; Voit, D; Gupta, JK; Hyde, C; Song, FJ; Khan, KS. Accuracy of hysteroscopy in the diagnosis of endometrial cancer and hyperplasia - A systematic quantitative review. *JAMA* 2002;288:1610-21.

[3] Rogerson, L; Duffy, S. A national survey of outpatient hysteroscopy. *Gynecol. Endosc.* 2001;10:343-7.

[4] Bradley, LD. Complications in hysteroscopy: prevention; treatment and legal risk. *Curr. Opin. Obstet. Gynecol.* 2002;14:409-15.

[5] Elfayomy, AK; Habib, FA; Alkabalawy, MA. Role of hysteroscopy in the detection of endometrial pathologies in women presenting with postmenopausal bleeding and thickened endometrium. *Arch. Gynecol. Obstet.* 2012;285:839-43.

[6] Tabor, A; Watt, HC; Wald, NJ. Endometrial thickness as a test for endometrial cancer in women with postmenopausal vaginal bleeding. *Obstet. Gynecol.* 2002;99:663-70.

[7] Litta, P; Merlin, F; Saccardi, C; Pozzan, C; Sacco, G; Fracas, M; et al. Role of hysteroscopy with endometrial biopsy to rule out endometrial cancer in postmenopausal women with abnormal uterine bleeding. *Maturitas* 2005; 50: 117-23.

[8] Dijkhuizen, FPHLJ; Mol, BWJ; Brolmann, HAM; Heintz, APM. The accuracy of endometrial sampling in the diagnosis of patients with endometrial carcinoma and hyperplasia - A meta-analysis. *Cancer* 2000;89: 1765-72.

[9] Triolo, O; Antico, F; Palmara, V; Benedetto, V; Panama, S; Nicotina, PA. Hysteroscopic findings of endometrial carcinoma. Evaluation of 104 cases. *Eur. J. Gynecol. Oncol.* 2005;26:434-6.

[10] Clark, TJ; Mann, CH; Shah, N; Khan, KS; Song, F; Gupta, JK. Accuracy of outpatient endometrial biopsy in the diagnosis of endometrial hyperplasia. *Acta Obstet. Gynecol. Scand.* 2001;80:784-93.

[11] Surico, D; Vigone, A; Bonvini, D; Tinelli, R; Leo, L; Surico, N. Narrow-band imaging in diagnosis of endometrial cancer and hyperplasia: a new option? *J. Minim. Invasive Gynecol.* 2010;17:620-5.

[12] Lalchandani, S; Phillips, K. Evaluation of endometrial cavity investigation option. *Rev. Gynecol. Prac.* 2003;3:165-70.

[13] Mariani, A; Webb, MJ; Keeney, GL; Calori, G; Podratz, KC. Role of wide/radical hysterectomy and pelvic lymph node dissection in endometrial cancer with cervical involvement. *Gynecol. Oncol.* 2001;83:72-80.

[14] Manfredi, R; Mirk, P; Maresca, G; Margariti, PA; Testa, A; Zannoni, GF; et al. Local-regional staging of endometrial carcinoma: Role of MR imaging in surgical planning. *Radiology* 2004;231:372-8.

[15] Toki, T; Oka, K; Nakayama, K; Oguchi, O; Fujii, S. A comparative study of pre-operative procedures to assess cervical invasion by endometrial carcinoma. *BJOG* 1998;105:512-6.

[16] Kietlinska, Z; Stelmachow, J; Antczak-Judycka, A; Timorek, A; Sawicki, W; Tyminska, B. Fractional curettage, hysteroscopy and imaging techniques: transvaginal sonography (TVS), magnetic resonance imaging (MRI) and computed tomography (CT) in the diagnosis of cervical canal involvement in cases of endometrial carcinoma. *Eur. J. Gynecol. Oncol.* 1998;19:561-4.

[17] Cowles, TA; Magrina, JF; Masterson, BJ; Capen, CV. Comparison of clinical and surgical staging in patients with endometrial carcinoma. *Obstet Gynecol.* 1985;66: 413-6.

[18] Kikuchi, A; Sultana, J; Okai, T; Kobayashi, K; Taketani, Y. Intrauterine sonography for preoperative assessment of cervical invasion in endometrial carcinoma. *Gynecol. Oncol.* 1997;65:415-20.

[19] Frei, KA; Kinkel, K. Staging endometrial cancer: Role of magnetic resonance imaging. *J. Magn. Reson. Imaging* 2001;13:850-5.

[20] Lo, KWK; Cheung, TH; Yim, SF; Chung, TKH. Preoperative hysteroscopic assessment of cervical invasion by endometrial carcinoma: A retrospective study. *Gynecol. Oncol.* 2001;82:279-82.

[21] Avila, ML; Ruiz, R; Cortaberria, JR; Rivero, B; Ugalde, F. Assessment of cervical involvement in endometrial carcinoma by hysteroscopy and directed biopsy. *Int. J. Gynecol. Cancer* 2008;18:128-31.

[22] Cicinelli, E; Marinaccio, M; Barba, B; Tinelli, R; Colafiglio, G; Pedote, P; et al. Reliability of diagnostic fluid hysteroscopy in the assessment of cervical invasion by endometrial carcinoma: A comparative study with transvaginal sonography and MRI. *Gynecol. Oncol.* 2008;111:55-61.

[23] Maggino, T; Romagnolo, C; Landoni, F; Sartori, E; Zola, P; Gadducci, A. An analysis of approaches to the management of endometrial cancer in North America: A CTF study. *Gynecol. Oncol.* 1998;68:274-9.

[24] Zerbe, M; Zhang, JY; Bristow, RE; Grumbine, FC; Abularach, S; Montz, FJ. Retrograde seeding of malignant cells during hysteroscopy in presumed early endometrial cancer. *Gynecol. Oncol.* 2000;79:55-8.

[25] Duan, H.; Deng, XH. The diagnosis of endometrial cancer and the effect of malignant cells disseminating during hysteroscopy. *J. Pract. Obstet. Gynecol.* 2007;23:17-9.

[26] Rose, PG; Mendelsohn, G; Konabluth, I. Hysteroscopic dissemination of endometrial carcinoma. *Gynecol. Oncol.* 1998;71:145-6.

[27] Ben-Arie, A; Tamir, S; Dubnik, S; Gemer, O; Ben Shushan, A; Dgani, R; et al. Does hysteroscopy affect prognosis in apparent early-stage endometrial cancer? *Int. J. Gynecol. Cancer* 2008;18:813-9.

[28] Selvaggi, L; Cormio, G; Ceci, O; Loverro, G; Cazzolla, A; Bettocchi, S. Hysteroscopy does not increase the risk of microscopic extrauterine spread in endometrial carcinoma. *Int. J. Gynecol. Cancer* 2003;13:223-7.

[29] Chang, Y; Kay, N; Chen, YH; Chen, HS; Tsai, EM. Resectoscopic treatment of ectopic pregnancy in previous cesarean delivery scar defect with vasopressin injection. *Fertil. Steril.* 2011;96:E80-2.

[30] Solima, E; Brusati, V; Ditto, A; Kusamura, S; Martinelli, F; Hanozet, F; et al. Hysteroscopy in endometrial cancer: new methods to evaluate transtubal leakage of saline distension medium. *Am. J. Obstet. Gynecol.* 2008;198:214.e1.

[31] Biewenga, P; de Blok, S; Birnie, E. Does diagnostic hysteroscopy in patients with stage I endometrial carcinoma cause positive peritoneal washings? *Gynecol. Oncol.* 2004;93:194-8.

[32] Fadare, O; Mariappan, MR; Hileeto, D; Wang, S; Mcalpine, JN; Rimm, DL. Upstaging based solely on positive peritoneal washing does not affect outcome in endometrial cancer. *Mod. Pathol.* 2005;18:673-80.

[33] Pecorelli, S. Revised FIGO staging for carcinoma of the vulva, cervix, and endometrium. *Int. J. Gynaecol. Obstet.* 2009;105:103-4.

[34] Creasman, WT; Morrow, CP; Bundy, BN; Homesley, HD; Graham, JE; Heller, PB. Surgical pathological spread patterns of endometrial cancer – a gynecologic oncology group-study. *Cancer* 1987;60(Suppl 8):2035-41.

[35] Holub, Z; Jabor, A; Kliment, L. Comparison of two procedures for sentinel lymph node detection in patients with endometrial cancer: A pilot study. *Eur. J. Gynaecol. Oncol.* 2002;23:53-7.

[36] Mariani, A; Webb, MJ; Galli, L; Podratz, KC. Potential therapeutic role of para-aortic lymphadenectomy in node-positive endometrial cancer. *Gynecol. Oncol.* 2000;76: 348-56.

[37] Kilgore, LC; Partridge, EE; Alvarez, RD; Austin, JM; Shingleton, HM; Noojin, F; et al. Adenocarcinoma of the endometrium: survival comparison of patients with and without pelvic node sampling. *Gynecol. Oncol.* 1995;56: 29-33.

[38] Niikura, H; Okamura, C; Utsunomiya, H; Yoshinaga, K; Akahira, J; Ito, K; et al. Sentinel lymph node detection in patients with endometrial cancer. *Gynecol. Oncol.* 2004;92:669-74.

[39] Maccauro, M; Lucignani, G; Aliberti, G; Villano, C; Castellani, MR; Solima, E; et al. Sentinel lymph node detection following the hysteroscopic peritumoural injection of Tc-99m-labelled albumin nanocolloid in endometrial cancer. *Eur. J. Nucl. Med. Imaging* 2005;32:569-74.

[40] Raspagliesi, F; Ditto, A; Kusamura, S; Fontanelli, R; Vecchione, F; Maccauro, M; et al. Hysteroscopic injection of tracers in sentinel node detection of endometrial cancer: A feasibility study. *Am. J. Obstet. Gynecol* 2004;191:435-9.

[41] Gien, LT; Kwon, JS; Carey, MS. Sentinel node mapping with isosulfan blue dye in endometrial cancer. *J. Obstet. Gynecol. Can.* 2005;27:1107-12.

[42] Fersis, N; Gruber, I; Relakis, K; Friedrich, M; Becker, S; Wallwiener, D; et al. Sentinel node identification and intraoperative lymphatic mapping. First results of a pilot study in patients with endometrial cancer. *Eur. J. Gynecol. Oncol.* 2004;25:339-42.

In: Endometrial Cancer: Prevention, Diagnosis and Treatment ISBN: 978-1-62257-740-8
Editor: Stefano Greggi

Chapter V

Pre-Operative Staging: What Is the Cost-Effective Workup?

Roberto Angioli*, Francesco Plotti, Corrado Terranova, Carlo De Cicco Nardone, Michela Angelucci, Irma Oronzi, Patrizio Damiani, Roberto Montera and Giuseppe Scaletta

Obstetrics and Gynecology, "Campus Bio-Medico" University, Rome, Italy

Abstract

Carcinoma of the endometrium is among the most common female pelvic malignancies and may develop in normal, atrophic, or hyperplastic endometrium. Most of the cancers are detected at an early stage, with the tumor confined to the uterine corpus in 75% of patients. Endometrial biopsy, usually using an aspiration-type curet or other device, is generally accepted as the first-step office procedure. Many investigators have demonstrated that dilatation and curettage (D&C) lacks accuracy and reliability compared with other diagnostic methods. Recent studies have investigated the role of hysteroscopy in the diagnosis of endometrial cancer, a role that today is not yet clear. Ultrasonography (US) is the modality of choice for the initial imaging evaluation of female pelvic organs. US is widely available in many regions of the world, is relatively inexpensive, is noninvasive and does not use ionizing radiation. Transvaginal sonography (TVS) is superior to computed tomography (CT) and approaches magnetic resonance imaging (MRI) in its ability to depict endometrial carcinoma and to provide information regarding myometrial, cervical and, perhaps, parametrial tumor invasion. However, US is unable to depict the entire intra-pelvic or intra-abdominal anatomic regions adequately. CT and MRI are more accurate staging modalities than US. Both techniques allow the survey of the entire pelvis, abdomen, thorax and brain. MRI, which is superior to CT for visualizing uterus and pelvic tissues, is recommended as knowledge of extrauterine spread or cervix

* E-mail address: r.angioli@unicampus.it.

involvement by tumor. There are no differences in the ability of MRI or positron emission tomography (PET)/CT to detect lymph node metastases.

Introduction

About 75% of endometrial cancers are diagnosed in early stage because early symptoms include vaginal spotting or bleeding [1,2]. The prognosis of endometrial carcinoma depends on the depth of myometrial invasion and the presence of lymph node metastasis. Myometrial extension is a reliable index of lymphatic spread. Preoperative assessment of myometrial invasion is important in planning the surgical procedure and determining whether to perform lymph node sampling [1-3]. Patients with lymph node metastases have a significantly higher recurrence rate and a lower 5-year survival rate than those without lymph node metastases [4]. The histologic examination of the cancer and grade can be evaluated preoperatively after biopsy or dilatation and curettage (D&C).Numerous studies have evaluated the use of computed tomography (CT), magnetic resonance imaging (MRI), and transabdominal, transvaginal and intrauterine ultrasonography (US) in assessing the depth of myometrial invasion, sometimes giving contradictory results [5-9].

Invasive Methods

Dilatation and Curettage (D&C) and Endometrial Biopsy

These procedures are traditionally considered the standard for investigation of abnormal uterine bleeding and intrauterine disorders, procedures which Mengert and Slate called "the most expensive test in the entire medical field" [10].

Many investigators have demonstrated that D&C lacks accuracy and reliability compared with other diagnostic methods. Since 1958, studies have been published comparing histologic findings on D&C with those on subsequent hysterectomy in patients with abnormal uterine bleeding [11,12].

These studies revealed the inadequacy of curettage for diagnosis of intrauterine disorders, especially endometrial polyps and submucous myomas [12].

Furthermore, D&C is considered a low-yield procedure for exclusion of endometrial cancer, with a high rate of false-negative results [13].

Stovall et al. described 407 patients who had D&C that missed endometrial hyperplasia or carcinoma found on hysterectomy in 23 cases (5.7%) [14].

The sensitivity and specificity of D&C cannot be calculated from most of these reports owing to inadequate information [12]. A variety of instruments (the Pipelle, the Pipette, the Tis-U-Trap and the Z-sampler) has been developed over the last decade for using in the office as alternatives to the expense, risk, and inconvenience of fractional D&C. With the use of these devices, the sensitivity for detecting endometrial cancer ranges from 67% to 96%.

Hysteroscopy and Direct Biopsy

Some consider this method as the standard for the diagnosis of abnormal uterine bleeding. However, a recent study of 373 patients which retrospectively compared hysteroscopy and D&C, concluded that hysteroscopy did not improve upon the sensitivity of D&C in the detection of endometrial hyperplasia or carcinoma. On the contrary, Clark et al. found that hysteroscopy is highly accurate and useful in diagnosing, rather than excluding, endometrial cancer in women with abnormal uterine bleeding [15].

A recent study performed by Bedner and Rzepka-Gorska compared the effectiveness of D&C with hysteroscopy and guided biopsy in perimenopausal women at risk of endometrial hyperplasia or cancer. They found that hysteroscopy with directed biopsy was more sensitive than D&C for detecting all types of uterine lesions [16.]

Several retrospective studies have found increased positive peritoneal cytology in women who underwent hysteroscopy, but recent studies have indicated that there is currently no evidence to suggest that diagnostic hysteroscopy increases the risk of malignant cells spreading into the peritoneal cavity or worsens the prognosis in women with endometrial cancer.

Noninvasive Methods

Ultrasonography (US)

Transvaginal sonography (TVS) is useful for the evaluation of myometrial invasion by endometrial carcinoma. The demonstration of partial or total disruption of the hypoechoic subendometrial halo, formed by the compact and vascular inner myometrial region, usually reflects the presence of myometrial invasion, although depiction of intact subendometrial halo may be associated with superficial invasion or lack of invasion. The depth of myometrial invasion can be estimated by measuring, on sagittal images, the thickness of the tumor extending beyond the outer margin of the endometrium and dividing it by the entire thickness of the adjacent intact myometrium. TVS is superior to CT and approaches MRI in its ability to provide information regarding myometrial, cervical, and perhaps parametrial invasion by endometrial carcinoma [17]. TVS is reasonably accurate (70-90% PPV) in the prediction of deep myometrial invasion and is inexpensive in comparison to CT and MRI [18-20].

Van Doorn et al. considered TVS to be only moderately reliable in the prediction of deep myometrial invasion, but when combined with patient age and degree of tumour differentiation in the curettings, it was possible to preoperatively select women at high risk of lymph node metastases with sufficient reliability [21]. No US feature can reliably differentiate between malignant and benign endometrial pathology in the absence of identifiable myometrial invasion. The reported overall accuracy of US in detecting myometrial invasion and distinguishing between superficial and deep myometrial invasion by endometrial carcinoma ranges from 69-90%. The reported sensitivity and specificity of US evaluation of the depth of myometrial invasion are 50-100% and 65-100%, respectively. The reported sensitivity and specificity of US evaluation of cervical invasion by endometrial carcinoma are 66.7-80% and 95.2-100%, respectively [17,22].

Computed Tomography (CT)

Several retrospective studies have suggested that pelvic and abdominal CT scanning has limited utility in the preoperative assessment of women with endometrial carcinoma [23-26]. CT showed poor prediction of nodal disease and depth of myometrial invasion though it was suggested it could have some utility in high-risk histologic types such as clear cell and serous papillary [23,24]. In the largest and most recent series, Bansal reviewed the records of 762 women with uterine malignancies between 1990-2006. Abdomino-pelvic CT scans were performed preoperatively in 250 women (32 sarcoma and 218 with carcinoma) and CT findings were correlated with intraoperative and histopathologic data. The analysis focused on extranodal metastatic disease and any other incidental findings, and their capacity to alter the planned management. Extra nodal disease was found in 22 (9%) of women (adnexa 10, omentum 4, bowel 3, ascites 1) but patient management was altered in only seven (3%). Of these seven women, four had grade 3 endometrial endometrioid adenocarcinoma (EEA), one had a sarcoma and the other two had grade 1 EEA. Incidental findings were noted in 43 (17%) and management altered in only seven (3%) of these women in whom the findings were considered important, namely renal mass in five, severe diverticular disease requiring resection in one and a retroperitoneal mass with hydronephrosis due to squamous carcinoma in one patient. Further analysis based on preoperative histologic diagnosis showed that CT findings were more likely to alter management (10.7%) in women with high-risk serous papillary and clear cell histologic subtypes. They concluded that routine CT scanning of women with EEA is costly, of limited value and rarely alters treatment, but may have some utility in women with high-risk histology [25].

Magnetic Resonance Imaging (MRI)

MRI has been shown to be an accurate tool for the measurement of the depth of myometrial invasion by endometrial carcinoma though an isointense junctional zone, polypoid tumours or presence of leiomyomas may lead to an underestimate of myometrial invasion. This study showed 83.3% accuracy in differentiating deep from superficial invasion in 100 of 120 cases [27].

In a comprehensive literature review of the conservative management of endometrial cancer in young women, Erkanli suggested that MRI may be of assistance specifically in assessing the absence of invasion [28]. In a recent Australian study, Cade reported on progestogen treatment options for early endometrial cancer and considered an MRI scan negative for myometrial invasion or extension to the cervix an essential prerequisite to conservative treatment [29].

In contrast, Nakao has reported that although MRI is good at determining deep myometrial invasion it is not as accurate in assessing the absence of microscopic myometrial invasion [30].

This view is supported by an Australian study in which Cade questions whether radiological staging is sufficient for planning conservative treatment. This study compared MRI scans and final histopathological diagnoses of 111 patients with endometrioid adenocarcinoma over a six year period at a tertiary centre. They reported that MRI had a high negative predictive value (NPV) for the presence of deep invasion (87% overall and 95% for grade 1 disease), but a poor NPV for the presence of any myometrial invasion, making it less reliable in predicting the absence of invasion. However, if the new revised 2008 FIGO staging system was used then stage IA (no invasion or up to 50% invasion) was more accurately predicted using MRI, making it very useful if clinicians were to consider all patients with stage IA disease to be eligible for conservative treatment when fertility was desired [31].

In a retrospective review of 182 women diagnosed with clinical stage 1 disease, Cho et al. studied the accuracy of preoperative investigations. They found that MRI correctly differentiated stage 1A, IB and 1C disease in 58.2% (150/182) of patients but that the sensitivity and specificity of MRI in detecting lymph node metastases was only 45% and 80.8% respectively. They concluded that the inaccuracy of MRI would lead to incorrect surgical treatment in a substantial number of patients and that full systematic lymphadenectomy was necessary to determine the stage of the disease and tailor subsequent adjuvant therapy [32].

MRI has been shown to be accurate in the prediction of cervical stromal involvement with a positive predictive value of 89.8% in a study of 135 consecutive women [33].

This is important as it will allow for an informed decision regarding the type of hysterectomy to be performed: radical rather than simple.

Celik evaluated cervical involvement in endometrial cancer by comparing TVS, MRI and intraoperative frozen section in 64 consecutive patients. The accuracy rates of TVS, MRI and frozen section were 90.6%, 92.2% and 95.5%, respectively. Obviously frozen section does not allow for alteration of the type of hysterectomy to be offered but will suggest the need for lymphadenectomy in patients without other high-risk prognostic factors. MRI was noted to be more time consuming and expensive than TVS but could be recommended in cases where the TVS was of poor quality [20].

MRI was found to be more reliable than diagnostic fluid mini-hysteroscopy and TVS in predicting cervical involvement with a positive predictive value of 71%, a negative predictive value of 94% and an accuracy rate of 91% [34].

A meta-analysis of radiologic staging in patients with endometrial cancer was reported by Kinkel [35].

There were insufficient studies of CT and TVS for meaningful meta-analysis in regard to cervical involvement, but MRI showed equal specificity and sensitivity of 92% for prediction of cervical involvement. Most authors have suggested that gadolinium contrast enhanced MRI is better for prediction of deep myometrial invasion [36-37], but others have found no difference between T2 weighted and contrast enhanced MRI [38-39].

MRI may be used to assess the depth of myometrial invasion in order to predict women with deep invasion greater than 50% of myometrial thickness and this finding has utility as a surrogate for the likelihood of lymph node metastases and to determine appropriate surgical treatment [27,35-38].

It should be noted that nearly all of the MRI literature relates to the old FIGO 1988 staging. There is only one report regarding the efficiency of MRI in FIGO 2009 staged cases compared with FIGO 1988 staging. Ballester reported that MRI staging was more accurate using FIGO 2009 but only moderately better [40]. It is possible that as more work is reported using FIGO 2009, the role of routine MRI will be clearer but at present the evidence is lacking.

MRI may be used in subspecialist tertiary Centres for the assessment of cervical stromal involvement and appropriate surgical planning.

Positron Emission Tomography (PET) and PET/CT

The use of positron emission tomography using fluoro-2-deoxyglucose (FDG-PET) has been studied in the preoperative evaluation of endometrial cancer [41-43].

FDG-PET has a sensitivity of 83.3% in detecting extrauterine lesions (excluding retroperitoneal nodes) and was useful in providing additional information regarding lesions detected on CT/MRI that were of uncertain significance. FDG-PET was not able to identify any lymph node metastasis less than 1 cm in diameter, and therefore a negative finding is not a reason to omit retroperitoneal lymph node dissection [41].

Park retrospectively compared the validity of MRI and PET/CT in the preoperative evaluation of 53 women with endometrial cancer. There was no difference in the ability of MRI or PET/CT to detect lymph node metastases and it was concluded that PET/CT could not replace surgical staging, but because of its high negative predictive value in predicting lymph node and distant metastases, it could be helpful in the assessment of patients who are unsuited for full surgical staging [42].

Signorelli prospectively studied FDG-PET/CT in 37 fully surgically staged women confirming the results of other authors and the limitation in detecting nodal lesions of 5 mm or less, probably related to the limited spatial resolution of PET/CT scanners used in the study. They noted an accuracy of 94.4% in detecting nodal disease and concluded that the high NPV of 93.1% may be useful in selecting patients who may benefit from lymphadenectomy [43].

PET or PET/CT may be used in subspecialist tertiary Centres for the assessment of some patients and appropriate surgical planning. It is more commonly used post operatively, when the surgico-pathological findings show locally advanced disease or pelvic node involvement, in order to direct appropriate adjuvant therapy.

Conclusion

Endometrial biopsy, usually using an aspiration-type curet or other device, is generally accepted as the first-step office procedure. US is the most used and widespread for initial evaluation of initial imaging evaluation of gynecologic cancer. TVS is superior to CT and approaches MRI in its ability to depict endometrial carcinoma and to provide information regarding myometrial, cervical, and, perhaps, parametrial tumor invasion.

CT is clinically advocated in the evaluation of patients with poorly differentiated or high-grade tumor, serous papillary carcinoma, or clear cell carcinoma because of the high risk for advanced disease and metastatic lymphadenopathy at the time of presentation. CT also is advised for patients who have abnormal liver function test results, elevated serum CA125 levels, clinical suggestion of advanced disease, or inconclusive clinical evaluation.

MRI, with its exquisite soft tissue contrast and multiplanar capability, is superior to US and CT in helping assess the depth of myometrial invasion, cervical invasion, and early parametrial invasion. MRI is approximately equivalent to CT in detecting enlarged lymph nodes, but CT is considerably superior to MRI in detecting and distinguishing intraperitoneal, omental, and mesenteric metastases from bowel. Table 1 summarizes CT and MRI limitations.

Although MRI is superior to CT in evaluating myometrial and cervical invasion and is the best alternative for patients with significant contrast allergies or renal malfunction, CT is more sensitive than MRI in the overall detection of tumor spread outside the uterus. In addition, CT remains the imaging modality used most frequently in clinical practice for comprehensive preoperative evaluation of the extent of disease.

There are no difference in the ability of MRI or PET/CT to detect lymph node metastases.

Table 1. CT and MRI limitations

CT Limitations
Understaging cancers presenting with microscopic tumor spread
Diminished accuracy in evaluating myometrial invasion in elderly women, particularly in the setting of atrophic myometrium and polypoid endometrial tumors
Overlap with the appearances of other malignant uterine masses and leiomyomata
Similarity in the appearances of the irregular uterine contours and adjacent soft tissue stranding produced by parametrial tumor invasion and by parametritis secondary to fractional curettage or endometrial biopsy
Inability to differentiate lymph node enlargement resulting from benign causes from that resulting from metastases
MRI Limitations
Understaging cancers presenting with microscopic tumor spread
Difficulty in consistently differentiating endometrial cancer from benign pathologic findings
Diminished accuracy in evaluating myometrial invasion in the setting of polypoid tumor or blood distending the uterine cavity, resulting in the appearance of a thin myometrium
Difficulty in assessing the depth of myometrial invasion in elderly/postmenopausal patients with an ill-defined or nonvisible myometrial junctional zone or in those who have atrophic myometrium

References

[1] Berman, ML; Ballan, SC; LaGasse, LK; Watring, WG. Prognosis and treatment of endometrial cancer. *Am. J. Obstet. Gynecol.* 1980;136:679-88.

[2] Palter, SF; Olive, DL. Uterine cancer. In: Berek, JS; eds. *Novak's gynecology*. 12th ed. Baltimore: Williams and Wilkins; 1996.

[3] DiSaia, P; Creasman, W. *Clinical gynecologic oncology*. St Louis: Mosby; 1981.

[4] Lurain, JR; Rice, BL; Rademaker, AW; Poggensee, LE; Schink, JC; Miller, DS. Prognostic factors associated with recurrence in clinical stage I adenocarcinoma of the endometrium. *Obstet. Gynecol.* 1991;78:63-9.

[5] Hirai, Y; Kaku, S; Teshima, H; Chen, JT; Hamada, T; Fujimoto, I; et al. Use of angio computed tomography to evaluate extent of endometrial cancer. *Gynecol. Oncol.* 1989;33:372-5.

[6] Kinkel, K; Kaji, Y; Yu, KK; Segal, MR; Lu, Y; Powell, CB; et al. Radiologic staging in patients with endometrial cancer: A meta-analysis. *Radiology* 1999;212:711-8.

[7] Fleischer, AC; Dudley, BS; Entman, SS; Baxter, JW; Kalemeris, GC; James; AE Jr. Myometrial invasion by endometrial carcinoma: Sonographic assessment. *Radiology* 1987;162:307-10.

[8] Lee, EJ; Byun, JY; Kim, BS; Koong, SE; Shinn, KS. Staging of early endometrial carcinoma: Assessment with T2-weighted and gadolinium-enhanced T1-weighted MR imaging. *Radio Graphics* 1999;19:937-45.

[9] Tsuda, H; Murata, K; Kawabata, M; Yamamoto, K. Preoperative assessment of myometrial invasion of endometrial cancer by MR imaging and intrauterine

ultrasonography with a high-frequency probe: Preliminary study. *J. Ultrasound Med.* 1997;16:545-8.

[10] Mengert, WF; Slate, WG. Diagnostic dilatation and curettage as an outpatient procedure. *Am. J. Obstet. Gynecol.* 1960;79:727-9.

[11] Word, B; Gravlee, LC; Wideman, GL. The fallacy of simple uterine curettage. *Obstet. Gynecol.* 1958;12:642-3.

[12] Emanuel, MH; Wamsteker, K; Lammes, FB. Is dilatation and curettage obsolete for diagnosing intrauterine disorders in premenopausal patients with persistent abnormal uterine bleeding? *Acta Obstet. Gynecol. Scand.* 1997;76:65-8.

[13] Stock, RJ; Kanbour, A. Prehysterectomy curettage. *Obstet. Gynecol.* 1975;45:537-41.

[14] Stovall, TG; Solomon, SK; Ling, FW. Endometrial sampling prior to hysterectomy. *Obstet. Gynecol.* 1989;73:405-9.

[15] Clark, TJ; Voit, D; Gupta, JK; Hyde, C; Song, F; Khan, KS. Accuracy of hysteroscopy in the diagnosis of endometrial cancer and hyperplasia: a systematic quantitative review. *JAMA* 2002;288:1610-21.

[16] Bedner, R; Rzepka-Gorska, I. Hysteroscopy with directed biopsy versus dilatation and curettage for the diagnosis of endometrial hyperplasia and cancer in perimenopausal women. *Eur J Gynaecol Oncol* 2007;28:400-2.

[17] Gordon, AN; Fleischer, AC; Reed, GW. Depth of myometrial invasion in endometrial cancer: preoperative assessment by transvaginal ultrasonography. *Gynecol. Oncol.* 1990;39:321-7.

[18] Ruangvutilert, P; Sutantawibul, A; Sunsaneevithayakul, P; Boriboonhirunsarn, D; Chuenchom, T. Accuracy of transvaginal ultrasound for the evaluation of myometrial invasion in endometrial carcinoma. *J. Med. Assoc. Thai.* 2004;87:47-52.

[19] Takac, I. Transvaginal ultrasonography with and without saline infusion in assessment of myometrial invasion of endometrial cancer. *J. Ultrasound Med.* 2007;26:949-55.

[20] Celik, C; Ozdemir, S; Kiresi, D; Emlik, D; Tazegül, A; Esen, H. Evaluation of cervical involvement in endometrial cancer by transvaginal sonography; magnetic resonance imaging and frozen section. *J. Obstet. Gynaecol.* 2010;30:302-7.

[21] van Doorn, HC; van der Zee, AG; Peeters, PH; Kroeks, MV; van Eijkeren, MA. Preoperative selection of patients with low-stage endometrial cancer at high risk of pelvic lymph node metastases. *Int. J. Gynecol. Cancer* 2002;12:144-8.

[22] Tsuda, H; Kawabata, M; Yamamoto, K; Inoue, T; Umesaki, N. Prospective study to compare endometrial cytology and transvaginal ultrasonography for identification of endometrial malignancies. *Gynecol. Oncol.* 1997;65:383-6.

[23] Connor, JP; Andrews, JI; Anderson, B; Buller, RE. Computed tomography in endometrial carcinoma. *Obstet. Gynecol.* 2000;95:692-6.

[24] Zerbe, MJ; Bristow, R; Grumbine, FC; Montz, FJ. Inability of preoperative computed tomography scans to accurately predict the extent of myometrial invasion and extracorporal spread in endometrial cancer. *Gynecol. Oncol.* 2000;78:67-70.

[25] Bansal, N; Herzog, TJ; Brunner-Brown, A; Wethington, SL; Cohen, CJ; Burke, WM; et al. The utility and cost effectiveness of preoperative computed tomography for patients with uterine malignancies. *Gynecol Oncol* 2008;111:208-12.

[26] Gien, LT; Barbera, L; Kupets, R; Saskin, R; Paszat, L. Utilization of preoperative imaging in uterine cancer patients. *Gynecol. Oncol.* 2009;115:226-30.

[27] Chung, HH; Kang, SB; Cho, JY; Kim, JW; Park, NH; Song, YS; et al. Accuracy of MR imaging for the prediction of myometrial invasion of endometrial carcinoma. *Gynecol. Oncol.* 2007;104:654-9.

[28] Erkanli, S; Ayhan, A. Fertility-sparing therapy in young women with endometrial cancer: 2010 update. *Int. J. Gynecol. Cancer* 2010;20:1170-87.

[29] Cade, TJ; Quinn, MA; Rome, RM; Neesham, D. Progestogen treatment options for early endometrial cancer. *BJOG* 2010;117:879-84.

[30] Nakao, Y; Yokoyama, M; Hara, K; Koyamatsu, Y; Yasunaga, M; Araki, Y; et al. MR imaging in endometrial carcinoma as a diagnostic tool for the absence of myometrial invasion. *Gynecol. Oncol.* 2006;102:343-7.

[31] Cade, TJ; Quinn, MA; McNally, OM; Neesham, D; Pyman, J; Dobrotwir, A. Predictive value of magnetic resonance imaging in assessing myometrial invasion in endometrial cancer: is radiological staging sufficient for planning conservative treatment? *Int. J. Gynecol. Cancer* 2010;20:1166-9.

[32] Cho, H; Kim, YT; Kim, JH. Accuracy of preoperative tests in clinical stage I endometrial cancer: the importance of lymphadenectomy. *Acta Obstet. Gynecol. Scand.* 2010;89:175-81.

[33] Nagar, H; Dobbs, S; McClelland, HR; Price, J; McCluggage, WG; Grey, A. The diagnostic accuracy of magnetic resonance imaging in detecting cervical involvement in endometrial cancer. *Gynecol. Oncol.* 2006;103:431-4.

[34] Cicinelli, E; Marinaccio, M; Barba, B; Tinelli, R; Colafiglio, G; Pedote, P; et al. Reliability of diagnostic fluid hysteroscopy in the assessment of cervical invasion by endometrial carcinoma: a comparative study with transvaginal sonography and MRI. *Gynecol. Oncol.* 2008;111:55-61.

[35] Kinkel, K; Kaji, Y; Yu, KK; Segal, MR; Lu, Y; Powell, CB; et al. Radiologic staging in patients with endometrial cancer: a meta-analysis. *Radiology* 1999;212:711-8.

[36] Frei, KA; Kinkel, K; Bonél, HM; Lu, Y; Zaloudek, C; Hricak, H. Prediction of deep myometrial invasion in patients with endometrial cancer: clinical utility of contrast-enhanced MR imaging-a meta-analysis and Bayesian analysis. *Radiology* 2000;216:444-9.

[37] Sala, E; Crawford, R; Senior, E; Shaw, A; Simcock, B; Vrotsou, K; et al. Added value of dynamic contrast-enhanced magnetic resonance imaging in predicting advanced stage disease in patients with endometrial carcinoma. *Int. J. Gynecol. Cancer* 2009;19:141-6.

[38] Rockall, AG; Meroni, R; Sohaib, SA; Reynolds, K; Alexander-Sefre, F; Shepherd, JH; et al. Evaluation of endometrial carcinoma on magnetic resonance imaging. *Int. J. Gynecol. Cancer* 2007;17:188-96.

[39] Takahashi, S; Murakami, T; Narumi, Y; Kurachi, H; Tsuda, K; Kim, T; et al. Preoperative staging of endometrial carcinoma: diagnostic effect of T2-weighted fast spin-echo MR imaging. *Radiology* 1998;206:539-47.

[40] Ballester, M; Koskas, M; Coutant, C; Chéreau, E; Seror, J; Rouzier, R; et al. Does the use of the 2009 FIGO classification of endometrial cancer impact on indications of the sentinel node biopsy? *BMC Cancer* 2010;10:465.

[41] Suzuki, R; Miyagi, E; Takahashi, N; Sukegawa, A; Suzuki, A; Koike, I; et al. Validity of positron emission tomography using fluoro-2-deoxyglucose for the preoperative evaluation of endometrial cancer. *Int. J. Gynecol. Cancer* 2007;17:890-6.

[42] Park, JY; Kim, EN; Kim, DY; Suh, DS; Kim, JH; Kim, YM; et al. Comparison of the validity of magnetic resonance imaging and positron emission tomography/computed tomography in the preoperative evaluation of patients with uterine corpus cancer. *Gynecol. Oncol.* 2008;108:486-92.

[43] Signorelli, M; Guerra, L; Buda, A; Picchio, M; Mangili, G; Dell'Anna, T; et al. Role of the integrated FDG PET/CT in the surgical management of patients with high risk clinical early stage endometrial cancer: detection of pelvic nodal metastases. *Gynecol. Oncol.* 2009;115:231-5.

In: Endometrial Cancer: Prevention, Diagnosis and Treatment ISBN: 978-1-62257-740-8
Editor: Stefano Greggi

Chapter VI

The Surgical Treatment in the Early Disease

***Andrea Tinelli*[1*], *Giorgio Giorda*[2], *Sarah Gustapane*[3], *Roberta Montefrancesco*[4], *Marilena Greco*[5], *Daniele Vergara*[6], *Michele Maffia*[6], *Marianna Giampaglia*[7], *Vito Lorusso*[7] *and Antonio Malvasi*[8]**

[1]Gynecology and Obstetrics, "Vito Fazzi" Hospital, Lecce, Italy
[2]Gynecologic Oncology, Centro di Riferimento Oncologico, Aviano (PN), Italy
[3]Gynecology and Obstetrics, "SS. Annunziata" Hospital, Chieti, Italy
[4]Radiology, "Vito Fazzi" Hospital, Lecce, Italy
[5] Laboratory of Genetics and Genomics, Vito Fazzi Hospital, Lecce, Italy
[6]Biological and Environmental Sciences and Technologies, University of Salento, Lecce, Italy
Clinical Proteomic, "Giovanni Paolo II" Hospital, Lecce, Italy
[7]Oncology, Oncological Hospital, Lecce, Italy
[8] Gynecology and Obstetrics, "Santa Maria" Hospital, Bari, Italy

Abstract

Each year endometrial cancer affects lots of women in industrialized societies. The diagnosis of endometrial carcinoma requires histopathological confirmation. This diagnosis is made according to the World Health Organisation (WHO) pathological classification. About 80% of endometrial carcinomas are of endometrioid type. Endometrial carcinoma is a surgically staged disease. Operation is the therapy of choice in the primary treatment of patients with endometrial cancer. The type of surgery and postoperative therapy depends on the stage and other clinical-pathological risk factors. The traditional abdominal approach, vaginal, laparoscopic and robotic-assisted methods

[*] E-mail address: andreatinelli@gmail.com.

are available for the surgical treatment of endometrial cancer. This chapter discusses these different treatment options. With a rising incidence of obesity, number of patients with endometrial cancer will also increase. However, operations in obese patients are more challenging. Laparotomy as a standard therapy in endometrial cancer patients stage I and II should be replaced by laparoscopic approaches. Laparoscopy is oncologically adequate to open procedures and offers many advantages to patients. Robotic surgery in the treatment of endometrial cancer is still under evaluation. Most controversial points of treatment today are an indication and an extension of lymphadenectomy in different stages. Most recurrences will occur within the first 3 years after treatment and 3- to 4-montly evaluations with history. Physical and gynecological examination are usually recommended. Follow-up intervals of 6 months are recommended during the fourth and fifth years, and annually thereafter. No impact on survival of a routine follow-up strategy has been demonstrated.

Introduction

Endometrial cancer is the most common invasive gynecologic malignancy in developed countries and the eighth leading cause of cancer death in women; it typically arises in the sixth or seventh decade of life. The crude incidence of endometrial carcinoma in the European Union is 16 cases/100,000 women/year (range 13-24). The mortality rate is 4-5 cases/100,000/year.

The lifetime risk of developing endometrial carcinoma is about 1.7-2% and age-standardized incidence rates continue to rise in most developed countries [1]. The American Cancer Society's most recent estimates for uterus cancer (both endometrial cancer and uterine sarcomas) in the United States are from 2010: about 43,470 new cases of uterus cancer and 7,950 deaths from uterus cancer [2]. In comparison 41,200 women were diagnosed with EC in the United States in 2006, a substantial increase from 35,000 in 1987 [3]. The most important risk factors for the development of endometrial cancer are obesity, postmenopausal status, excessive fat consumption, body mass index (BMI) of 25 kg/m^2 or more, nulliparity, anovulation and unopposed estrogen use (Type I endometrial cancer). Despite the lack of systematic data for the steady rise of overweight patients in Europe there seems to be a similar trend for the incidence of adiposity comparable to America. More than 80% are, fortunately, detected in the prognostic favorable stages I and II. Fewer patients with endometrial cancer are rather thin, have no history of exogenous estrogen exposure (Type II endometrial cancer), or are perimenopausal (20-25% or younger than 40 years). The average age of women with endometrial cancer is 68 years. Therefore many patients are affected by additional relevant co-morbidities [4]. Combination of uterine corpus cancer with adiposity, hypertension, diabetes, coronary heart disease and/or other internal diseases increases surgical-anaesthesiologic risk are the major gynecological oncologic challenges in the current century.

However, chronological age by itself is not a reason for higher perioperative morbidity and mortality [5]. In addition to the traditional abdominal approach, vaginal, laparoscopic and robotic-assisted methods are also available for the surgical treatment of endometrial cancer today.

Endometrial Cancer in Young Women: Optional Surgical Treatments

Approximately 5% of the patients affected by endometrial cancer are younger than 40 years. Even if this neoplasia appears uncommonly in young patients; it probably includes less than 5% of all cases. Some of the patients wish to preserve fertility. The question of sparing fertility emerges as a challenge in some cases, especially in those that have been diagnosed in a very early stage and have not already had children [6,7].

However there is not, so far, enough experience worldwide of the conservative management of early endometrial cancer in young patients [8,9].

There are some questions that must be raised when this conservative management is evaluated:

1. Is it possible to take a conservative approach when facing an endometrial cancer?
2. In which cases?
3. How should we treat these patients?
4. What will their reproductive outcome be?
5. Do we know the risks they run?

The decision for uterus conservation is complicated by the fact that in patients with endometrial cancer stage grading 1 one can find in 10-45% synchronous ovarian tumors. Additionally, in up to 10% of cases myometrial infiltration is histological confirmed in spite of a negative Magnetic Resonance Imaging (MRI) and a higher grading than in the Dilatation and Curettage is detected in nearly 20% of cases. The accuracy of MRI to detect myometrial invasion is 70% [10].

After reviewing the international literature, the most important conclusion that can be drawn is that selecting patients correctly for conservative treatment is absolutely crucial for success. The first criterion for conservative treatment would be an accurate diagnosis of a well differentiated endometrial carcinoma, done by an expert pathologist. Only well differentiated tumors can be selected for conservative treatment.

The second important criterion for patient selection is the clinical absence of myometrial invasion. Only superficial tumors can be selected for conservative treatment.

These are criteria for conservative management:

- A well differentiated carcinoma
- The tumor does not deeply invade the myometrium, as demonstrated by MRI
- Absence of suspicious pelvic or pre-aortic nodes (Figure 1)
- Absence of synchronous ovarian tumor, meaning that we should consider performing a diagnostic laparoscopy before including the patient in the protocol
- No contraindications for medical treatment
- Patient understands and accepts that this is not a standard treatment
- The patient should show her desire to complete the follow-up protocol.

Until today there are only a few case series or case reports available. All patients described in these publications were staged by imaging systems, as ultrasonography (Figure

2), even though PET-CT has been shown (in a small study) to have a sensitivity for detection of pelvic lymph node metastasis of only 67% [11].

A meta-analysis on the assessment of myometrial invasion by radiologic imaging. They demonstrated that MRI offered the best sensitivity for a specific false positive rate using ROC curves [2].

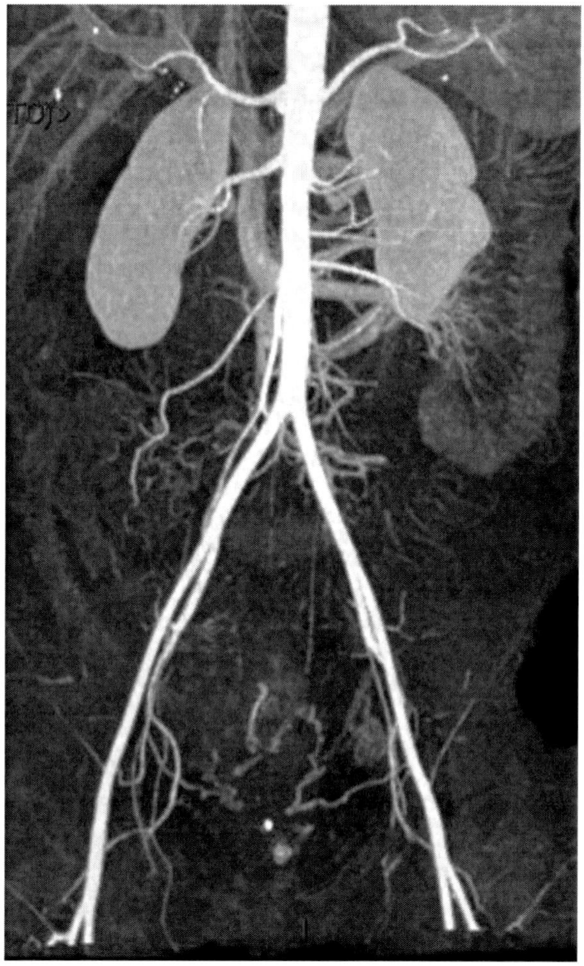

Figure 1. A reconstruction of abdomino-pelvic vascular tree, without evidence of suspicious pelvic or pre-aortic nodes in a women with endometrial cancer in stage IA.

Probably PET-CT will be the standard staging tool in the future; Yoshida has just published his first experience with fluorestradiol as a nuclear marker to follow the response in these patients.

The range of described conservative therapy modalities is broad and comprises gestagen therapy, intrauterine insertion of levonorgestrel-releasing system, oral application of aromatase inhibitors, GnRH analogue or hysteroscopic resection of endometrial cancer in combination with hormonal treatment.

It is important to advise these patients carefully about individual treatment, thus high compliance and understanding are paramount. After informed consent has been obtained, following criteria must be fulfilled: grading 1 carcinoma, no myometrial infiltration in MRI or sonography, no detection of suspicious pelvic or para-aortic lymph nodes, no evidence of adnexal tumors, no contraindication for hormonal treatment, agreement for close follow-up (curettage every 3 month), stage adjusted therapy after finishing desire for childbearing.

Chiva et al. summarized data of 133 women with fertility preserving therapy in endometrial cancer; 76% of patients responded to hormonally therapy. However, 34% of women developed recurrence after a mean of 20 months. In 24% of patients there was no response to hormonal therapy: 53 pregnancies occurred but also 4 treatments related deaths [12].

It is advisable, that young patients with clinical stage IA G1 endometrial cancer should undergo staging laparoscopy after informed counseling to exclude secondary ovarian neoplasia and lymph node metastases before starting hormonal therapy.

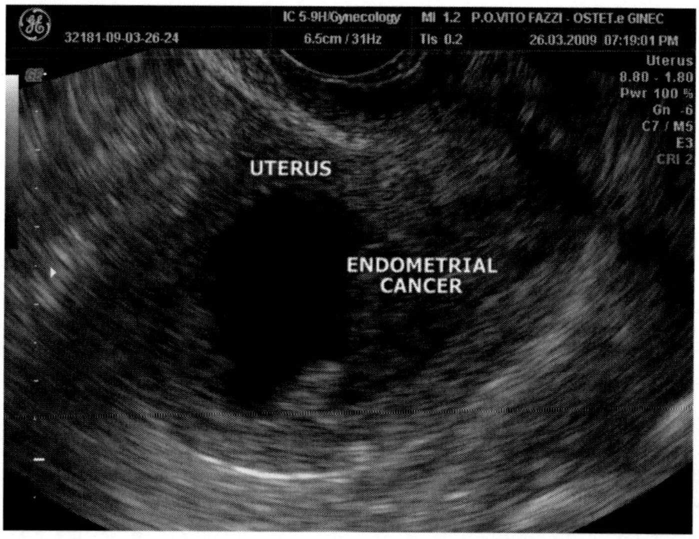

Figure 2. Transvaginal ultrasonographic section of a post-menopausal uterus with a dilated cavity and an endometrial cancer growing on the posterior wall.

After finishing family planning stage-adjusted operative (and radiation) therapy has to be initiated, frequently resulting in the discovery of higher tumor stages than initially diagnosed [13].

Ovarian preservation during surgical management of early stage endometrial cancer is still under debate and should be done only individually after extensive discussion and informed consent with the patient [14-16].

Clinical Recommendation Guidelines for Endometrial Cancer in International Federation of Gynecology and Obstetrics (FIGO) Stage I

The recent clinical recommendation guidelines of the European Society for Medical Oncology (ESMO) for diagnosis, treatment and follow-up of endometrial cancer, in line with many international guidelines, include the acquisition of peritoneal fluid or washings, a thorough exploration of the abdominal cavity and (at least 15 lymph nodes) and para-aortic (at least 10 lymph nodes) nodal areas, and a total hysterectomy with bilateral salpingo-oophorectomy.

In high risk cases retroperitoneal lymph node dissection and omentectomy (for serous carcinomas) are often recommended, though the effect of these procedures on survival is debated. In case of uterine papillary-serous carcinoma or clear cell carcinoma it is mandatory to extract multiple peritoneal samples as well as to perform omentectomy [17].

In clinical stages IA G1 and G2 and IB G1 and G2 lymphadenectomy is optional. In patients with relevant co-morbidities it is acceptable to omit lymphadenectomy, even in higher clinical stages.

Systematic surgical staging, including simple hysterectomy with bilateral salpingo-oophorectomy and pelvic lymphadenectomy (Figure 3) is for most of the women affected by endometrial cancer the baseline therapy and allows clear decision for stage-related adjuvant therapy. More extensive parametrial resection (radical hysterectomy) does not improve oncologic outcome in patients with stage I endometrial cancer [18].

However, definitive histological grading, myometrial invasion and lymph node involvement differ in a substantial rate from intraoperative gross assessment (up to 15%) and frozen section result (up to 25%) [19,20]. Therefore decision on comprehensiveness of surgical treatment is challenging.

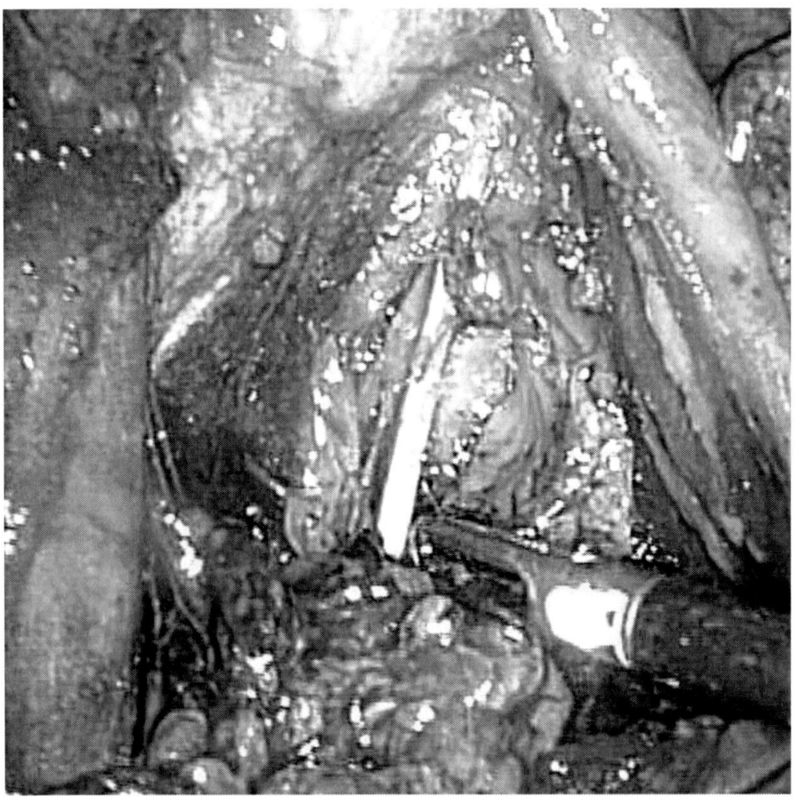

Figure 3. Left pelvic laparoscopic lymphadenectomy with obturator nerve and lymph nodes exposing in obturator fossa.

Total Abdominal Hysterectomy with Bilateral Salpingo-Oophorectomy (TAH-BSO)

Most patients affected by histological proven endometrial cancer today still undergo surgical treatment by surgical abdominal approach (Figure 4).

In most cases a midline longitudinal laparotomy is performed that starts above the pubic symphysis and (depending on the extension of the lymphadenectomy) expands until the xiphoid. Alternative ways of laparotomies are a wide Pfannenstiel incision (optionally with Kustner incision) or laparotomy including a panniculectomy [21].

With increasing BMI rate of successful lymphadenectomy is however significantly decreasing. The estimated blood loss rises and duration of surgery extends [22]. In morbidly obese patients, noninfectious wound breakdown occurs in up to 10% [23].

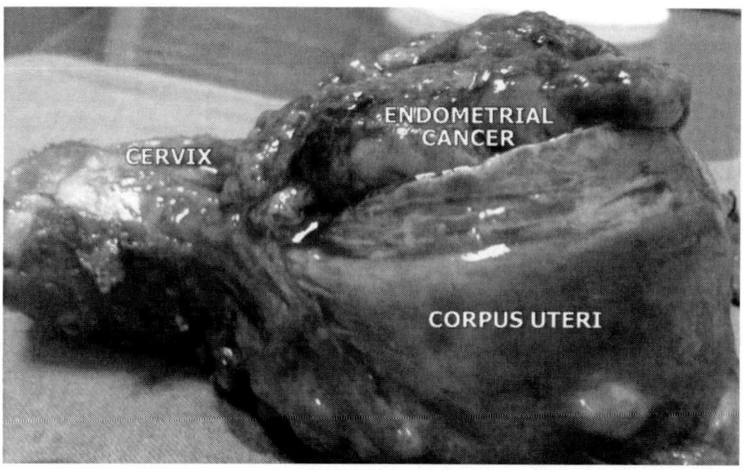

Figure 4. An endometrial cancer perforating serosa tissue of uterine body.

Vaginal Hysterectomy (VH)

In cases of considerable limited operability, vaginal hysterectomy is a feasible alternative to abdominal approach. Lelle et al. demonstrated in 60 patients with EC undergoing vaginal hysterectomy 5- and 10-year survival rates of 91% and 87%, respectively [24]. Despite refraining from bilateral salpingo-oophorectomy in 50% of the women treated with vaginal hysterectomy, Chan et al. published similar oncologic results with respect to 5-year survival [25].

The disadvantage of the exclusive vaginal approach is the impossibility of performing a lymphadenectomy. A possible combination of vaginal hysterectomy and open extraperitoneal lymphadenectomy was described by Massi et al., though without demonstrating oncologic results [26]. Dowdy et al. [27] successfully performed laparoscopic extraperitoneal para-aortic lymphadenectomy as second procedure in 90% of women with high risk endometrial cancer after previous vaginal hysterectomy.

Laparoscopic Assisted Vaginal Hysterectomy (LAVH) and Total Laparoscopic Hysterectomy (TLH)

While laparoscopic approach is already the standard approach in treating benign gynecological diseases, it is only more recently used in gynecological oncology, including in the therapy of endometrial cancer [28]. This was possible following secure ability to perform laparoscopic pelvic and para-aortic lymphadenectomy at the end of the last century [29,30]. The trocar placement is standardized.

So far, the results of laparoscopic therapy of endometrial cancer have been evaluated in about 50 prospective and retrospective, studies, predominantly designed as monocenter studies. More important data are available from 5 prospective randomized trials. One major argument against laparoscopic treatment of endometrial cancer, occurrence of port-side metastasis, could be invalidated. Martinez et al. found after 1216 laparoscopic procedures, including 295 for endometrial cancer, an incidence of trocar metastasis of 0.33%. Excluding patients with peritoneal carcinomatosis rate drops down to 0.16% [31].

All studies performing either laparoscopic assisted vaginal hysterectomy or total laparoscopic hysterectomy with or without lymphadenectomy report similar and consistent results, demonstrating that laparoscopic approach is a safe and oncologic adequate way of surgical treatment in patients with endometrial cancer stage I.

Laparoscopic staging in endometrial cancer provides substantial benefits for the patients, as reported in Table 1.

Disadvantages are the longer duration of surgery, especially when lymphadenectomy is performed, and the overcoming of the learning curve [32-43]. Conversion rate in the randomized studies varies between 7-20%. Nevertheless it could be shown that particular older patients with additional co-morbidity [44] and obese patients [45] benefited mostly from laparoscopic approach.

The advantages lasting at least six months [46]. More importantly, oncologic results (OS, DFS) of the laparoscopic surgery are equivalent to conventional abdominal surgery. This has been shown with the highest evidence level in 5 prospective randomized studies and related meta-analyses [47-53].

Table 1. Substantial benefits for the patients affected by endometrial cancer laparoscopically staged

LESS BLOOD LOSS
LESS TRANSFUSION RATE
REDUCED DURATION OF HOSPITAL STAY
FASTER RECOVERY TO NORMAL DAILY ACTIVITY
LESS POSTOPERATIVE DEMAND ON ANALGESICS
HIGHER OR EQUAL NUMBER OF REMOVED LYMPH NODES
LESS COMPLICATIONS

Unfortunately these 5 studies include only 238 patients in the groups that underwent laparoscopic surgery. If the results of further randomized studies like the Dutch multicenter trial NTR 821 and Gynecologic Oncology Group (GOG) LAP2 study should confirm these results, every patient affected by endometrial cancer stage I should be offered a laparoscopic surgical therapy, and abdominal approach should only be chosen and accepted in cases of severe contraindications [54,55].

Laparoscopic Treatment

Given the advancement of minimally invasive surgical techniques over the last decade, the prospect of endoscopic treatment of endometrial cancer is attractive and featuring. Since early studies by Childers et al., it was already demonstrated the feasibility of incorporating laparoscopy into the surgical management of early stage endometrial cancer. They demonstrated that laparoscopy appeared to be a reasonable alternative to laparotomy, with a similar complication rate and surgical time [56].

Subsequent studies have confirmed the safety and efficacy of the laparoscopic approach to endometrial cancer, even suggesting that a minimally invasive approach to early endometrial cancer may be preferable over the standard laparotomy, with equivalent or superior lymph node yields, quicker patient recovery and decreased postoperative complications [57].

Most recently the Gynecologic Oncology Group published operative results and complications of their LAP2 study evaluating laparoscopy compared to laparotomy in the surgical staging of Stage I- Stage II (occult) endometrial cancer [58].

Not surprisingly, laparoscopy was associated with a superior quality of life at six weeks post operatively. Other endpoints, including short-term outcomes, complication rates and length of hospital stay, favor laparoscopy. The length of surgery time was significantly longer in the laparoscopy arm of the study, but the conclusion of the study was that laparoscopy is safe, feasible, results in fewer complications, shorter hospital stay, and should be considered a standard of care for uterine cancer.

Moreover, at the 2010 Society of Gynecologic Oncologists annual meeting, survival results of this study were presented which demonstrated no difference in recurrence or survival between the two surgical modalities: specifically, estimated three-year overall survival was 89.8% for the laparoscopy group and 89.9% for the laparotomy group (p=NS) [59].

Robotic-Assisted Treatment

With approval of the DaVinci Surgical System (Intuitive Surgical Inc., Sunnyvale, CA, USA) by the FDA in 2005 (Figure 5), a new era of laparoscopic technique in gynecology began. This technique will potentially be able to overcome prejudices and resistances against laparoscopic oncological surgery.

Robotic-assisted laparoscopy offers substantial advantages such as a three-dimensional view that improves visualization of the surgical field, allowing greater precision and accuracy.

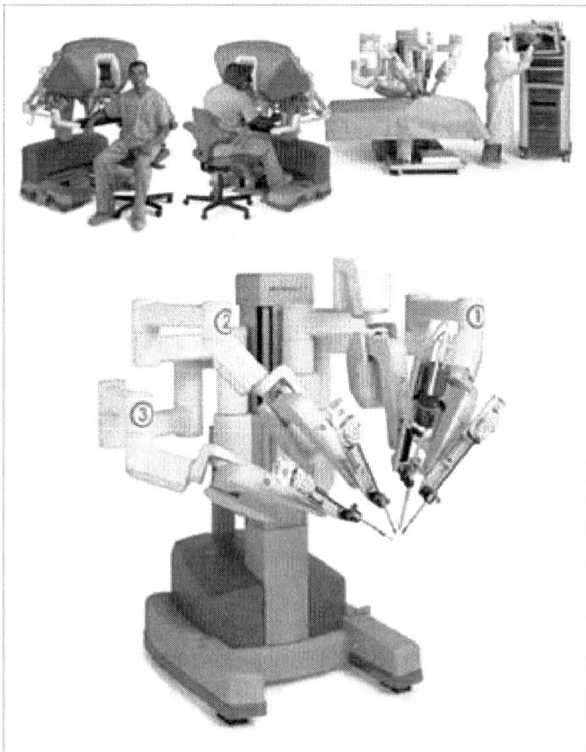

Figure 5. The DaVinci Surgical System by Intuitive Surgical Inc.

While operating the robotic operative instruments, the surgeon is capable of manipulating, repositioning, grasping, retracting, cutting, dissecting, coagulating, and suturing. Another advantage is the wrist-like motion of the robotic arm which provides finer and more dexterous movements, enabling surgical procedures which were impossible with the conventional laparoscopy. The only currently available surgical robot employs two magnifying, wide-angle cameras that when aligned provide three-dimensional vision to the console surgeon with an available high-definition vision system. This enhanced visualization gives the gynecologic surgeon an improved ability to identify the tissue planes, blood vessels, and nerves while performing the surgical procedures [60,61].

The improved dexterity and control allow for finer, more delicate, tremor-free manipulation, dissection, removal, or reconstruction of tissue.

The main disadvantages of robotic surgery across applications are the high costs, the large size of the robot and console, lack of tactile feedback or haptic, the increased operating time associated with equipment set up and docking, the inability to reposition the patient once the robot arms are attached and the need to train residents, attending surgeons and operating room personnel on the use of this technology. The costs associated with robotic surgery include the costs of the unit that can range from 1.6 million Euros, annual maintenance fees, and the cost of instrumentation that has limited patient uses [60-62].

Moreover, costs for robotic staging of endometrial cancer patients are significant higher, approximately 1,300$ per operation, due to longer operating room time and disposable instruments compared to traditional laparoscopy [63]. After passing the learning curve of about 20 operations [64] many authors consider robotic-assisted surgery to be an ideal combination of the advantages of abdominal and laparoscopic approach [64-67].

In endometrial cancer, Hoekstra et al. evaluated the impact of a new robotic surgery program on perioperative outcomes for endometrial cancer, comparing, in a prospective study, demographic data and perioperative outcomes between 65 cases performed via laparotomy, laparoscopy and robotics (LAP-26, LSC-7, ROB-32). No difference in surgical volume in the year before vs. after robotics was identified.

Median operative time for robotics and laparotomy was significantly less than for laparoscopy ($p=0.023$). There was no significant difference in lymph nodes yield between the three groups ($p=0.92$). Robotics was associated with significantly less blood loss ($p<0.0001$). Complication rates were significantly lower in the robotic group compared to the laparotomy group ($p=0.05$). Median hospital stay was 1 day for the minimally invasive groups. Total number of perioperative inpatient days decreased from 331 to 150 in one year. Practice management of endometrial cancer transitioned from a predominantly open approach (5.6% LSC) to robotics (11% LSC, 49% ROB) within 12 months. In the conclusion, the authors reported that robotic surgery was associated with a significant improvement in several perioperative outcomes when compared to laparotomy and laparoscopy, in endometrial cancer [68].

Bell et al analyzed outcomes and cost for endometrial cancer staging via traditional laparotomy, standard laparoscopy and robotic techniques on one hundred and ten patients and concluded that Robotic hysterectomy provides comparable node retrieval to laparotomy and laparoscopic procedures in the case of the experienced laparoscopic surgeon. While robotic hysterectomy takes longer to perform than hysterectomy completed via laparotomy, it is equivalent to laparoscopic hysterectomy and provides the patient with a more expeditious return to normal activity with reduced post-operative morbidity. Additionally, the average cost for hysterectomy and staging was highest for laparotomy, followed by robotic, and least for standard laparoscopy [69].

This new method of surgery is advantageous in comparison to the conventional abdominal approach and might even perform better than the conventional-laparoscopic surgery in relation to operative times, blood loss and postoperative hospital stay [70-72], which has however still to be confirmed by further studies.

De Nardis et al. compared 2008 the surgical morbidity of 56 patients affected by endometrial cancer clinical stage I after undergoing robotic-assisted laparoscopic hysterectomy with lymphadenectomy with a group of 106 patients who underwent abdominal approach. Three (5.4%) originally planned robotic-assisted operations needed to be converted to abdominal approach. Intraoperative blood loss, rate of perioperative complications (3.6% vs. 20.8%) and duration of hospital stay were significantly favorable in the DaVinci-group, but operative times were substantially longer. The lymph node yields were comparable. These results have to be interpreted cautiously because of differences in the characteristics of the groups of patients, with the group achieving robotic-assisted surgery containing younger and slimmer women with less co-morbidities and earlier clinical stages of endometrial cancer [70].

Veljovich et al. performed a similar study and compared 118 patients after robotic operations with 131 women undergoing an open abdominal surgery and could demonstrate longer operative times for robotic surgery but also a significantly lower blood loss and a considerably shorter hospital stay. The lymph node yields were as well comparable [72].

Boggess et al. compared three possible ways to performing an extensive endometrial cancer staging: abdominal approach (n=138), conventional laparoscopic (n=81) und robotic-assisted (n=103). The blood loss was lowest in the DaVinci-group, the lymph node yields were significantly higher and the hospital stays shortest. The operative times were comparable in the robotic-assisted and conventional laparoscopy, but longer than by laparotomy. Boggess inserted five trocars for his operation; a placement, that is now used by many other centers. The complication rates of the robotic-assisted operations were significantly lower than in the laparotomy group (5.9% vs. 29.7%). There was no difference in the conversion rates between conventional and robotic-assisted laparoscopy [73].

Analyzing the subgroup of obese and morbid obese patients, there is a considerable advantage in using the robot compared to conventional laparoscopy, including shorter operative times, less blood loss and higher lymph node yields [74].

Comparable favorable results were demonstrated by Seamon et al. 2008. Only 12.4% of the originally planned 105 robotic-assisted operations had to be converted, especially in morbid obese patients. The mean operative time was 242 minutes, the blood loss 99 cc, the lymph node yields 29. 24 hours later most of the patients were in the condition to get discharged [75].

More recently Cardenas-Goicoechea and co-workers demonstrated similar results by analyzing 102 patients with endometrial cancer after robotic-assisted staging [76].

Up to now there are no oncologic follow-up date after robotic assisted staging in endometrial cancer patients available. Ultimately, the 5-year survival rate must be the decisive oncologic criterion for robotic surgery [77].

A recent systematic review described clinical outcomes of robotic-assisted surgeries compared with traditional laparoscopic or laparotomy techniques for the treatment of endometrial cancer. This study indicates that robotic surgery can be considered at least as adequate as laparotomy and laparoscopy for the staging of endometrial cancer from the perspective of lymph node counts and morbidity. Considering that data from robotic hysterectomy case-series represents “the learning curve”, it is possible that more mature data will reflect a larger reduction in perioperative morbidity for robotic hysterectomy.

Conversely, it is possible that experienced surgeons will attempt more difficult cases and increase the reported morbidities with robotic hysterectomy.

There are no long-term studies reporting recurrence rates and survival for patients with endometrial cancer treated with the robotic approach, but there is no reason to believe it will be different than laparoscopy. Retrospective comparison trials uniformly indicate that perioperative outcomes are similar for robotic hysterectomy and laparoscopy with the exception of less blood loss, possibly fewer transfusions, and laparotomy conversions for robotic hysterectomy cases. Future prospective multi-institutional trials are required to more accurately survey for postoperative complications and verify the long-term oncologic outcomes and associated costs with this new technology [78].

Comparison between Laparoscopy and Robotic-Assisted Surgery

Increasingly, robotic assisted laparoscopy is being utilized for the management of patients with endometrial cancer. As more gynecologic oncologists incorporate robotic assisted laparoscopy into their clinical practice, data addressing the adequacy of this surgical approach in the management of endometrial cancer is becoming available. Building on experience from clinical practice and trials such as the LAP2 study, it appears that the advantages of robotic assisted surgery may help to overcome the limitations of traditional laparoscopy, including improved optics, improved range of motion of the instruments lending to increased surgical dexterity, operator control of the camera and improved ergonomics decreasing surgeon fatigue [70].

Moreover, several studies have attempted to compare outcomes between laparotomy, laparoscopy and robotic hysterectomy in the management of early stage endometrial cancer. Recently published data comparing different surgical techniques for the management of endometrial cancer has focused on surgical length, blood loss, and complications including conversion from laparoscopy to laparotomy, recovery time, and lymph node dissection yield. Although mature data regarding intermediate survival in laparoscopically staged patients was recently presented (by Walker JPM at GOG Meeting 2010 in San Francisco, USA), we currently lack data on long term outcomes and recurrence rates pertaining to robotic hysterectomies for the management of endometrial cancer patients. While there are variations between groups, it has been consistently reported that when compared to laparotomy, robotically assisted laparoscopic hysterectomies take longer to perform, but with a decrease in estimated blood loss, transfusion rate, intra- and post-operative complications, and length of hospital stay [57,70,73].

When compared to standard laparoscopy, there was a consistent decrease in estimated blood loss, although the true clinical impact of this may be debated. The rate of conversion to laparotomy was variable between groups. Estimated blood loss is an interesting marker for the advocates of robotic surgery. While studies have demonstrated that blood loss is consistently, significantly lower in robotic hysterectomies, the question remains as to its clinical significancc. Onc can arguc that transfusion rate is a better indicator of superiority. In two of the largest studies directly comparing TLH to Total Robotic Hysterectomy (TRH) there is conflicting data about transfusion rate following surgery.

Boggess et al. showed no difference in transfusion rates between TLH and TRH [73], while Seamon and colleagues demonstrated a significantly increased risk of transfusion with TLH [71].

Studies have also documented that robotic assisted lymphadenectomy lymph node yield is similar to laparotomy [57,70,73].

It is somewhat uncertain how to evaluate nodal yield data as the performance of a lymph node dissection was not standardized between all groups and only the cases that underwent a lymph node dissection were used for comparison. With the recent publication of the ASTEC trial, there continues to be ongoing debate about the utility of a pelvic, and to a lesser degree para-aortic, lymph node dissection in the complete staging of endometrial cancer and without the long term outcome data on recurrence and survival, its usefulness and indicates will likely continue to be debated [80,81].

Other than the oncologic outcome of survival, potentially the most important comparison between management strategies is the overall complication rate between the different surgical approaches. Since TRH is an extension of traditional laparoscopic surgery it is reasonable to anticipate similar complications and complication rates to TLH. Published data support this, with intra- and post-operative complication rates and types of complications being similar between TRH and TLH [73].

As with TLH, the rate of complications is significantly decreased when comparing TRH to TAH [73].

Conversion from laparoscopy to laparotomy is also a significant factor when comparing TLH to TRH. A majority of studies show a significant decrease in conversion rate when a TRH is performed compared to TLH [71,73].

The most common factor sited for the increase conversion rate associated with TLH is poor visualization which proponents of robotic surgery argue is overcome by using the robot [59,73].

Finally, and not unique to TRH performed for malignancy, vaginal cuff dehiscence remains a concern that continues to be evaluated and addressed [82,83].

Obesity is historically cited as a relative contraindication for laparoscopic surgery. Given that the average woman with endometrial cancer is overweight it is important to include this group in any comparison between the different surgical procedures. Fortunately, in most recent reviews of TRH in the management of endometrial cancer, the BMI was comparable between the TLH and TRH cohorts [71,73].

Reflecting the fact that the average patient with endometrial cancer is overweight, almost all cohorts had a BMI in excess of 30. As previously stated the conversion rate of TRH to TAH is lower than that of TLH with comparable BMI. Given these results, it may be reasonable to consider robotic surgery preferentially over standard laparoscopy in overweight patients. Another consideration is length of the surgical procedure. It is generally accepted that minimally invasive surgery takes longer to perform than an equivalent open procedure. We must weigh the risks of prolonged anesthesia for the initial procedure versus the benefit of a shorter recovery time. Given the propensity for the average patient with endometrial cancer to be obese this should not be overlooked. It is known that during pneumoperitoneum, obese patients have less efficient ventilation [84]. When compared to TAH, TLH and TRH took longer to perform [57,70,71,73].

Interestingly in the studies that directly compared TLH to TRH, it consistently took less time to perform TRH [71,73].

In the Veljovich et al. study who evaluated the outcomes during the initial year of implementing a robotic surgery platform, although it did not reach statistical significance, they found that the operative times for the second half of the year were shorter than for the first half of the year [72].

A final important consideration in the comparison of surgical techniques for endometrial cancer is cost. Bell et al. compared the direct and indirect costs at their institution for performing laparotomy, laparoscopy and robotic staging of endometrial cancer [69].

Interestingly, because of the significantly decreased hospital stay and the quicker return to normal activity, the laparoscopic and robotic staging appear to cost less in the long run than laparotomy. Concluding the reported experience with robotic assisted laparoscopy appears to be equivalent, if not better than, most clinical aspects when compared to standard laparoscopy or exploratory laparotomy. In light of the recently released GOG-LAP2 data demonstrating no increase in recurrence or survival, minimally invasive surgery for the treatment of endometrial cancer is a viable and likely superior surgical procedure for eligible patients. Although no randomized trials have evaluated laparoscopy with or without robotic assistance, the published studies to date would suggest that TRH is non-inferior to TLH. If randomized trials are not undertaken, it is imperative that additional studies continue to evaluate the utility of these modalities and ultimately include survival.

Debate on the Role of Lymphadenectomy

The role of pelvic (Figure 6) and para-aortic lymphadenectomy (Figure 7) is currently the most controversial and internationally most inconsistently used element of the surgical approach to endometrial carcinoma.

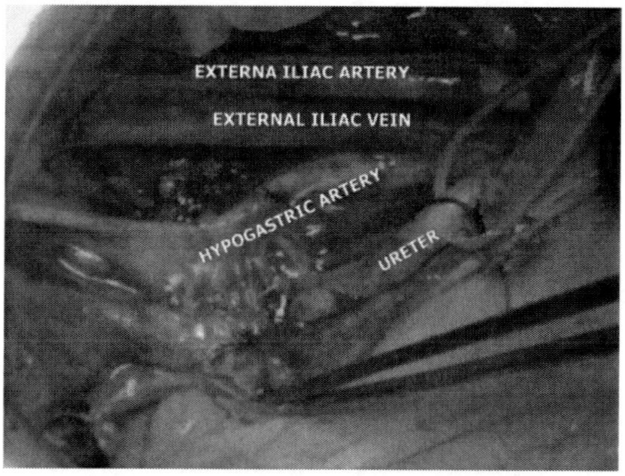

Figure 6. A right pelvic systematic lymphadenectomy with a clip on hypogastric artery and highlighting of right ureter by Liga-Loop.

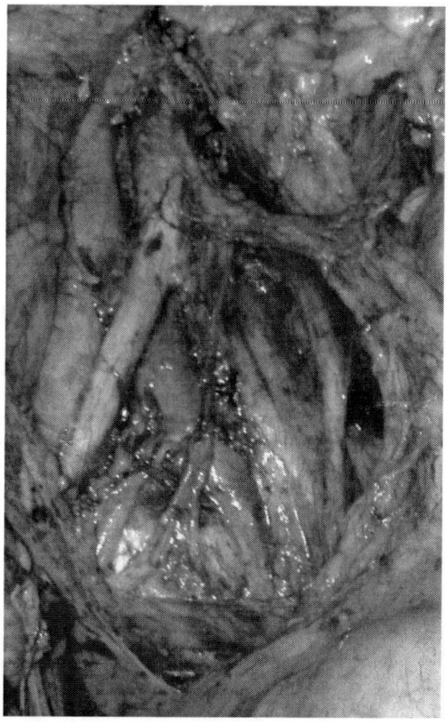

Figure 7. Lombo-aortic laparotomic infra renal lymphadenectomy with nerve sparing; it is well showed the inferior mesenteric artery on the right side of picture.

Following FIGO women with histological confirmed endometrial cancer requires comprehensive staging that includes total hysterectomy, bilateral salpingo-oophorectomy, peritoneal washing and loco regional lymphadenectomy. This is the only way stage IIIC (nodal positive) can be identified and the appropriate radiation therapy can be subsequently initiated or avoided. In addition, systematic lymphadenectomy seems to have a therapeutic effect in women with endometrial cancer [85,86].

However, extend (sampling or complete) and level (only pelvic, pelvic and para-aortic inframesenteric / infrarenal) of lymphadenectomy and are not mandatorily defined.

Guidelines for surgical treatment of endometrial cancer vary between countries. ESMO recommendation is to perform comprehensive pelvic and para-aortic lymphadenectomy up to the renal vessels in all patients except stage IA G1 [13,87].

In stages IB G1, IA G2 and IB G2 lymph node dissection is optional, an all other cases obligatory according to retrospective Mayo data, that demonstrated a high percentage of pelvic and (sometimes isolated) para-aortic lymph node metastasis [88]. These results could, however, not be confirmed in other analysis.

In the last FIGO Report (2006) pelvic lymph node metastases are detected in stage I endometrial cancer in 1.4-37.2% of patients and para-aortic lymph node metastases in 0.3-12.6% (in correlation to grading and myometrial invasion) [89].

A similar distribution of lymph node metastases in 349 patients was found by Chi at al. 2008 in a retrospective monoinstitutional analysis [90].

All together one can expect lymph node metastases in 10-12% of women affected by stage I endometrioid endometrial carcinoma [88-90].

Additionally, pelvic and infrarenal para-aortic lymphadenectomy in patients with relevant co-morbidities and obesity is often associated with increased rate of early and late postoperative complications or cannot be performed at all [91]. Furthermore, lymph node metastases of endometrial carcinoma are often not macroscopically enlarged [92].

In contrast there are the results of two prospective randomized studies including more than 2000 patients that could not demonstrate an oncological advantage (OS, DSF) comparing patients that had a pelvic lymphadenectomy with those having not [89-92].

Though these two studies (with a high evidence level) reach identical conclusions, the results have to be interpreted carefully. In both studies only pelvic lymphadenectomy was performed. In the ASTEC study the mean lymph node yield was just 12 lymph nodes. A systematic para-aortic lymph node dissection was not required. The adjuvant therapy was inconsistent (due to a lack of definition) and the participating centers had discretion in choosing the right adjuvant therapy. In addition, statistical assumptions are justifiable to only a limited extent.

A comparison of other two important studies, GOG-99 and Postoperative Radiation Therapy in endometrial cancer (PORTEC), seems to suggest that lymphadenectomy does not affect disease-related and recurrence free survival in patients with intermediate-risk tumors confined to the uterus [93-94].

However, 60% of the patients enrolled in the PORTEC trial were actually grade 1 (thus their prognosis was even more favorable) whereas doubts have been raised concerning the adequacy of surgical staging performed in the GOG-99 trial. When the endometrial cancer presents a cervical extension (FIGO stage II), a radical hysterectomy, with an extensive dissection to expose the ureter and secure the uterine vessels at the origin rather than at their entry into the uterus, may be considered. This type of surgery allows removing the parametrial tissue and facilitates safe dissection of the bladder away from the uterus and cervix such that a significant cuff of upper vagina can be removed [95]. Parametrial metastasis does not form part of the FIGO staging system, but their involvement is associated with a poor prognosis [96].

Therefore the possible spectrum of lymph node staging comprises no lymphadenectomy, exclusive pelvic lymph node sampling, and additional inframesenteric para-aortic sampling and complete pelvic and infrarenal para-aortic lymphadenectomy. The incidence of isolated para-aortic lymph node metastasis in case of negative pelvic nodes is very low [97].

In summary it can be said, therefore, that these differing research results might rather increase the level of confusion than clarifying the evidence for performing pelvic and para-aortic lymphadenectomy in patients with endometrioid endometrial cancer stage I and II. Further research, in particular prospective randomized studies are required to evaluate the significance of systematic para-aortic lymphadenectomy in correlation to pelvic lymph node status as part of surgical treatment of endometrial carcinoma to be able to indicate appropriate adjuvant therapy [87-90]. Outside of studies lymphadenectomy is not adequate in low and intermediate risk endometrial cancer patients because risk-benefit balance seems rather in favor of not performing surgical staging. In contrast high-risk patients seem to profit from complete pelvic and para-aortic lymphadenectomy [98].

Clinical Recommendation Guidelines for Endometrial Cancer in FIGO Stage II

In case of confirmed infiltration of the cervix uteri (stage pTIIb) in an endometrial carcinoma the few available studies demonstrate an increased survival rate when performing a radical hysterectomy so that the parametria also should be resected as the guidelines recommend [12].

Several studies [99-104] have reported the superiority of radical hysterectomy in the treatment of FIGO stage II uterine endometrial cancer with cervical involvement. Currently, parametrial spread was predicted only by cervical involvement, and radical hysterectomy should be performed only for uterine endometrial cancer with cervical involvement.

Watanabe et al. retrospectively evaluated parametrical spread by histopathological analysis of surgically resected specimens in 334 individuals with uterine endometrial cancer. Parametrial spread occurred not only in individuals with cervical involvement but also in individuals with more than half myometrial invasion, retroperitoneal (pelvic, para-aortic, or both), lymph node metastasis, ovarian metastasis, positive peritoneal cytology results and lymphovascular space invasion. Although several previous studies have reported that radical hysterectomy improved the prognosis for uterine cancer with positive parametrial spread, the accuracy of preoperative examination to determine cervical involvement has remained within 29.6% to 45%. Therefore, the majority of individuals with clinical stage II have undergone surgical overtreatment. This study showed that parametrial spread cannot be predicted by cervical involvement alone but may be predicted by various lymphovascular space invasion-related histopathological factors. Further, parametrial spread may not be an independent prognostic factor in individuals with uterine endometrial cancer [105].

Sartori et al. retrospectively compared 135 patients receiving a simple hysterectomy to 68 patients undergoing radical hysterectomy in stage pTIIb.

They detected a significant difference in the 10-year-survival in favor of radical hysterectomy (94% versus 74%), while adjuvant radiation was without effect [106].

Almost the same results were demonstrated by Cohn et al. They retrospectively evaluated 162 patients affected by endometrial cancer stage II. 75% were treated with simple hysterectomy and 25% with radical hysterectomy. 5-year-survival rate was 94% in the radical hysterectomy group and 76% (p=0.05) in the simple hysterectomy group [107]. However, other study groups demonstrated only marginal differences in survival rate [108].

Sentinel Node (SN) Detection

Ditto et al. evaluated the sensitivity, the specificity, the positive and negative predicting value of hysteroscopic injection technetium 99m (Tc) in the detection of SN in endometrial cancer patients by lymphoscintigraphy and radio-guided surgery. Seventy-seven patients with endometrial cancer were submitted to hysteroscopic injection of 111 MBq of Tc. After hysterectomy and frozen section assessment of surgical specimen, a hand-held gamma-ray detector probe was used to locate and remove the sentinel lymph nodes. Systematic pelvic and para-aortic lymphadenectomy was further carried out. Histological results of sentinel node and non sentinel node were analyzed to assess the diagnostic accuracy of this method. In all but three cases at least one sentinel node was detected using radio-guided surgery. In the entire cases more than one site was positive to Tc. In four patients sentinel nodes and non sentinel nodes where histological positive for cancer, in 6 cases sentinel nodes where histological positive and no sentinel nodes where negative. In 45 cases no cancer cells where found in removed lymph nodes. The hysteroscopic injection of Tc99 labeled human albumin colloid particles in the detection of sentinel node(s) in endometrial cancer is a feasible technique. The authors confirm the good sensitivity and specificity of this technique [109].

The role of 18F-FDG-PET/CT in the management of endometrial cancer is not well defined due to the lack of consistent data in the literature, and due to this reason uterine corpus cancer is not included among appropriate applications in oncology. In endometrial cancer, the most relevant indications obtained by PET are: the possibility of detecting disease recurrence in asymptomatic patients presenting an increase of the CA125 serum levels; the ability in distinguishing fibrotic tissue from viable lesions after the treatment; the metabolic definition of the radiotherapy treatment planning. Encouraging results are also available in the assessment of lymph nodes and distant metastasis during the disease staging [110].

Few small studies assessed the validity of PET alone in the evaluation of primary endometrial cancer, showing good levels of sensitivity (range 83.3-96.7%) [111-113]. Park et al. concluded that there are two main advantages of 18F-FDG- PET/CT in the preoperative assessment of endometrial cancer: the good negative predictive value in predicting lymph node metastasis that allows avoidance of surgical staging in poor candidates for such procedure; the high accuracy in detecting distant metastasis [114].

As indicated [114,115], in endometrial cancer the major contribution of 18F-FDG-PET/CT could be in the early assessment of disease recurrence after therapy. The good performance of 18F-FDG-PET/CT has been confirmed by Kitajima et al. in a recent paper including 30 patients that showed an overall patient-based sensitivity, specificity and accuracy of 93% [116].

Common Complications of Surgical Treatments in Early Stage Disease

Lymphocele

In the literature the most frequently recorded postoperative complication of pelvic lymph node dissection is the development of a symptomatic lymphocele (Figure 8) and, afterwards, other complications as hemorrhage, hematoma, and postoperative ileus [117].

Lymphocele, also known as lymphocysts, consists of a collection of lymphatic fluid and dense fibrotic tissue, especially along the iliac vessels, containing a low concentration of clotting factors and has no platelets, as a consequence of surgical dissection and the inadequate closure of afferent lymphatic vessels. Lymphocele can be detected by clinical examination, ultrasonography, intravenous urography, CT scan or MRI.

Lymphocele usually appear 7 to 15 days after pelvic node dissection and most of them represent incidental findings without clinical significance, usually resolving spontaneously when lymph reabsorbs and new lymphatic vessels develop [118].

When symptoms do occur, they are typically related to compression of surrounding structures, resulting in pelvic pain, leg edema, gastrointestinal obstruction, obstructive uropathy, and deep vein thrombosis. Furthermore, severe and potentially life-threating complications can arise including sepsis, chylous ascites, lymphatic fistula formation and pulmonary embolism.

Endometrial carcinoma is a surgically staged disease and lymphadenectomy is accounted in endometrial cancer treatment [119]. To evaluate lymph nodes involving by endometrial cancer, pelvic lymphadenectomy (PL) is necessary since to date no imaging study equals PL for sensitivity and specificity in the detection of lymph node metastasis [120].

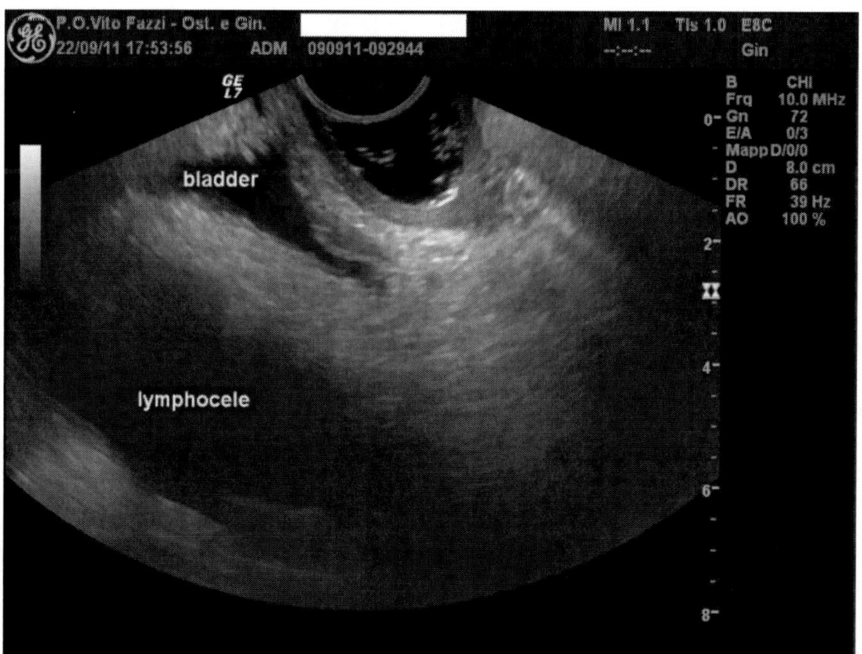

Figure 8. A right pelvic lymphoceledetected by transvaginal ultrasonography on 15th day after pelvic node dissection, as a consequence of surgical dissection and the inadequate closure of afferent lymphatic vessels.

However, this potential benefit must be weighed against the additional morbidity and costs associated with PL, since studies have shown that patients with low-risk factors such as those with grade 1 or 2 and no myometrial invasion, would not derive a benefit from lymphadenectomy given the low risk of lymph node metastases in this patient population [119].

The incidence of lymphocele after PL ranges from 1 to 49% and the time to lymphocele development may be unpredictable. Mori reported an average incidence of 48.5%, Ilancheran et al. noted an incidence of 25.3% in clinically diagnosable lymphocele with cervical cancer, Conte et al. noted an incidence of 22% in cervical cancer, Logmans et al. an incidence of 20-32% in gynecologic cancer and Benedetti Panici et al. an incidence of 10-25% in gynecologic cancer [121-124].

Several factors may contribute to this varied/broad incidence. Lymphocele developmental factors are thought to include: the extent of lymphadenectomy, the number of lymph nodes removed no ligation of lymph vessels, pre/postoperative radiation therapy and the presence of metastases to the lymph nodes [125].

Ghezzi et al. [126] evaluated the incidence of lymphocele, lymphorrhea, and lymphedema after systematic pelvic lymphadenectomy in patients who underwent laparoscopic or open abdominal staging for endometrial cancer. They used a postoperative screening for lymphadenectomy-related complications by ultrasound. In the results, the incidence of perioperative complications was lower in cases than in control subjects. Overall, lymphocele were diagnosed in 19 (15.4%) and 2 (1.4%) patients who had open and laparoscopic staging, respectively ($p<0.0001$). Symptomatic lymphocele were more frequent after open staging than after laparoscopy ($p=0.028$). Their findings suggested that laparoscopic endometrial cancer staging was associated with a lower occurrence of both asymptomatic and symptomatic lymphocelescompared to open surgery [126]. Similarly, symptomatic lymphocelesare eight times less common when a minimally invasive approach is adopted, and a tendency toward a protective effect of the endoscopic approach has been identified for lymphorrhea.

In literature, reported risk factors for the occurrence of lymphocysts are: the number of lymph nodes removed, the presence of metastatic disease in the lymph nodes, postoperative radiotherapy, the prophylactic administration of perioperative heparin and extraperitoneal surgery, and the presence of drainage. Lymphocele likely occur as a result of tissue trauma or surgery, after the leakage of lymph from afferent lymphatic channels. Their incidence can be minimized by meticulous surgical techniques and attention to sealing the LV during node dissection, by blocking lymphatic drainage from the lower extremities and preventing lymph accumulation in the pelvic cavity. In particular, the treatment- associated morbidity can be reduced when all lymphatic channels lateral to the external artery are saved or clamped. [127]

Kim et al. evaluated the incidence and risk factors of lymphocele development after pelvic lymphadenectomy on 264 patients. Among the 264 patients, a total of 50 patients (18%) developed lymphocele. The BMI and number of resected lymph nodes were higher in the lymphocele group, and the use of postoperative radiotherapy was associated with a higher risk of lymphocele. The treatment of lymphocele should be individualized. If they are asymptomatic, they should be monitored for spontaneous regression. In the majority of cases this will lead to successful resolution, as in the present series. However, regression may be a slow process; occurring over several months [128]. There are several preventive strategies proposed to reduce lymphocele development, such as fibrin application, omentoplasty, omission of peritoneal closure, avoidance of preoperative heparin use and, finally, the placement of retroperitoneal drainage at the end of surgery [129].

Percutaneous catheter drainage is safe and effective for treatment of symptomatic postoperative lymphocele; and this is confirmed by the study conducted by Kim et al. where there was no statistical correlation between the size of the lymphocele and the duration of drainage and percutaneous catheter results in a high success rate in the treatment of symptomatic lymphocele after radical pelvic lymphadenectomy [130].

In a recent randomized, prospective study on fifty-eight patients with endometrial cancer treated by surgery, the prevention of lymphocele was tested using collagen patch coated with the human coagulation factors (TachoSil®, Nycomed, Linz, Austria).

Authors demonstrated that intraoperative application of TachoSil® reduced rate of postoperative lymphocysts after PL, and it seems to provide a useful additional treatment option for reducing drainage volume and preventing lymphocele development after PL [131].

Another Italian study compared the use of the Ligaclip® (Ethicon Endo-Surgery, Cincinnati, USA) with bipolar coagulation in preventing lymphocele after laparoscopic pelvic lymphadenectomy for gynecologic cancer. Authors showed that the use of the Ligaclip® to close lymphatic vessels may reduce the incidence of lymphocele in patients undergoing laparoscopic pelvic lymphadenectomy [127].

Urinary Tract Injuries

Iatrogenic injuries to the urinary tract may occur during gynecological surgery. The bladder and distal ureters (Figure 9) are the most frequently involved organs. Injuries comprise advertent cystostomy, ureteral angulations, occlusion by improperly placed sutures, and direct ureteral damage (e.g., crush, ischemia, and partial or complete transaction) [132-134].

Early identification of the injury and repair during primary surgery most often result in less morbidity for the patient, a more successful outcome, and increased ease of repair [132,135].

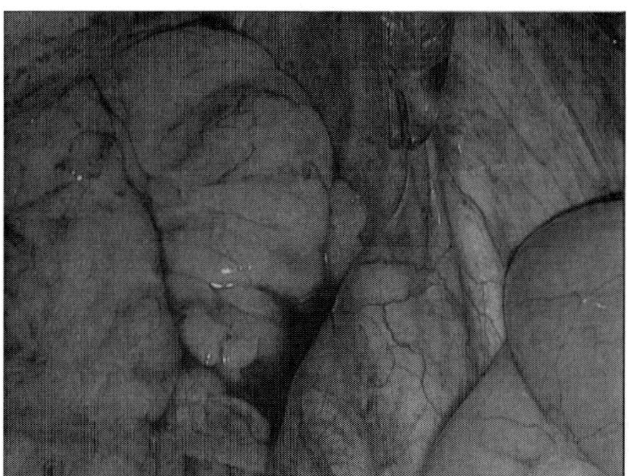

Figure 9. A right pelvic ureter detected by trans-peritoneal vision during laparoscopy.

The most important factor for correct management of urologic injury during gynecological surgery is prompt damage control. Despite their rare occurrence, every effort must be made to identify and treat all injuries intraoperatively. If left unrecognized and not repaired during surgery, injuries to the bladder or ureter may lead to late complications. The most frequent complications are renal damage and genitourinary fistulas [136-138]. The next step is damage assessment.

Anticipated findings are a bladder tear, ureteral angulations, occlusion by improperly placed sutures, or direct ureteral damage. An isolated small bladder tear at the dome can be sutured and no additional evaluation required. A larger tear may be associated with a concomitant injury to the ureter, particularly if damage involves the posterior bladder wall, approximates the ureteral orifice, or is associated with lateral extension of the uterine incision. In these cases ureteral catheterization is suitable, even at the cost of expanding the primary bladder tear toward the trigone in order to clearly identify the orifices.

When injury to the ureter is supposed and the bladder is undamaged, assessment strategies may include cystoscopy or fluoroscopy. Open dissection and exploration of the ureters may cause more risk than benefit. Then, introducing a ureteral catheter in a retrograde manner through the cystoscope or directly into the ureteral orifices following anterior cystostomy is most likely the preferred diagnostic method. To avoid damage to the ureter while introducing the catheter, stent advancement over a hydrophilic guidewire is recommended [139,140]. The risk of injuries especially to the ureter is increased with the laparoscopic approach and mainly with gynecologic laparoscopic procedures. The reason for the higher risk with laparoscopy may be explained on the basis of lack of tactile sensation, decreased mobility, reduced vision, especially depth perception and panoramic view, reluctance of the gynecologist to open into the retroperitoneal space, suboptimal knowledge of pelvic anatomy, and reliance on haemostatic devices, which increase the risk for urinary tract injury. Baggish analyzes a series of 75 patients who sustained urinary tract injuries in the course of a variety of laparoscopic operations Thirty-three bladder injuries and 42 ureteral injuries were identified. Twelve entry (trocar) complications damaged the bladder but only 1 ureteral injury could be attributed to this factor. Virtually every ureteral injury was related to the operative procedure as were 21 of the 33 bladder incidents. Only 27% complications were identified intraoperatively, whereas 50% were diagnosed in the late postoperative period or in the remote postoperative follow-up period. Three vesicovaginal fistulas and two ureterovaginal fistulas were diagnosed in the late postoperative period. Adhesions secondary to prior operative procedures or prior infections and adhesiolysis were the most significant etiological factors associated with both bladder and ureteral damage. Energy devices and stapling tools accounted for the majority of urological injuries (28 ureteral and 13 bladders). Clinical symptoms and signs pointing to urinary tract disruption ranged widely from dysuria, urgency, abdominal pain, bloating, nausea, fever and flank pain, to no symptoms or signs (11 of 75). The locations of injuries to the ureter within the pelvis varied relative to the type of surgical procedure and nature of the complications (e.g., 5 of 8 stapling injuries occupied at the infundibulopelvic ligament), whereas thermal injuries were more or less evenly distributed relative to location. Transection and ligation injuries were more common at or below the uterine vessels [141]. When radical hysterectomy and lymph node dissection are needed, the urinary tract injures are more frequent and serious. The effects of radical hysterectomy and lymph node dissection on normal bladder function are frequents and comprise voiding difficulties, storage problems and incontinence. The degree of these complications is related to the radicality of the procedure, preservation of the pelvic nerve bundles results in fewer and less severe complications [142]. Due to its close proximity to the cervix the ureter is at risk of inadvertent intraoperative trauma. This may be due to revascularization, crush injuries or transection. Recognized trauma can be repaired quickly with no long-term effects. Reported incidences of such trauma are low; Wertheim [143] reported 11 injuries in 500 cases (2.2%) in his series. Improvements in operative techniques with emphasis on preservation of the urethral sheath, the routine use of prophylactic antibiotics and the use of pelvic suction drainage have almost eradicated the above urethral complications. More recent series have reported fistula rates and intraoperative injury rates of less than 1% [144-147].

Direct bladder injury and postoperative fistula formation are unusual and as with ureteral complications are in the order of 1% or less [145,147]. The most frequent site of injury is the trigone, which is adherent to the anterior wall of the vagina. Meticulous surgical technique and intra- and postoperative bladder drainage [148] can help to reduce the incidence of bladder trauma to a minimum.

Long-term bladder dysfunction is reported in over 50% of women following radical surgery [146,150-152] and over 10% may be severely handicapped by their symptoms. In a study reported by Fishman et al. [149] in the late 1980s, 35% of women were unhappy with their bladder function after surgery.

Obesity and Endometrial Cancer

The rate of obesity also increases around the world. As the cancer most associated with obesity and the most common gynecologic cancer, uterine cancer management may be affected significantly by patient's obesity.

Obesity is a significant risk factor in developing endometrial cancer. As obesity is becoming more endemic, is necessary to evaluate the impact of obesity on perioperative outcomes in patients undergoing uterine cancer surgery. Obesity increases surgical blood loss and operative time.

However, obesity does not affect length of hospital stay, number of lymph nodes harvested, or perioperative complications in uterine cancer staging surgery.

Some studies have suggested that obesity increases the difficulty of surgical staging in the uterine cancer. Obesity has been traditionally considered a relative contraindication to laparoscopic surgery. Obesity complicates laparoscopic surgery by making entry into the peritoneal cavity difficult, limiting the amount of Trendelenburg positioning the patient can tolerate, and interfering with visualization of the pelvic and abdominal vessels during lymphadenectomy.

Although there is an increased risk of procedure conversion to laparotomy in obese women, the incidence of operative complications, blood loss, operative times, postoperative complications, and lengths of hospital stay was similar to that among thin women undergoing laparoscopic surgery [153]. Some authors [154-156] have reported no significant difference in the number of lymph nodes removed through laparoscopic surgery and those removed by laparotomy.

The small incisions needed for laparoscopic surgery and the absence of bowel manipulation decrease postoperative pain and ileus and allow early ambulation, feeding, and hospital discharge [157].

Controversies in the Management of Endometrial Cancer

Controversies exist in the management of endometrial cancer regarding the surgical staging, the role of lymphadenectomy and radiotherapy in patients with intermediate-risk tumors confined to the uterus, the diagnostic strategies for postmenopausal bleeding, the follow-up, and the use of novel target therapy.

There are no prospective randomized data available to aid general consensus about an appropriate management of women with advanced endometrial cancer. The appropriate extent of surgery in this setting of patients and the true value of radical surgery in advanced disease are still not clear.

Pliskow et al. published a retrospective study of 41 women with clinical stage III and IV endometrial cancer, and suggested that the extent of disease and tumor bulk have greater prognostic value than histological subtype, grading, or depth of myometrial invasion. Other recent studies propose that the primary cytoreductive surgery for advanced endometrial cancer offers a survival benefit as in epithelial ovarian cancer [115,159].

Regarding the role of lymphadenectomy in women with disease that clinically seems to be confined to the uterus, there has been much debate. Although lymphadenectomy forms part of the FIGO surgical staging system [160], evidence from a large randomized controlled trial, A Study in the Treatment of Endometrial Cancer (ASTEC), showed that this approach does not provide therapeutic benefit [60].

Panici et al. conducted a randomized clinical trial to determine whether the addition of pelvic systemic lymphadenectomy to standard hysterectomy with bilateral salpingo-oophorectomy improves overall and disease-free survival. They found that significantly it improved only surgical staging and neither overall nor disease-free survival [112]. Accurate preoperative risk stratification can guide to the appropriate type of surgery by selecting patients who benefit of lymphadenectomy. However, available preoperative and intraoperative investigations are not highly accurate methods to detect lymph nodes and a complete surgical staging remains the most precise method to evaluate extra uterine spread of the disease [162].

A great challenge in surgical management of endometrial cancer is standardization of pelvic and para-aortic lymphadenectomy strategies, in order to avoid unnecessary procedures and to offer complete staging with high survival rates.

Laparotomy has always been considered the standard approach for endometrial cancer surgical staging. Traditional and robotic assisted laparoscopic techniques seem to provide equivalent results in terms of disease-free survival and overall survival compared to laparotomy, even if they are not without risk (Figure 10).

These minimally invasive approaches demonstrated additional benefits as shorter hospital stay, less use of pain killers, lower rate of complications and improved quality of life.

Regarding the postmenopausal bleeding, the best diagnostic strategy for diagnosing endometrial carcinoma in patients with postmenopausal bleeding still remains controversial. Sensitivity of transvaginal sonography endometrial thickness measurement in women with postmenopausal bleeding is still controversial. Future research should aim at achieving a higher accuracy of the diagnostic strategy applied. Such higher accuracy might be achieved by incorporation of patient's characteristics (e.g., age, presence of diabetes, BMI, presence of hypertension) in the diagnostic work-up. The incorporation of transvaginal sonography with patient's characteristics in a diagnostic strategy has been studied and resulted in higher diagnostic accuracy [163-165].

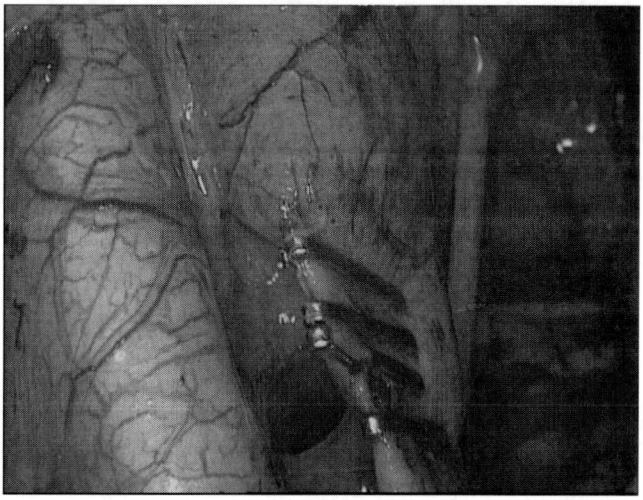

Figure 10. A vascular lesion of external iliac vein during pelvic laparoscopic lympadenectomy; from the left side, in sequence they appear: left iliac artery, left iliac vein repaired by clips and obturator nerve.

The goal of screening endometrial cancers is to identify all patients who have a risk for developing this disease. Therefore clarification of the molecular and genetic mechanisms of development or progression of this disease is required. Understanding the genetic changes underlying cancer development or progression in the different histological subtypes is important for discovery of new targets for both diagnosis and therapy for individual patients [166].

Conclusion

Surgical treatment is the goal therapy in the primary treatment of patients with endometrial cancer. With rising incidence of obesity number of patients with endometrial cancer, it will also increase complications and difficulties. However, operations in obese patients are more challenging. Laparotomy as standard therapy could be replaced by laparoscopic or robotic assisted surgical approaches in endometrial cancer patients stage I and II. Laparoscopy, at the moment, is oncological adequate to open procedures and offers many advantages to patients–less blood loss, lower complication rate, shorter hospital stay and better quality of life, especially those with relevant co-morbidity. In the next future, robotic surgery in the treatment of endometrial cancer will be the gold standard. Most controversial points of treatment today regard the indication and the extension of pelvic lymphadenectomy to abdomen in different stages. In advanced endometrial cancers' stages, an optimal debulking therapy should be performed in order to improve effectiveness of adjuvant chemotherapeutic and/or radiation therapy.

References

[1] Tinelli, A; Vergara, D; Martignago, R; Leo, G; Malvasi, A; Tinelli, R. Hormonal carcinogenesis and socio-biological development factors in endometrial cancer: a clinical review. *Acta Obstet. Gynecol. Scand.* 2008;87:1101-13.

[2] Ries, LAG; Eisner, MP; Kosary, CL; Hankey, BF; Miller, BA; Clegg, L; et al (eds). SEER Cancer Statistics Review, 1975-2001, National Cancer Institute. Bethesda, MD, *http://seer.cancer.gov/csr/1975_2001/*, 2004.

[3] Bakkum-Gamez, JN; Gonzales-Bosquet, J; Laack, NN; Mariani, A; Dowdy, S. Current issues in the management of endometrial cancer. *Mayo. Clin. Proc.* 2008;83(2):97-112.

[4] Kennedy, AW; Austin, JM; Look, KY; Munger, CB. The society of gynecologic oncologists task force study of endometrial cancer initial experience. *Gynecol. Oncol.* 2000;79:379-88.

[5] Vaknin, Z; Ben-Ami, I; Schneider, D; Pansky, M; Halperin, R. A comparison of perioperative morbidity, perioperative mortality, and disease-specific survival in elderly women (>70 years) versus younger women (<70 years) with endometriod endometrial cancer. *Int. J. Gynecol. Cancer* 2009;19:879-83.

[6] Jemal A, Murray T, Ward E, Samuels A, Tiwari RC, Ghafoor A, et al. Cancer statistics, 2005. *CA Cancer J. Clin.* 2005;55:10-30.

[7] Ron, E; Lunenfeld, B; Menczer, J; Blumstein, T; Katz, L; Oelsner, G; Serr, D. Cancer incidence in a cohort of infertile women. *Am. J. Epidemiol.* 1987;125:780-90.

[8] Meirow, D; Schenker, JG. The link between female infertility and cancer: epidemiology and possible aetiologies. *Hum. Reprod. Update* 1996;2:63-75.

[9] Creasman WT, Morrow CP, Bundy BN, Homesley HD, Graham JE, Heller PB. Surgical pathologic spread patterns of endometrial cancer. *Cancer* 1987;60:2035-41.

[10] Sato, S; Itamochi, H; Shimada, M; Fujii, S; Naniwa, J; Uegaki, K; et al. Preoperative and intraoperative assessment of depth of myometrial invasion in endometrial cancer. *Int. J. Gynecol. Cancer* 2009;19:884-7.

[11] Signorelli, M; Guerra, L; Buda, A; Picchio, M; Mangili, G; Dell'Anna, T; et al. Role of the integrated FDG PET/CT in the surgical management of patients with high risk clinical early stage endometrial cancer: detection of pelvic nodal metastasis. *Gynecol. Oncol.* 2009;115:231-5.

[12] Chiva, L; Lapuente, F; Gonzales-Cortijo, L; Carballo, N; Garcia, JF; Rojo, A; et al. Sparing fertility in young patients with endometrial cancer. *Gynecol. Oncol.* 2008;111:101-4.

[13] Signorelli, M; Caspani, G; Bonazzi, C; Chiappa, V; Perego, P; Mangioni, C. Fertility-sparing treatment in young women with endometrial cancer or atypical complex hyperplasia: a prospective single-institution experience of 21 cases. *Int. J. Obstet. Gynaecol.* 2009;116:114-8.

[14] Richter, CE; Qian, B; Martel, M; Yu, H; Azodi, M; Rutherford, TJ; et al. Ovarian preservation and staging in reproductive-age endometrial cancer patients. *Gynecol. Oncol.* 2009;114;99-104.

[15] Zivanovic, O; Carter, J; Kauff, ND; Barakat, RR. A review of the challenges faced in the conservative treatment of young women with endometrial carcinoma and risk of ovarian cancer. *Gynecol. Oncol.* 2009;115:504-9.

[16] Lee, TS; Kim, JW; Kim, TJ; Cho, CH; Ryu, SY; Ryu, HS; et al; the Korean Gynecologic Oncology Group. Ovarian preservation during the surgical treatment of early stage endometrial adenocarcinoma: unraveling a mystery. *Gynecol. Oncol.* 2009;115:26-31.
[17] Baekelandt, MM; Castiglione, M; ESMO Guidelines Working Group. Endometrial carcinoma: ESMO clinical recommendations for diagnosis, treatment and follow-up. *Ann. Oncol.* 2009;20(Suppl4):29-31.
[18] Han, CH; Lee, KH; Lee, HN; Kim, CJ; Park, TC; Park JS. Does the type of hysterectomy affect the prognosis in clinical stage I endometrial cancer? *J. Obstet. Gynaecol. Res.* 2010;36:581-7.
[19] Furukawa, N; Takekuma, M; Takahashi, N; Hirashima, Y. Intraoperative evaluation of myometrial invasion and histological type and grade in endometrial cancer: diagnostic value of frozen section. *Arch. Gynecol. and Obstet.* 2010;281:913-7.
[20] Pristauz, G; Bader, AA; Regitnig, P; Haas, J; Winter, R; Tamussino, K. How accurate is frozen section histology of pelvic lymph nodes in patients with endometrial cancer? *Gynecol. Oncol.* 2009;115:12-7.
[21] Fagotti, A; Ferrandina, G; Longo, R; Mancuso, S; Scambia, G. Minilaparotomy in early stage endometrial cancer: an alternative to standard and laparoscopic treatment. *Gynecol Oncol* 2002;86:177-83.
[22] Foley, K; Lee, RB. Surgical complications of obese patients with endometrial carcinoma. *Gynecol. Oncol.* 1990;39:171-4.
[23] Pavelka, JC; Ben-Shachar, I; Fowler, JM; Ramirez, NC; Copeland, LJ; Eaton, LA; et al. Morbid obesity and endometrial cancer: surgical, clinical and pathologic outcomes in surgically managed patients. *Gynecol. Oncol.* 2004;95:588-92.
[24] Lelle, RJ; Morley, GW; Peters, WA. The role of vaginal hysterectomy in the treatment of endometrial carcinoma. *Int. J. Gynecol. Cancer* 1994;4:342-7.
[25] Chan, JK; Lin, YG; Monk, BJ; Tewari, K; Bloss, JD; Berman, ML. Vaginal hysterectomy as primary treatment of endometrial cancer in medically compromised women. *Obstet. Gynecol.* 2001;97:707-11.
[26] Massi, G; Susini, T; Amunni, G. Extraperitoneal pelvic lymphadenectomy to complement vaginal operations for cervical and endometrial cancer. *Int. J. Obstet. Gynecol.* 2000;69:27-35.
[27] Dowdy, SC; Aletti, G; Cliby, WA; Podratz, KC; Mariani, A. Extra-peritoneal laparoscopic para-aortic lymphadenectomy – A prospective cohort study of 293 patients with endometrial cancer. *Obstet. Gynecol.* 2008;111:418-24.
[28] Capmas, P; Bats, AS; Bensaid, C; Huchon, C; Scarabin, C; Nos, C; et al. Surgical treatment of early endometrial cancer: what are the benefits of laparoscopy? *J. Obstet. Gynecol. Reprod. Biol.* 2009;38:537-44.
[29] Köhler, C; Klemm, P; Schau, A; Possover, M; Krause, N; Tozzi, R; et al. Introduction of transperitoneal lymphadenectomy in a gynecologic oncology center: analysis of 650 laparoscopic pelvic and/or paraaortic transperitoneal lymphadenectomies. *Gynecol. Oncol.* 2004;95:52-61.
[30] Querleu, D; Leblanc, E; Cartron, G; Narducci, F; Ferron, G; Martel, P. Audit of preoperative and early complications of laparoscopic lymph node dissection in 1000 gynecologic cancer patients. *Arch. Gynecol. Obstet.* 2006;195:1287-92.

[31] Martinez, A; Querleu, D; Leblanc, E; Narducci, F; Ferron, G. Low incidence of port-side metastases after laparoscopic staging of uterine cancer. *Gynecol. Oncol.* 2010;118:145-50.

[32] Ghezzi F; Cromi, A; Bergamini, V; Uccella, S; Beretta, P; Franchi, M; et al. Laparoscopic-assisted vaginal hysterectomy versus total laparoscopic hysterectomy for the management of endometrial cancer: a randomized clinical trial. *J. Minim. Invasive Gynecol.* 2006;13:114-20.

[33] O'Hanlan, KA; Huang, GS; Garnier, AC; Dibble, SL; Reuland, ML; Lopez, L; et al. Total laparoscopic hysterectomy versus total abdominal hysterectomy: cohort review of patients with uterine neoplasia. *J. Soc. Laparoendsc. Surg.* 2005;9:277-86.

[34] Pellegrino, A; Signorelli, M; Fruscio, R; Villa, A; Buda, A; Beretta, P; et al. Feasibility and morbidity of total laparoscopic radical hysterectomy with or without pelvic lymphadenectomy in obese women with stage I endometrial cancer. *Arch. Gynecol. Obstet.* 2009;279:655-60.

[35] Wong, CK; Wong, YH; Lo, LS; Tai, CM; Ng, TK. Laparoscopy compared with laparotomy for the surgical staging of endometrial carcinoma. *J. Obstet. Gynaecol. Res.* 2005;31:286-90.

[36] Zapico, A; Fuentes, P; Grassa, A; Arnanz, F; Otazua, J; Cortes-Prieto, J. Laparoscopic-assisted vaginal hysterectomy versus abdominal hysterectomy in stages I and II endometrial cancer. Oparating Data; Follow-up and Survival. *Gynecol. Oncol.* 2005;98:222-7.

[37] Volpi, E; Ferrero, A; Jacomuzzi, ME; Carus, AP; Fuso, L; Martra, F; et al. Laparoscopic treatment of endometrial cancer: feasibility and results. *Eur. J. Obstet. Gynecol. Reprod. Biol.* 2006;124:232-6.

[38] Kim, DY; Kim, MK; Suh, DS; Kim, YM; Kim, YT; Mok, JE; et al. Laparoscopic-assisted vaginal hysterectomy versus abdominal hysterectomy in patients with stage I and II endometrial cancer. *Int. J. Gynecol. Cancer* 2005;15:932-7.

[39] Frigerio, L; Gallo, A; Ghezzi, F; Trezzi, G; Lussanna, M; Franchi, M. Laparoscopic-assisted vaginal hysterectomy versus abdominal hysterectomy in endometrial cancer. *Int. J .Obstet. Gynecol.* 2006;93:209-13.

[40] Tollund, L; Hansen, B; Kjer, JJ. Laparoscopic-assisted vaginal vs. abdominal surgery in patients with endometrial cancer stage I. *Acta Obstet. Gynecol. Scan.* 2006;85:1138-41.

[41] Seracchioli, R; Venturoli, S; Ceccarin, M; Cantarelli, M; Ceccaroni, M; Pignotti, E; et al. Is total laparoscopic surgery for endometrial carcinoma at risk of local recurrence? A long term survival. *Anticancer Res.* 2005;25:2423-8.

[42] Fader, AN; Michener, CM; Frasure, HE; Giannios, N; Belinson, JL; Zanotti, KM. Total laparoscopic hysterectomy versus laparoscopic-assisted vaginal hysterectomy in endometrial cancer: surgical and survival outcomes. *J. Minim. Invasive Gynecol.* 2009;16:333-9.

[43] Eisenkop, SM. Total laparoscopic hysterectomy with pelvic/aortic lymph node dissection for endometrial cancer – a consecutive series without case selection and comparison to laparotomy. *Gynecol. Oncol.* 2010;117:216-23.

[44] Tozzi, R; Malur, S; Köhler, C; Schneider, A. Analysis of morbidity in patients with endometrial cancer: is there a commitment to offer laparoscopy. *Gynecol. Oncol.* 2005;97:4-9.

[45] Obermair, A; Manolitsas, TP; Leung, Y; Hammond, IG; McCartney, AJ. Total laparoscopic hysterectomy versus total abdominal hysterectomy for obese women with endometrial cancer. *Int. J. Gynecol. Cancer* 2005;15:319-24.
[46] Zullo, F; Palomba, S; Russo, T; Falbo, A; Costantino, M; Tolino, A; et al. A prospective randomized comparison between laparoscopic and laparotomic approaches in women with early stage endometrial cancer: a focus on the quality of live. *Am. J. Obstet. Gynecol.* 2005;193:1344-52.
[47] Zorlu, CG; Simsek, T; Ari, ES. Laparoscopy or laparotomy for the management of endometrial cancer. *J. Soc. Laparoendsc. Surg.* 2005;9:442-6.
[48] Tozzi, R; Malur, S; Koehler, C; Schneider, A. Laparoscopy versus laparotomy in endometrial cancer: first analysis of survival of a randomized prospective study. *J. Minim. Invasive Gynecol.* 2005;12:130-6.
[49] Fram, KM. Laparoscopically assisted vaginal hysterectomy versus abdominal hysterectomy in stage I endometrial cancer. *Int. J. Gynecol. Cancer* 2002;12:57-61.
[50] Malzoni, M; Tinelli, R; Cosentino, F; Perone, C; Rasile, M; Iuzzolino, D; et al. Total laparoscopic hysterectomy versus abdominal hysterectomy with lymphadenectomy for early-stage endometrial cancer: a prospective randomized study. *Gynecol. Oncol.* 2009;112:126-33.
[51] Nezhat, F; Yadav, J; Rahaman, J; Gretz, H; Cohen, C. Analysis of survival after laparoscopic management of endometrial cancer. *J. Min. Inv. Gyn.* 2008;15:181-7.
[52] Palomba, S; Falbo, A; Mocciaro, R; Russo, T; Zullo, F. Laparoscopic treatment for endometrial cancer: a meta-analysis of randomized controlled trials (RCTs). *Gynecol. Oncol.* 2009;112:415-21.
[53] Lin, F; Zhang, QJ; Zheng, FY; Zhao, HQ; Zeng, QQ; Zheng, MH; et al. Laparoscopically assited versus open surgery for endometrial cancer – A meta-analysis of randomized controlled trials. *Int. J. Gynecol. Cancer* 2008;18:1315-25.
[54] Bijen, CB; Briet, JM; de Bock, GH; Arts, HJ; Bergsma-Kadijk, JA; Mourits, MJ. Total laparoscopic hysterectomy versus abdominal hysterectomy in the treatment of patients with early stage endometrial cancer: A randomized multi center study. *BMC Cancer* 2009;15:9-23.
[55] Walker, J; Mannel, R; Piedmonte, M; Schlaerth, J; Spirtos, N; Spiegel, G. Phase III trial of laparoscopy versus laparotomy for surgical resection and comprehensive surgical staging of uterine cancer: A GOG study founded by the national cancer institute. *Gynecol Oncol* 2006;101:177.
[56] Childers, JM; Brzechffa, PR; Hatch, KD; Surwit, EA. Laparoscopically assisted surgical staging (LASS) of endometrial cancer. *Gynecol. Oncol.* 1993;51:33-8.
[57] Palomba, S; Falbo, A; Mocciaro, R; Russo, T; Zullo, F. Laparoscopic treatment for endometrial cancer: a meta-analysis of randomized controlled trials (RCTs). *Gynecol. Oncol.* 2009;112:415-21.
[58] Walker, JL; Piedmonte, MR; Spirtos, NM; Eisenkop, SM; Schlaerth, JB; Mannel, RS; et al. Laparoscopy compared with laparotomy for comprehensive surgical staging of uterine cancer: Gynecologic Oncology Group Study LAP2. *J. Clin. Oncol.* 2009;27:5331-6.
[59] Walker, JPM; Spirtos, N; Eisenkop, S; Spiegel, G; Mannel, R; Barakat, R; et al. Recurrence and Survival after Randomization to Laparoscopy versus Laparotomy for

Comprehensive Surgical Staging of Uterine Cancer (Gynecologic Oncology Group LAP2). *Society of Gynecologic Oncologist;* 2010; San Francisco; USA.

[60] Visco, AG; Advincula, AP. Robotic gynecologic surgery. *Obstet. Gynecol.* 2008;112:1369-84.

[61] Tinelli, A; Malvasi, A; Gustapane, S; Buscarini, M; Gill, I; Stark, M; et al. Robotic assisted surgery in gynecology: current insights and future perspectives. *Recent Pat Biotechnol* 2011; 5(1):12-24.

[62] Nezhat, F. Minimally invasive surgery in gynecologic oncology: laparoscopy versus robotics. *Gynecol. Oncol.* 2008;111(2):29-32.

[63] Holtz, DO; Miroshnichenko, G; Finnegan, MO; Chernick, M; Dunton, CJ. Endometrial cancer surgery costs: robot versus laparoscopy. *J. Minim. Invasive Gynecol.* 2010;17:500-3.

[64] Seamon, LG; Fowler, JM; Richardson, DL; Carlson, M J; Valmadre, S; Phillips GS; et al. A detailed analysis of the learning curve: robotic hysterectomy and pelvic-aortic lymphadenectomy for endometrial cancer. *Gynecol. Oncol.* 2009;114:162-7.

[65] Pareja, R; Ramirez, PT. Robotic radical hysterectomy in the management of gynecologic malignancies. *J. Minim. Invasive Gynecol.* 2008;15:673-6.

[66] Mettler, L; Schollmeyer, T; Boggess, J; Magrina, JF; Oleszczuk, A. Robotic assistance in gynecological oncology. *Curr. Opin. Oncol.* 2008;20:581-9.

[67] Peiretti, M; Zanagnolo, V; Bocciolone, L; Landoni, F; Colombo, N; Minig, L; et al. Robotic surgery: changing the surgical approach for endometrial cancer in a referral cancer center. *J. Minim. Invasive Gynecol.* 2009;16:427-31.

[68] Hoekstra, AV; Jairam-Thodla, A; Rademaker, A; Singh, DK; Buttin, BM; Lurain, JR. The impact of robotics on practice management of endometrial cancer: transitioning from traditional surgery. *Int. J. Med. Robot.* 2009;5:392-7.

[69] Bell, MC; Torgerson, J; Seshadri-Kreaden, U; Suttle, AW; Hunt, S. Comparison of outcomes and cost for endometrial cancer staging via traditional laparotomy; standard laparoscopy and robotic techniques. *Gynecol. Oncol.* 2008;111:407-11.

[70] DeNardis, SA; Holloway, RW; Bigsby, GEt; Pikaart, DP; Ahmad, S; Finkler, NJ. Robotically assisted laparoscopic hysterectomy versus total abdominal hysterectomy and lymphadenectomy for endometrial cancer. *Gynecol. Oncol.* 2008;111:412-7.

[71] Seamon, LG; Cohn, DE; Henretta, MS; Kim, SH; Carlson, MJ; Phillips, GS; et al. Minimally invasive comprehensive surgical staging for endometrial cancer: robotics or laparoscopy? *Gynecol. Oncol.* 2009;113:36-41.

[72] Veljovich, DS; Paley, PJ; Drescher, CW; Everett, EN; Shah, C; Peters, WA. Robotic surgery in gynecologic oncology: program initiation and outcomes after the first year with comparison with laparotomy for endometrial cancer staging. *Am. J. Obstet. Gynecol.* 2008;198:1-9.

[73] Boggess, JF; Gehrig, PA; Cantrell, L; Shafer, A; Ridgway, M; Skinner, EN; et al. A comparative study of 3 surgical methods for hysterectomy with staging for endometrial cancer: robotic assistance; laparoscopy; laparotomy. *Am. J. Obstet. Gynecol.* 2008;199:1-9.

[74] Gehrig, PA; Cantrell, LA; Shafer, A; Abaid, LN; Mendivil, A; Boggess, JF. What is the optimal minimally invasive surgical procedure for endometrial cancer staging in the obese and morbidly obese woman. *Gynecol. Oncol.* 2008;111:41-5.

[75] Seamon, GL; Cohn, DE; Richardson, DL; Valmadre, S; Carlson, MJ; Phillips, GS; et al. Robotic hysterectomy and pelvic-aortic lymphadenectomy for endometrial cancer. *Obstet. Gynecol.* 2008;112:1207-13.

[76] Cardenas-Goicoechea, J; Adams, S; Bhat, SB; Randall, TC. Surgical outcomes of robotic-assisted surgical staging for endometrial cancer are equivalent to traditional laparoscopic staging at Minimally Invasive Surgical Center. *Gynecol. Oncol.* 2010;117:224-8.

[77] Field, JB; Benoit, MF; Dinh, TA; Diaz-Arrastia, C. Computer-enhanced robotic surgery in gynecologic oncology. *Surg Endosc* 2007;21:244-6.

[78] Cragun, JM; Havrilesky, LJ; Calingaert, B; Synan, I; Secord, AA; Soper, JT; et al. Retrospective analysis of selective lymphadenectomy in apparent early-stage endometrial cancer. *J .Clin. Oncol.* 2005;23:3668-75.

[79] Aalders, JG; Thomas, G. Endometrial cancer--revisiting the importance of pelvic and para aortic lymph nodes. *Gynecol. Oncol.* 2007;104:222-31.

[80] Kitchener, H; Swart, AM; Qian, Q; Amos, C; Parmar, MK. Efficacy of systematic pelvic lymphadenectomy in endometrial cancer (MRC ASTEC trial): a randomised study. *Lancet* 2009;373:125-36.

[81] Robinson, BL; Liao, JB; Adams, SF; Randall, TC. Vaginal cuff dehiscence after robotic total laparoscopic hysterectomy. *Obstet. Gynecol.* 2009;114:369-71.

[82] Kho, RM; Akl, MN; Cornella, JL; Magtibay, PM; Wechter, ME; Magrina, JF. Incidence and characteristics of patients with vaginal cuff dehiscence after robotic procedures. *Obstet. Gynecol.* 2009;114:231-5.

[83] Sprung, J; Whalley, DG; Falcone, T; Warner, DO; Hubmayr, RD; Hammel, J. The impact of morbid obesity; pneumoperitoneum; and posture on respiratory system mechanics and oxygenation during laparoscopy. *Anesth. Analg.* 2002;94:1345-50.

[84] Gaia, G; Holloway, RW; Santoro, L; Ahmad, S; Di Silverio, E; Spinillo, A. Robotic-assisted hysterectomy for endometrial cancer compared with traditional laparoscopic and laparotomy approaches. *Obstet. Gynecol.* 2010;116:1422-31.

[85] Chan, JK; Wu, HW; Cheung, MK; Shin, JY; Osann, K; Kapp, DS. The outcomes of 20.063 women with unstaged endometroid uterine cancer. *Gynecol. Oncol.* 2007;106:282-8.

[86] Smith, DC; Macdonald, OK; Lee, CM; Gaffney, DK. Survival impact of lymph node dissection in endometrial adenocarcinoma: a surveillance; epidemiology and end result analysis. *Int. J. Gynecol. Cancer* 2008;18:255-61.

[87] Mariani, A; Dowdy, SC; Cliby, WA; Gostout, BS; Jones, MB; Wilson, TO; et al. Prospective assessment of lymphatic dissemination in endometrial cancer: a paradigm shift in surgical staging. *Gynecol. Oncol.* 2008;109:11-8.

[88] Creasman, WT; Odicino, F; Maisonneuve, P; Quinn, MA; Beller, U; Benedet, JL; et al. Carcinoma of the corpus uteri in 26th annual report on the results of treatment in gynaecologic cancer. *Int. J. Gynecol. Obstet.* 2006;95:S105-43.

[89] Chi, DS; Barakat, RR; Palayekar, MJ; Levine, DA; Sonoda, Y; Alektiar, K; et al. The incidence of pelvic lymph node metastasis by FIGO staging for patients with adequately surgically staged endometrial adenocarcinoma of endometroid histology. *Int. J. Gynecol. Cancer* 2008;18:269-73.

[90] Benedetti Panici, P; Basile, S; Maneschi, F; Lissoni, A; Signorelli, M; Scambia, G; et al. Systematic pelvic lymphadenectomy vs. no lymphadenectomy in early-stage

endometrial carcinoma: randomized clinical trail. *J. Natl. Cancer Institute* 2008;100:1707-16.

[91] Creasman, WT; Morrow, CP; Bundy, BN; Homesley, HD; Graham, JE; Heller, PB. Surgical pathologic spread patterns of endometrial cancer. A gynecologic oncology group study. *Cancer* 1987;60:2035-41.

[92] ASTEC Study Group; Kitchener, H; Swart, AM; Qian, Q; Amos, C; Parmar, MK. Efficacy of systematic pelvic lymphadenectomy in endometrial cancer (MRC ASTEC Trail): a randomised study. *Lancet* 2009;373:125-36.

[93] Klip, H; Burger, CW; Kenemans, P; Van Leeuwen, FE. Cancer risk associated with subfertility and ovulation induction: a review. *Cancer Cause Control* 2000;11:319-44.

[94] Creutzberg, CL; van Putten, WLJ; Koper, PCM; Lybeert, ML; Jobsen, JJ; Wárlám-Rodenhuis, CC; et al. Surgery and postoperative radiotherapy versus surgery alone for patients with stage-1 endometrial carcinoma: multicentre randomised trial. *Lancet* 2000;355:1404-11.

[95] Piver, MS; Rutledge, F; Smith, JP. Five classes of extended hysterectomy for women with cervical cancer. *Obstet. Gynecol.* 1974;44:265-72.

[96] ASTEC/EN.5 Study Group. Adjuvant external beam radiotherapy in the treatment of endometrial cancer (MRC ASTEC and NCIC CTG EN.5 randomised trials): pooled trial results; systematic review; and meta-analysis. *Lancet* 2009;373:137-46.

[97] Boronow, RC. Endometrial cancer and lymph node surgery: the spins continue – A case for reason. *Gynecol. Oncol.* 2008;111:3-6.

[98] Aalders, J; Abeler, V; Kolstad, P; Onsrud, M. Post-operative external irradiation and prognostic parameter in stage I endometrial carcinoma: clinical and histopathologic study of 540 patients. *Obstet. Gynecol.* 1980;56:419-27.

[99] Creutzberg, CL; Van Putten, WL; Koper, PC; Lybeert, ML; Jobsen, JJ; Wárlám-Rodenhuis, CC; et al. Surgery and postoperative radiotherapy versus surgery alone for patients with Stage-1 endometrial carcinoma: multicentre randomised trial. PORTEC Study Group. Post operative radiation therapy in endometrial carcinoma. *Lancet* 2000;355:1404-11.

[100] Keys, HM; Roberts, JA; Brunetto, VL; Zaino, RJ; Spirtos, NM; Bloss, JD; et al.; Gynecologic Oncology Group. A phase III trial of surgery with or without adjunctive external pelvic radiation therapy in intermediate risk endometrial adenocarcinoma: A Gynecologic Oncology Group study. *Gynecol. Oncol.* 2004;92:744-51.

[101] ASTEC/EN.5 Study Group; Blake, P; Swart, AM; Orton, J; Kitchener, H; Whelan, T; Lukka, H; et al. Adjuvant external beam radiotherapy in the treatment of endometrial cancer (MRC ASTEC and NCIC CTG EN.5 Randomised Trials): pooled trial results; systematic review; and meta-analysis. *Lancet* 2009;373:137-46.

[102] Delpech, Y; Barranger, E. Management of lymph nodes in endometrioid uterine cancer. *Curr. Opin. Oncol.* 2010;22:487-91.

[103] Boothby, RA; Carlson, JA; Neiman, W; Rubin, MM; Morgan, MA; Schults, D; et al. Treatment of stage II endometrial carcinoma. *Gynecol. Oncol.* 1989;33:204-8.

[104] Boente, MP; Jr Yordan, EL; McIntosh, DG; Jr Grendys, EC; Orandi, YA; Davies S; et al. Prognostic factors and long-term survival in endometrial adenocarcinoma with cervical involvement. *Gynecol. Oncol.* 1993;51:316-22.

[105] Boente, MP; Orandi, YA; Yordan, EL; Miller, A; Graham, JE; Kirshner, C; et al. Recurrence patterns and complications in endometrial adenocarcinoma with cervical involvement. *Ann. Surg. Oncol.* 1995;2:138-44.
[106] Sartori, E; Gadducci, A; Landoni, F; Lissoni, A; Maggino, T; Zola, P; et al. Clinical behavior of 203 stage II endometrial cancer cases: the impact of primary surgical approach and of adjuvant radiation therapy. *Int. J. Gynecol. Cancer* 2001;11:430-7.
[107] Bristow, RE; Zerbe, MJ; Rosenshein, NB; Grumbine, FC; Montz, FJ. Stage IVB endometrial cancer: the role of cytoreductive surgery and determinants of survival. *Gynecol. Oncol.* 2000;78:85-91.
[108] Ayhan, A; Taskiran, C; Celik, C; Yuce, K. The long-term survival of women with surgical stage II endometrioid type endometrial cancer. *Gynecol. Oncol.* 2004;93:9-13.
[109] Ditto, A; Martinelli, F; Hanozet, F; Reato, C; Solima, E; Zanaboni, F; et al. Class III NSRH: oncological outcome in 170 cervical cancer patients. *Gynecol. Oncol.* 2010;119:192-7.
[110] Pirro, V; Skanjeti, A; Pelosi, E. PET in uterine malignancies. *Health* 2010;2:652-60
[111] Torizuka, T; Nakamura, F; Takekuma, M; Toshihiko, K; Ogusu, T; Yoshikawa, E; et al. 18F-FDG PET for the assessment of myometrial infiltration in clinical stage I uterine corpus cancer. *Nuc. Med. Commun.* 2006;27:481-7.
[112] Chao, A; Chang, TC; Ng, KK; Hsueh, S; Huang, HJ; Chou, HH; et al. 18F-FDG PET in the management of endometrial cancer. *Eur. J. Nucl. Med. Mol. Imaging* 2006;33:36-44.
[113] Suzuki, R; Miyagi, E; Takahashi, N; Sukegawa, A; Suzuki, A; Koike, I; et al. Validity of positron emission to-mography using fluoro-2-deoxyglucose for the preoperative evaluation of endometrial cancer. *Int J. Gynecol. Cancer* 2007;17:890-6.
[114] Park, JY; Kim, EN; Suh, DS; Kim, JII; Kim, YM; Kim, YT; et al. Comparison of the validity of magnetic resonance imaging and positron emission tomography/ computed tomography in the preoperative evaluation of patients with uterine corpus cancer. *Gynecol. Oncol.* 2008;108:486-92.
[115] Sironi, S; Picchio, M; Landoni, F; Galimberti, S; Signorelli, M; Bettinardi, V; et al. Post-therapy surveillance of patients with uterine cancers: Value of integrated 18F-FDG-PET/CT in the detection of recurrence. *Eur. J. Nucl. Med. Mol. Imaging* 2007;34:472-9.
[116] Kitajima, K; Murakami, K; Yamasaki, E; Hagiwara, S; Fukasawa, I; Inaba, N; et al. Performance of 18F-FDG-PET/CT in the diagnosis of recurrent endometrial cancer. *Ann. Nuc. Med.* 2008;22:103-9.
[117] Manchana, T; Sirisabya, N; Lertkhachonsuk, R; Worasethsin, P; Khemapech, N; Sittisomwong, T; et al. Long term complications after radical hysterectomy with pelvic lymphadenectomy. *J. Med. Assoc. Thai.* 2009;92:451-6.
[118] Conte, M; Benedetti Panici, P; Guariglia, L; Scambia, G; Greggi, S; Mancuso, S. Pelvic lymphocele following radical para-aortic and Lymphatic Complications and Endometrial Cancer pelvic lymphadenectomy for cervical carcinoma: incidence rate and percutaneous management. *Obstet. Gynecol.* 1990;76:268-71.
[119] Baekelandt, MM; Castiglione, M; ESMO Guidelines Working Group. Endometrial carcinoma: ESMO clinical recommendations for diagnosis; treatment and follow-up. *Ann. Oncol.* 2009;20(Suppl4):29-31.

[120] Cho, H; Kim, YT; Kim, JH. Accuracy of preoperative tests in clinical stage I endometrial cancer: the importance of lymphadenectomy. *Acta Obstet. Gynecol. Scand.* 2010;89:175-81.

[121] Mori, N. Clinical and experimental studies on the so-called lymphocyst which develops after radical hysterectomy in cancer of the uterine cervix. *J. Jpn. Obstet. Gynecol. Soc.* 1955;2:178-203.

[122] Ilancheran, A; Monaghan, JM. Pelvic lymphocyst – a 10-year experience. *Gynecol. Oncol.* 1988;29:333-6.

[123] Logmans, A; Kruyt, RH; de Bruin, HG; Cox, PH; Pillay, M; Trimbos, JB. Lymphedema and lymphocysts following lymphadenectomy may be prevented by omentoplasty: A pilot study. *Gynecol. Oncol.* 1999;75:323-7.

[124] Benedetti Panici, P; Maneschi, F; Cutillo, G. Pelvic and aortic lymphadenectomy. *Surg. Clin. North Am.* 2001;81:841-58.

[125] Shingleton, HM; Orr, HW. Cancer of the cervix: Diagnosis and Treatment in Current reviews in obstetrics and gynecology. Vol. 5; Churchill Livingstone; Edinburgh; 1993.

[126] Ghezzi, F; Uccella, S; Cromi, A; Bogani, G; Robba, C; Serati, M; et al. Lymphoceles; lymphorrhea; and lymphedema after laparoscopic and open endometrial cancer staging. *Ann. Surg. Oncol.* 2011 Jun 22. [Epub ahead of print]

[127] Gallotta V; Fanfani, F; Rossitto, C; Vizzielli, G; Testa, A; Scambia, G; et al. A randomized study comparing the use of the Ligaclip with bipolar energy to prevent lymphocele during laparoscopic pelvic lymphadenectomy for gynecologic cancer. *Am. J. Obstet. Gynecol.* 2010 Nov;203(5):483.e1-6.

[128] Kim, HY; Kim, JW; Kim, SH; Kim, YT; Kim, JH. An analysis of the risk factors and management of lymphocele after pelvic lymphadenectomy in patients with gynecologic malignancies. *Cancer Res. Treat.* 2004;36:377-83.

[129] Charoenkwan, K; Kietpeerakool, C. Retroperitoneal drainage versus no drainage after pelvic lymphadenectomy for the prevention of lymphocyst formation in patients with gynaecological malignancies. *Cochrane Database Syst. Rev.* 2010;1:CD007387.

[130] Kim, HY; Kim, JW; Kim, SH; Kim, YT; Kim, JH. An analysis of the risk factors and management of lymphocele after pelvic lymphadenectomy in patients with gynecologic malignancies. *Cancer Res. Treat.* 2004;36:377-83.

[131] Tinelli, A; Giorda, G; Manca, C; Pellegrino, M; Prudenzano, R; Guido, M; et al. Prevention of lymphocele in female pelvic lymphadenectomy by a collagen patch coated with the human coagulation factors: A pilot study. *J. Surg. Oncol.* 2012; 105(8):835-40.

[132] Kaskarelis, D; Sakkas, K; Aravantinos, D; Michalas, S; Zolotas, J. Urinary tract injuries in gynecological and obstetrical procedures. *Int. Surg.* 1975;60:40-3.

[133] Kritchevsky, SB; Braun, BI; Gross, PA; Newcomb, CS; Kelleher, CA; Simmons, BP. Definition and adjustment of Cesarean section rates and assessments of hospital performance. *Int. J. Qual. Health Care* 1999;11:283-91.

[134] Rajasekar, D; Hall, M. Urinary tract injuries during obstetric intervention. *Br. J. Obstet. Gynaecol.* 1997;104:731-4.

[135] Thomas, DP; Burgess, NA; Gower, RL; Peeling, WB. Ureteric injury at cesarean section. *Br. J. Urol.* 1994;74:122-3.

[136] Lenkovsky, Z; Pode, D; Shapiro, A; Caine, M. Vesicouterine fistula: a rare complication of cesarean section. *J. Urol.* 1988;139:123-5.

[137] Nabi, G; Hemal, AK; Kumar, M; Ansari, MS; Dorairajan, LN. Diagnosis and management of post-cesarean ureterouterine fistulae. *Int Urogynecol J. Pelvic Floor Dysfunct* 2000;11:389-91.

[138] Hemal, AK; Kumar, R; Nabi, G. Post-cesarean cervicovesical fistula: technique of laparoscopic repair. *J. Urol.* 2001;165:1167-8.

[139] Baniel, J; Schein, M. The management of penetrating trauma to the urinary tract. *J. Am. Coll Surg.* 1994;178:417-25.

[140] Shelbaia, AM; Hussein, A, El Rahman, SA. Lower urinary tract injuries during gynecological operations. *UroToday Int. J.* 2010;3:doi:10.3834/uij.1944-5784.2010.02.04

[141] Baggish, MS. Urinary Tract Injuries Secondary to Gynecologic Laparoscopic Surgery: Analysis of 75 Cases. *J. Gynecol. Surg.* 2010;26:79-92

[142] Byrom, J; Redman, C. Urinary function following radical hysterectomy (based on various types; Piver classification). *CME J. Gynecol. Oncol.* 2002;7:51-6.

[143] Wertheim, E. The extended operation for carcinoma of the cervix. *Am. J. Obstet. Gynecol.* 1912;6:169-81.

[144] Riss, P; Koelbl, H; Neunteufel, W; Janisch, H. Wertheim radical hysterectomy 1921-1986: Changes in urological complications. *Arch. Gynecol. Obstet.* 1988; 241:249-53.

[145] Magrina, JF; Goodrich ,MA; Weaver, AL; Podratz, KC. Modified radical hysterectomy: morbidity and mortality. *Gynecol. Oncol.* 1995;59:277-82.

[146] Kenter, GG; Ansink, AC; Heintz, APM; Aartsen, EJ; Delemarre, JFM; Hart, AAM. Carcinoma of the uterine cervix stage I and IIA: results of surgical treatment: complications; recurrence and survival. *Eur. J. Surg. Oncol.* 1989;15:55-60.

[147] Landoni, F; Maneo, A; Cormio, G; Perego, P; Milani, R; Caruso, O; et al. Class II versus class III radical hysterectomy in stage IB-IIA cervical cancer: a prospective randomized study. *Gynecol. Oncol.* 2001;80:3-12.

[148] van Nagell, JR Jr; Penny, RM Jr; Roddick, JW Jr. Suprapubic bladder drainage following radical hysterectomy. *Am. J. Obstet. Gynecol.* 1972;113:849-50.

[149] Fishman, IJ; Shabsigh, R; Kaplan, AL. Lower urinary tract dysfunction after radical hysterectomy for carcinoma of the cervix. *Urology* 1986; 28:462-68.

[150] Fraser, AC. The late effects of Wertheim's hysterectomy on the urinary tract. *J. Obstet. Gynaecol. Br. Common.* 1966;73:1002-7.

[151] Seski, JC; Diokno, AC. Bladder dysfunction after radical hysterectomy. *Am. J. Obstet. Gynecol.* 1977;128:643-51.

[152] Lin, HH; Yu, H-J; Sheu, BC; Huang, SC. Importance of urodynamic study before radical hysterectomy for cervical cancer. *Gynecol. Oncol.* 2001;81:270-2.

[153] Eltabbakh, GH; Piver, MS; Hempling, RE; Recio, FO. Laparoscopic surgery in obese women. *Obstet. Gynecol.* 1999;94:704-8.

[154] Childers, JM; Brzecheffa, PR; Hatch, KD; Surwit, EA. Laparoscopically-assisted surgical staging (LASS) of endometrial cancer. *Gynecol. Oncol.* 1993;51:33-8.

[155] Boike, G; Lurain, J; Burke, J. A comparison of laparoscopic management of endometrial cancer and traditional laparotomy. *Gynecol. Oncol.* 1994;52:105.

[156] Gemignani, ML; Curtin, JP; Zelmanovich, J; Patel, DA; Venkatraman, E; Barakat, RR. Laparoscopic-assisted vaginal hysterectomy for endometrial cancer: clinical outcomes and hospital charges. *Gynecol. Oncol.* 1999;73:5-11.

[157] Eltabbakh, GH; Shamonki, MI; Moody, JM; Garafano, LL. Hysterectomy for Obese Women with Endometrial Cancer: Laparoscopy or Laparotomy? *Gynecol. Oncol.* 2000;78:329-35.
[158] Chi, DS; Welshinger, M; Venkatraman, ES; Barakat, RR. The role of surgical cytoreduction in Stage IV endometrial carcinoma. *Gynecol. Oncol.* 1997;67:56-60.
[159] Bristow, RE; Zerbe, MJ; Rosenshein, NB; Grumbine, FC; Montz, FJ. Stage IVB endometrial carcinoma: the role of cytoreductive surgery and determinants of survival. *Gynecol. Oncol.* 2000;78:85-91.
[160] International Federation of Gynecology and Obstetrics. Corpus cancer staging. *Int. J. Gynecol. Obstet.* 1989;28;189-90.
[161] ASTEC/EN.5 Study Group. Adjuvant external beam radiotherapy in the treatment of endometrial cancer (MRC ASTEC and NCIC CTG EN.5 randomised trials): pooled trial results; systematic review; and meta-analysis. *Lancet* 2009;373:137-46.
[162] Panici, PB; Basile, S; Maneschi, F; Lissoni, A; Signorelli, M; Scambia, G; et al. Systematic pelvic lymphadenectomy vs no lymphadenectomy in early-stage endometrial carcinoma: randomized clinical trial. *J. Natl. Cancer Inst.* 2008;100;1707-16.
[163] Masciullo, V; Amadio, G; Lo Russo, D; Raimondo, I; Giordano, A; Scambia, G. Controversies in the management of endometrial cancer. *Obstet. Gynecol. Int.* 2010;2010:638165.
[164] Opmeer, BC; van Doorn, HC; Heintz, AP; Burger, CW; Bossuyt, PM; Mol, BW. Improving the existing diagnostic strategy by accounting for characteristics of the women in the diagnostic work up for postmenopausal bleeding. *BJOG* 2007;114:51-8.
[165] Bruchim, I; Biron-Shental, T; Altaras, MM; Fishman, A; Beyth, Y; Tepper, R; et al. Combination of endometrial thickness and time since menopause in predicting endometrial cancer in women with postmenopausal bleeding. *J. Clin. Ultrasound* 2004;32:219-24.
[166] Bachmann, LM; ter Riet, G; Clark, TJ; Gupta, JK; Khan, KS. Probability analysis for diagnosis of endometrial hyperplasia and cancer in postmenopausal bleeding: an approach for a rational diagnostic workup. *Acta Obstet. Gyn. Scan.* 2003;82:564-9.

In: Endometrial Cancer: Prevention, Diagnosis and Treatment ISBN: 978-1-62257-740-8
Editor: Stefano Greggi

Chapter VII

The Role of Laparoscopy/Robotics

Samar Nahas and Javier Magrina*
Medical and Surgical Gynecology, Mayo Clinic, Phoenix, AZ, US

Abstract

Endometrial cancer is the most common gynecological malignancy, most are diagnosed at an early stage, and in most cases the curative management is surgical. In the treatment of early stage endometrial cancer, minimally invasive approach, laparoscopic or robotic, has bccn shown to bc safc and fcasiblc, and prcfcrablc to laparotomy. Certainly it will become increasingly offered to patients as training programs evolve to teach its trainees laparoscopic and robotic skills.

In this chapter, the history, risks and benefits of minimally invasive approach will be presented and compared to traditional laparotomy.

Introduction

First laparoscopic assisted vaginal hysterectomy was performed in 1989 [1]. In the same year, Dargent et al. used the laparoscope to perform limited pelvic lymphadenectomy on women with cervical cancer [2]. Laparoscopic pelvic and para-aortic lymph node dissection for endometrial cancer was described by Childers et al. in 1992 [3].

Since then, laparoscopy evolved slowly for the treatment of endometrial cancer. However, since the advent of the robotic technology it has experienced a rapid growth. A recent survey of the Society of Gynecologic Oncologists has indicated that most of its members believe in the benefits of laparoscopy for their patients [4].

* E-mail address: jmagrina@mayo.edu.

Conventional Laparoscopy

Laparoscopic surgery for endometrial cancer started with laparoscopic assisted vaginal hysterectomy (LAVH) and progressed to total laparoscopic hysterectomy (TLH) and staging, with many proven advantages compare to laparotomy.

Obermair et al. did a retrospective review comparing TLH to open hysterectomy. Recurrence, disease free and overall survivals were similar. No port site metastases were noted in the TLH group [5].

Magrina et al. retrospectively reviewed 56 patients with clinical Stage I endometrial cancer treated laparoscopically. The mean follow-up was 6.4 years. Laparoscopic approach provided 5-year survival and recurrence rates similar to those previously attained by laparotomy in the same institution [6].

Magrina et al. reported a review of pertinent studies comparing laparoscopy to laparotomy for surgically manageable endometrial cancer. Similar results for recurrence and survival rates were noted for patients treated by laparoscopy and laparotomy, while laparoscopy patients had lower blood loss and shorter hospital stay. A similar or reduced cost was also noted for the laparoscopic approach [7].

In a small randomized trial, comparing LAVH to TLH in endometrial cancer with pelvic node dissection. The TLH had a shorter operative time and less operative complications, with no difference in port site metastasis [8].

The largest randomized trial comparing laparoscopic management of endometrial cancer to traditional open surgery was GOG LAP-2 trial. A total of 2616 patients with clinical stage I/IIA uterine cancer were randomized to laparotomy, or laparoscopy. There was a 23% conversion to laparotomy in the laparoscopy group. The laparoscopy group had a shorter hospital stay by average of one day, while the operating time was longer by one hour on average. Quality-of-Life (QoL) ratings were higher for the laparoscopy group at 6 weeks postoperatively. However, no differences were noted at 6 months. [9].

LACE was a two-stage randomized controlled trial, comparing TLH with total abdominal hysterectomy (TAH) for stage I endometrial cancer. The primary objective of the first stage of the study was to assess whether TLH resulted in equivalent or improved QoL up to 6 months after surgery compared with TAH. Three hundred sixty one participants were enrolled in the QoL study at 19 centers; 332 completed the QoL analysis. Results showed QoL improvements from baseline during early and later phases of recovery, and the adverse event profile favored TLH compared with TAH for treatment of stage I endometrial cancer. Stage 2 results are still pending [10].

Robotic-Assisted Laparoscopy

The surgical robot is a computer-controlled device that can be programmed to help in manipulating surgical instruments. The prototype was originally designed for use by the military to provide immediate operative care on the battlefield from a remote surgical station. Robotic telepresence technology became commercially available in 2000 (da Vinci® Surgical System, Intuitive Surgical inc., Sunnyvale, CA, USA). The system was developed by the

Stanford Research Institute, National Aeronautics and Space Administration [11]. The surgical robot is mainly used for laparoscopy instead of open procedures.

Surgical robotics were first used in 1985 in neurosurgery; application soon followed in urology and orthopedics [11,12]. In 1998, the first robotic assisted laparoscopic tubal anastomosis in live porcine was performed [13]. Diaz-Arrastia et al. published the first 10 case series reporting the use of a computer-enhanced surgical robot for performing hysterectomy in humans in 2002 [14].

Reynolds et al. attempted 7 robot-assisted laparoscopic staging procedures in gynecologic malignancies with no conversions to laparotomy. He concluded that robot-assisted laparoscopic staging is a feasible technique that may overcome the surgical limitations of conventional laparoscopy [15]. Bandera and Magrina et al. did a review of case series and concluded that robotic surgery is a minimally invasive alternative to laparoscopy for the surgical treatment of endometrial and cervical cancer [16]. Veljovich el at reported their first year experience in 1,188 patients, comparing robotic surgery to laparotomy in endometrial cancer staging, and concluded that robotic surgery is feasible in gynecologic oncology and facilitated a dramatic expansion in their minimally invasive surgical practice [17]. Boggess et al. compared the outcomes in women who underwent endometrial cancer staging by different surgical techniques. Three hundred twenty two women were included: 138 had laparotomy (TAH); 81 had laparoscopy (TLH) and 103 had robotic technique (TRH). They reported that TRH with staging is feasible and preferable over TAH and may be preferable over TLH in women with endometrial cancer [18]. Magrina et al. evaluated the results of robotic surgery for the primary treatment of endometrial cancer patients and compared them to a matched group of patients treated by laparoscopy, laparotomy, and vaginal- laparoscopy. Robotic, laparoscopy, and vaginal-laparoscopy techniques were preferable to laparotomy. Robotic was preferable to laparoscopy due to a shorter hospital stay and lower conversion rate, it was preferable to vaginal/laparoscopy due to a reduced hospitalization [19]. Paley et al. analyzed their first 1,000 robotic cases in gynecological oncology and found that robotic surgery is associated with favorable morbidity, conversion rates and outcome in an unselected cohort compared to laparotomy [20].

Lim et al. analyzed the learning curve and outcome for robotic assisted hysterectomy with lymphadenectomy in patients with endometrial cancer and compared it to laparoscopy. He observed that Robotic hysterectomy with lymphadenectomy had a faster learning curve in comparison to laparoscopy. The adequacy of surgical staging was comparable between the two surgical methods. The robotic surgery was associated with shorter hospitalization, less blood loss, less intraoperative and major complications, and lower rate of conversion to open procedure [21,22]. Seamon et al. studied the number of cases required in the learning curve for performing robotic hysterectomy with pelvic-aortic lymphadenectomy for endometrial cancer. The authors concluded that proficiency for robotic hysterectomy with pelvic-aortic lymphadenectomy for endometrial cancer was achieved after 20 cases; however, the number of procedures to gain efficiency varies for each portion of the case and continues to improve over time [23].

Barnett et al. did a cost comparison analysis between robotic, laparoscopic, and open hysterectomy for endometrial cancer. He found that laparoscopy is the least expensive surgical approach for the treatment of endometrial cancer. Robotics is less costly than abdominal hysterectomy when the societal costs associated with recovery time are accounted for and is most economically attractive if disposable equipment costs can be minimized [24].

Holtz et al. compared the cost of robotics vs. laparoscopy in endometrial cancer surgery in 33 patients. Robotic surgery costs were significantly higher than traditional laparoscopy costs for staging of endometrial cancer in a small cohort of patients [25]. Martino et al. compared the cost analysis of postoperative management for endometrial cancer between the robot and laparoscopy in 215 patients. Patients in the robotic surgery arm experienced less initial postoperative pain and had fewer drug interventions. The costs associated for their pain management represented a savings of greater than 50%, indicating the value of robotic surgery in regards to postoperative pain management by delivering higher quality care at a lower cost [26]. Bell et al. compared the outcome and cost of endometrial cancer surgery via laparotomy, robotics and laparoscopy. Robotic hysterectomy provided comparable node retrieval to laparotomy and laparoscopy in the case of an experienced laparoscopic surgeon. While robotic hysterectomy took longer to perform than via laparotomy, it was equivalent to laparoscopic approach and provided the patient with a faster return to normal activity and reduced post-operative morbidity. The average cost for hysterectomy and staging was highest for laparotomy, followed by robotic, and lowest for standard laparoscopy [27].

Minimally Invasive Surgery in the Elderly

The risk of gynecologic malignancy increases with age, 45% of endometrial cancers are diagnosed in women age 65 years or older [28]. With traditional open surgery, elderly patients are prone to have higher rate of postoperative cardiac, respiratory and thromboembolic complications, longer length of hospital stay, and greater risk for loss of independence after surgery [29].

Scribner et al. reported on the laparoscopic management of endometrial cancer in patients > 65 years. In their series of 67 patients, a shorter length of stay, less postoperative fever, less postoperative ileus and fewer wound complications were noticed in the laparoscopic group compared to laparotomy [29].

Vacnin et al. prospectively evaluated the perioperative data and postoperative quality-of-life survey of the first hundred robotic surgeries for endometrial cancer. Patients were divided in 2 groups based on age, 41 patients age ≥ 70 years and 59 patients age < 70 years. Elderly women had similar operative time, mean blood loss and perioperative complications compared with the younger group.

Median hospital stay tended to be longer in the elderly women (2 vs. 1 days), but it was not statistically significant. Quality-of-life was high in both groups. Robotics was safe and conferred an excellent quality-of-life for elderly patients [30]. Frey et al. compared the surgical outcome of elderly and younger patients undergoing laparoscopic or robotic surgical staging for endometrial cancer.

Sixty patients were > 65 years of age, and 69 patients were < 65 years of age. Among the 109 patients who underwent laparoscopic or robotic staging, there were no differences in estimated blood loss, lymph node count, surgical time, complications, rate of blood transfusion, conversion to laparotomy, and mean of postoperative stay between elderly and younger patients [31].

Minimally Invasive Surgery in the Obese Patient

Obesity is defined as a body mass index (BMI) ≥ 30 kg/m^2. Obese women have a higher risk of developing uterine and ovarian cancer [32]. According to the women's health initiative study, obese women who needed a hysterectomy were at a higher risk of having metabolic syndrome (hypertension, diabetes, hypercholesterolemia) and lower physical activity compared to women who did not have hysterectomy, with subsequence higher risks for cardiovascular events and mortality [33]. Therefore, it is important to be able to provide such women with a low risk surgical treatment. Laparoscopy in gynecologic surgery has consistently been demonstrated to improve the outcome over laparotomy for women regardless of BMI [34].

Eltabbakh et al. prospectively collected data on women with BMI 28-60 who underwent laparoscopy and compared their outcome to a controlled group of women who had a laparotomy 2 years prior. Laparoscopic surgery was successfully completed in 88% of patients. The laparoscopic group had a longer operative time. However surgeons were able to retrieve more pelvic lymph nodes in spite of less blood loss, less postoperative pain, and shorter hospital stay [35]. Scribner et al. compared the outcome of laparoscopic pelvic and para-aortic lymph node dissection to a historical control arm of obese patients who underwent laparotomy. Laparoscopy was successfully completed in 64% of patients. The laparoscopic group had a significantly shorter hospital stay, with similar blood loss and transfusion rates [36]. Eisenhauer et al. reported a higher node count in obese women with uterine cancer undergoing laparoscopy compared to laparotomy [37]. Gehrig et al. reported the outcome of robotic endometrial cancer staging in 36 obese and 13 morbidly obese patients and compared it to a matched group of laparoscopic patients. For both obese and morbidly obese patients, robotic surgery was associated with significantly shorter operative times, less blood loss, increased lymph node count, and shorter hospital stay [38].

Seamon et al. compared the outcome of 109 obese patients with a BMI ≥ 30 who underwent robotic staging for endometrial cancer to 162 matched laparotomy patients. Both groups had similar lymph node counts. The robotic group had statistically significant lower rates of complications, blood transfusion, and shorter hospital stay [39]. Subramaniam et al. reported a similar study comparing robotic staging in obese patients with endometrial cancer to a laparotomy group and reached similar conclusions. Robotic surgery is safe, efficient and feasible for obese women when compared to laparoscopy and laparotomy [40].

Complications

Incision Hernia

The American Association of Gynecologic Laparoscopists reported in their survey that the incidence of hernia was 21 per 100,000 laparoscopic procedures, 18% of these hernias occurred despite fascial closure [45]. The incidence of hernia in another study of 3,560 laparoscopic cases was 0.17%, with the greater risk in the extra-umbilical sites of ≥ 12 mm trocar (3.1%) than with a 10 mm trocar (0.23%) [46,47].

Vaginal Dehiscence

Hur et al. did an observational study of 7,039 hysterectomies done by different approaches. Laparoscopic hysterectomy had a significantly higher risk of vaginal dehiscence of 4.93% compared to vaginal hysterectomy of 0.29% and abdominal hysterectomy of 0.12% [52]. Kho et al. reviewed 510 post robotic hysterectomy cases. The incidence of vaginal cuff dehiscence was 4.1%. Coitus triggered 50% of vaginal deshiscences. Patients most commonly presented with vaginal bleeding or a sudden gush of watery vaginal discharge. Bowel evisceration was noted in only 28% of patients [53]. Nick et al. retrospectively studied 417 patients with laparoscopic or robotic hysterectomy for benign and malignant causes, 57 of those had radical hysterectomy. The overall risk of vaginal cuff complication was 1.7%. Radical hysterectomy was associated with a 9-fold increase in vaginal cuff complications [54].

Port Site Metastasis

It is very uncommon to have port site metastasis (PSM) post minimally invasive surgery for endometrial cancer. Nagarsheth et al. reviewed their own experience in 87 laparoscopic procedures in gynecological cancer, 39 of those patients had endometrial cancer. The rate of PSM was 2.3% (2 of 87 procedures); both were in advanced ovarian and peritoneal cancer patients.

There were no PSM in endometrial cancer patients [55]. Ramirez et al. did a midline search for laparoscopic PSM in gynecologic malignancy, 31 articles were found with a total of 58 patients. Majority of patients had an advanced ovarian cancer, 4 of 58 had endometrial cancer with a median age of 63 years, and a median time to diagnosis of 13.5 months. In three of the four patients, the PSM was not an isolated recurrence, at the time of re-exploration; evidence of disease was found at other sites [56].

Zivanovic et al. analyzed 2251 patients post laparoscopic procedure in women with underlying malignancy. Subdivided in two groups, 1694 patients underwent laparoscopic procedures for malignant intraabdominal condition, 505 were breast cancer patients undergoing risk-reducing, diagnostic or therapeutic laparoscopic procedures without intraabdominal disease. Port site metastases were documented in 20 of 1694 patients (1.18%) who underwent laparoscopic procedures for a malignant intraabdominal condition only. Of these, 15 patients had a diagnosis of epithelial ovarian or fallopian tube carcinoma, 2 had breast cancer, 2 had cervical cancer, and 1 had uterine cancer (0.05%). Nineteen of 20 patients (95%) had simultaneous carcinomatosis or metastases to other sites at the time of PSM [57].

Martínez et al. published a review of their own experience in PSM after laparoscopic procedures for cervical and uterine cancer. During the study period, 921 patients underwent laparoscopic staging for cervical cancer and 295 for endometrial cancer. The incidence of PSM after laparoscopy for cervical and endometrial cancer was 0.43% and 0.33%, respectively. The incidence of isolated PSM was 0%. They concluded that PSM is a rare complication of laparoscopic staging for endometrial and cervical cancer [58].

References

[1] Reich, H; DeCaprio, J; McGlynn, F. Laparoscopic hysterectomy. *J Gynecol Surg* 1989;5:213-6.

[2] Dargent, D; Salvat, J. *Envahissenent Ganglionnaire Pelvien: Place de la Pelviscopie Retroperitoneale*. Paris: McGraw-Hill; 1989.

[3] Childers, JM; Surwit, EA. Combined laparoscopic and vaginal surgery for the management of two cases of stage 1 endometrial cancer. *Gynecol Oncol* 1992;45:46-51.

[4] Frumovitz, M; Ramirez, PT; Greer, M. Laparoscopic training and practice in gynecologic oncology among Society of Gynecologic Oncologists members and fellows-in-training. *Gynecol Oncol* 2004;94:746-53.

[5] Obermair, A; Manolitsas, TP; Leung, Y; Hammond IG; McCartney AJ. Total laparoscopic hysterectomy for endometrial cancer. Patterns of recurrence and survival. *Gynecol Oncol* 2004;92:789-93.

[6] Magrina, JF; Weaver, AL. Laparoscopic treatment of endometrial cancer: five-year recurrence and survival rates. *Eur J Gynaecol Oncol* 2004;25:439-41.

[7] Magrina JF. Outcomes of laparoscopic treatment for endometrial cancer. *Curr Opin Obstet Gynecol* 2005;17:343-6.

[8] Ghezzi, F; Cromi, A; Uccella, S. Laparoscopy versus laparotomy for the surgical management of apparent early stage ovarian cancer. *Gynecol Oncol* 2007;10:409-13.

[9] Walker, JL; Piedmonte, M; Spirtos, N. Phase III trial of laparoscopy (scope) vs laparotomy (open) for surgical resection and comprehensive surgical staging of uterine cancer: a Gynecologic Oncology Group (GOG) Study funded by NCI. In: *Proceedings from the 37th Annual Meeting of the Society of Gynecologic Oncologists*; March 22-26, 2006; Palm Springs, CA. Abstract 22.

[10] Monika, J; Val, G; Alison, B. Quality of life after total laparoscopic hysterectomy versus total abdominal hysterectomy for stage I endometrial cancer (LACE): a randomized trial. *Lancet Oncol* 2010;11:772-80.

[11] Satava, RM. Robotic surgery: from past to future - a personal journey. *Surg Clin North Am* 2003;83:1491.

[12] Dharia, SP; Falcone, T. Robotics in reproductive medicine. *Fertile Steril* 2005;84:1-11.

[13] Margossian, H; Garcia-Ruiz, A; Falcone, T; Goldberg, JM; Attaran, M; Miller, JH; et al. Robotic assisted laparoscopic tubal anastomosis in a porcine model: A pilot study. *J Laparoendosc Adv Surg Tech A* 1998;8:69-73.

[14] Diaz-Arrastia, C; Jurnalov, C; Gomez, IG; Townsend, ZC. Laparoscopic hysterectomy using a computer-enhanced surgical robot. *Surg Endos* 2002;16:1271-3.

[15] Reynolds, RK; Burke, WM; Advincula, AP. Preliminary Experience with robot-assisted laparoscopic staging of gynecologic malignancies. *JSLS* 2005;9:149-58.

[16] Bandera, CA; Magrina, JF. Robotic surgery in gynecologic oncology. *Curr Opin Obstet Gynecol* 2009;21:25-30.

[17] Veljovich, DS; Paley, PJ; Drescher, CW. Robotic surgery in gynecologic oncology: program initiation and outcomes after the first year with comparison with laparotomy for endometrial cancer staging. *Am J Obstet Gynecol* 2008;198:679.e1-679.e10.

[18] Boggess, JF; Gehrig, PA; Cantrell, L. A comparative study of 3 surgical methods for hysterectomy with staging for endometrial cancer: robotic assistance, laparoscopy, laparotomy. *Am J Obstet Gynecol* 2008;199:360.e1-9.
[19] Magrina, JF; Zanagnolo, V; Giles, D; Noble BN; Kho, RM; Magtibay, PM. Robotic surgery for endometrial cancer: comparison of perioperative outcome and recurrence with laparoscopy, vaginal/laparoscopy and laparotomy. *Eur J Gynaecol Oncol* 2011;32:476-80.
[20] Paley, PJ; Veljovich, DS; Shah, CA. Surgical outcomes in gynecologic oncology in the era of robotics: analysis of first 1000 cases. *Am J Obstet Gynecol* 2011;204:551.e1-9.
[21] Lim, PC; Kang, E; PA-C; Park do, H. Learning curve and surgical outcome for Robotic-Assisted Hysterectomy with lymphadenectomy: Case-matched controlled comparison with laparoscopy and laparotomy for treatment of endometrial cancer. *J Minim Invasive Gynecol* 2010;17:739-48.
[22] Lim, PC; Kang, E; Park do, H. A comparative detail analysis of the learning curve and surgical outcome for robotic hysterectomy with lymphadenectomy versus laparoscopic hysterectomy with lymphadenectomy in treatment of endometrial cancer: a case-matched controlled study of the first one hundred twenty two patients. *Gynecol Oncol* 2011;120:413-8.
[23] Seamon, LG; Fowler, J; Richardson, D; Carlson, MJ; Valmadre, S; Phillips, GS; et al. A detailed analysis of the learning curve: Robotic hysterectomy and pelvic-aortic lymphadenectomy for endometrial cancer. *Gynecol Oncol* 2009;114:162-7.
[24] Barnett, JC; Judd, JP; Wu, JM; Scales, CD Jr; Mayers, ER; Havrilesky, LJ. Cost comparison among robotic, laparoscopic, and open hysterectomy for endometrial cancer. *Obstet Gynecol* 2010;116:685-93.
[25] Holtz, DO; Miroshnichenko, G; Finnegan, MO; Chernick, M; Dunton, CJ. Endometrial cancer surgery costs: robot vs laparoscopy. *J Minim Invasive Gynecol* 2010;17:500-3.
[26] Martino, MA; Shubella, J; Thomas, MB; Morcrette, RM; Schindler, J; Williams, S; et al. A cost analysis of postoperative management in endometrial cancer patients treated by robotics versus laparoscopic approach. *Gynecol Oncol* 2011;123:528-31.
[27] Bell, MC; Torgerson, J; Seshadri-Kreaden, U; Suttle, AW; Hunt, S. Comparison of outcomes and cost for endometrial cancer staging via traditional laparotomy, standard laparoscopy and robotic techniques. *Gynecol Oncol* 2008;111:407-11.
[28] Horner, M; Ries, L; Kraccho, M. *SEER Cancer Statistics Review 1975-2006*. Bethesda: National Cancer Institute; 2008.
[29] Scribner, DR Jr; Walker, JL; Johnson, GA. Surgical management of early stage endometrial cancer in the elderly: Is laparoscopy feasible? *Gynecol Oncol* 2001;83:563-8.
[30] Vaknin, Z; Perri, T; Lau, S; Deland, C; Drummond, FN; Rosberger, FZ; et al. Outcome and quality of life in a prospective cohort of the first 100 robotic surgeries for endometrial cancer, with focus on elderly patients. *Int J Gynecol Cancer* 2010;20:1367-73.
[31] Frey, MK; Ihnow, SB; Worley, MJ Jr; Heyman, KP; Kessler, R; Slomovitz, BM. Holcomb KM. Minimally invasive staging of endometrial cancer is feasible and safe in elderly women. *J Minim Invasive Gynecol* 2011;18:200-4.
[32] Anderson, B; Connor, JP; Andrews, JI. Obesity and prognosis in endometrial cancer. *Am J Obstet Gynecol* 1996;174:1171-78.

[33] Howard, BV; Kuller, L; Langer, R. Risk of cardiovascular diseases by hysterectomy status, with and without oophorectomy: The women's health initiative observational study. *Circulation* 2005;111:1462-70.

[34] O'Hanlan, KA; Lopez, L; Dibble, SL; Garnier, AC; Huang, GS. Leuchtenberger M. Total laparoscopic hysterectomy: Body mass index and outcomes. *Obstet Gynecol* 2003;102:1384-92.

[35] Eltabbakh, GH; Shamonki, MI; Moody, JM; Garafano, LL. Hysterectomy for obese women with endometrial cancer: Laparoscopy or laparotomy? *Gynecol Oncol* 2000;78:329-35.

[36] Scribner, DR Jr; Walker, JL; Johnson, GA. laparoscopic pelvic and paraaortic lymph node dissection in the obese. *Gynecol Oncol* 2002;84:426-30.

[37] Eisenhauer, EL; Wypych, KA; Mahrara, BJ. Comparing surgical outcomes in obese women undergoing laparotomy, laparoscopy, or laparotomy with panniculectomy for the staging of uterine malignancy. *Ann Surg Oncol* 2007;14:2384-91.

[38] Gehrig, PA; Cantrell, LA; Shafer, A; Abaid, LN; Mendivil, A; Boggess, JF. What is the optimal minimally invasive surgical procedure for endometrial cancer staging in the obese and morbidly obese woman? *Gynecol Oncol* 2008;111:41-5.

[39] Seamon, LG; Bryant, SA; Rheaume, PS; Kimball, KJ; Huh, WK; Fowler, JM; et al. Comprehensive Surgical Staging for Endometrial Cancer in Obese Patients Comparing Robotics and Laparotomy. *Obstet Gynecol* 2009;114:16-21.

[40] Subramaniam, A; Kim, KH; Bryant, SA; Zhang, B; Sikes, C; Kimball, KJ; et al. A cohort study evaluating robotic versus laparotomy surgical outcomes of obese women with endometrial carcinoma. *Gynecol Oncol* 2011;122:604-7.

[41] Magrina JF. Complications of laparoscopic surgery. *Clin Obstet Gynecol* 2002;45, 469-80.

[42] Jansen, FW; Kolkman, W; Bakkum, EA. Complication of laparoscopy: an inquiry about closed versus open entry technique. *Am J Obstet Gynecol* 2004;190:634-8.

[43] Chandler, JG; Conson, SL; Way, LW. Three spectra of laparoscopic entry access injuries. *J Am Coll Surg* 2001;192:478-90.

[44] Bhoyrul, S; Vierra, MA; Nezhat, CR. Trocar injuries in laparoscopic surgery. J AM Coll Surg, 2001;192:677-83.

[45] Montz, FJ; Holschneider, CH; Munro, MG. Incisional hernia following laparoscopy: a survey of the American Association of Gynecologic Laparoscopists. *Obstet Gynecol* 1994;84:881-4.

[46] Boike, GM; Miller, CE; Spirtos, NM. Incisional bowel herniation after operative laparoscopy: a series of nineteen cases and review of the literature. *Am J Obstet Gynecol* 1995;172:1726-31.

[47] Kadar, N; Reich, H; Liu, CY. Incisional hernias after major laparoscopic gynecologic procedures. *Am J Obstet Gynecol* 1993;168:1493-5.

[48] Jackson, SA; Laurence, AS; Hill, JC. Does post-laparoscopy pain related to residual carbon dioxide? *Anaesthesia* 1996;51:485-7.

[49] Phelps, P; Cakmakkaya, OS; Apfel, CC; Radke, OC. A Simple clinical maneuver to reduce laparoscopy-induced shoulder pain: a randomized controlled trial. *Obstet Gynecol* 2008;111:1155-60.

[50] Palmes, D; Rottgermann, S; Classen, C. Randomized clinical trail of the influence of intraperitoneal local anaesthesia on pain after laparoscopic surgery. *Br J Surg* 2007;94:824-32.
[51] Cunniffe, MG; McAnena, OJ; Dar, MA. A prospective randomized trail of intraoperative bupivacaine irrigation for management of shoulder-tip pain following laparoscopy. *Am J Surg* 1998;176:258-61.
[52] Hur, HC; Guido, RS; Mansuria, SM; Hacker, MR; Sanfilippo, JS; Lee, TT. Incidence and patient characteristics of vaginal cuff dehiscence after different modes of hysterectomies. *J Minim Invasive Gynecol* 2007;14:311-7.
[53] Kho, RM; Akl, MN; Cornella, JL; Magtibay, PM; Wechter, ME; Magrina, JF. Incidence and characteristics of patients with vaginal cuff dehiscence after robotic procedures. *Obstet Gynecol* 2009;114(Pt1):231-5.
[54] Nick, AM; Lange, J; Frumovitz, M; Soliman, PT; Schmeler, KM; Schlumbrecht, MP; et al. Rate of vaginal cuff separation following laparoscopic or robotic hysterectomy. *Gynecol Oncol* 2011;120:47-51.
[55] Nagarsheth, NP; Rahaman, J; Cohen, CJ; Gretz, H; Nezhat, F. The incidence of port-site metastases in gynecologic cancers. *JSLS* 2004;8:133-9.
[56] Ramirez, PT; Frumovitz, M; Wolf, JK; Levenback, C. Laparoscopic port-site metastases in patients with gynecological malignancies. *Int J Gynecol Cancer* 2004;14:1070-7.
[57] Zivanovic, O; Sonoda, Y; Diaz, JP; Levine, DA; Brown, CL; Chi, DS; et al. The rate of port-site metastases after 2251 laparoscopic procedures in women with underlying malignant disease. *Gynecol Oncol* 2008;111:431-7.
[58] Martínez, A; Querleu, D; Leblanc, E; Narducci, F; Ferron, G. Low incidence of port-site metastases after laparoscopic staging of uterine cancer. *Gynecol Oncol* 2010;118:145-50.

In: Endometrial Cancer: Prevention, Diagnosis and Treatment ISBN: 978-1-62257-740-8
Editor: Stefano Greggi

Chapter VIIIa

The Problem of Lymphadenectomy: Pro

Francesco Raspagliesi*[*], *Antonino Ditto and Fabio Martinelli
Gynecologic Oncology, National Cancer Institute,
Milan, Italy

Abstract

The role of lymphadenectomy in endometrial cancer is controversial even if part of the International Federation of Gynecology and Obstetrics (FIGO) staging. FIGO guidelines recommend pelvic and para-aortic lymphadenectomy. Despite these recommendations, controversy continues to exist regarding the recommended extent of lymph node dissection, as well as its utility in improving survival for endometrial cancer. Recently two randomized clinical studies favored the "no-lymphadenectomy" arm. However a lot of criticisms have been raised, starting from the thoroughness of lymphadenectomy. Moreover, the introduction of the sentinel node technique brought other issues to the debate. Sentinel node detection will compete with emerging technologies such as MRI, PET-TC, and Molecular Markers in the identification of subset of patients eligible for lymph node dissection. Whether or not a complete (pelvic and aortic) lymphadenectomy is superior to the evolving technique of sentinel node is under debate.

Up to date no definitive conclusions could be driven. Lymphadenectomy is not indicated in low-risk / negative nodes endometrial cancer. Lymphadenectomy seems to show therapeutic effects only in high-risk / positive nodes patients and could be used to tailor adjuvant therapies.

Introduction

The assessment of lymph node status has become the standard of care in the surgical staging of patients with endometrial cancer according to International Federation of

[*] E-mail address: francesco.raspagliesi@istitutotumori.mi.it.

Gynecology and Obstetrics (FIGO) since 1988, and represents a crucial parameter in decision making regarding further adjuvant therapies. Moreover the revised FIGO classification stresses the role of lymph nodes evaluation introducing two subcategories of node positivity according to the basin involved (pelvic IIIC1 / aortic IIIC2) [1].

Paul Morrow et al. referred about the relationship between surgical pathological risk factors and outcome in clinical stage I and II carcinoma of the endometrium in a Gynecologic Oncology Group (GOG) study and reported that the strongest predictor of recurrence is nodal status, the 5-yrs DFS was > 90% for node negative, 75% for pelvic node positive and 38% for para-aortic node positive; overall the 58% of patients with positive aortic lymph node recurred [2]. Data confirmed by Lurain: the 5-yrs DFS rate of clinical stage I patients with positive pelvic nodes has been reported to be 54% compared with 90% of those with negative nodes [3]. Creasman et al. in a GOG study reported about 621 patients clinically early stage (grade 1 excluded for the last 2 years), all underwent pelvic and para-aortic lymphadenectomy and the rate of lymphatic and extra-uterine disease was the following: extra uterine disease 22%, pelvic positive nodes 9%, para-aortic positive nodes 5%, pelvic and para-aortic positive nodes 11%, ovary metastases 5%.

Recurrence rate was 7% when the disease was confined to the uterus and 43%, in case of extrauterine disease. This study does confirm that a significant number of patients with Stage I disease can have extra-uterine disease. By applying this information to individual patients, appropriate therapy can be applied, and survival improved [4].

Which Clinico-Pathologic Factors Correlate with Lymphatic and Extra-Uterine Disease?

The risk factors for nodal involvement are tumor grade, lymph vascular invasion, and depth of myometrial invasion (GOG Study, Creasman et al., 1987) [4].

How Radical should Lymphadenectomy Be during the Surgical Staging?

In literature, the status of lymph node after surgical staging has been referred as: lymph node sampling, selective lymphadenectomy, or systematic lymph node dissection. Nodes counts is used as surrogates for assessing the radicality of lymphadenectomy, but the number of removed nodes vary significantly and depends on anatomic variations and on the pathologist's evaluation. Chan et al. analyzing the SEER data on 12,333 patients found that the survival increase with the increase of lymph nodes removed [5]. Most surgeons employ either complete or selective pelvic and para-aortic lymphadenectomy as their staging procedure. However a recent survey among Society of Gynecologic Oncologists (SGO) members raised the question about the upper limit of aortic dissection (50% of respondents use the inferior mesenteric artery as the upper border and only 11% reach the renal vessels) [6]. Whether complete lymphadenectomy provides more accurate information than selective procedure about the node status is still unclear. Nevertheless, the ability to identify the specific nodes that drain the uterus in the retroperitoneal space could enhance the reliability of staging lymphadenectomy. Moreover, the development of a selective node dissection method with a high negative predictive value could be helpful to reduce the invasiveness of the dissection required and the related complications.

Vascular and neural injuries, lymphocysts, and adhesion formation are all well documented complications in patients undergoing this procedure. The addition of radiotherapy may further increase the risk of lymph edema [7,8].

Site of Lymph Node Metastases

The most frequent nodal involvement locations in the pelvis are superficial obturatory, common, and external iliac nodes. More than 50% of patients with pelvic lymph node metastasis have aortic involvement, and up to 16% of node positive patients had isolated aortic involvement.

Site of Recurrence

Creasman reported a recurrence rate of 7% when the disease was confined to the uterus and 43% in the presence of extrauterine disease [4]. Furthermore, McMeekin: 5% for pelvic and 33% for distant disease [9]; Mariani: 25% for pelvic and 27% for distant [10,11]; Klopp: 20% for pelvic and 28% for distant [12]; Hoekstra: 1% for pelvic and 24% for distant [13].

Adjuvant Radiotherapy

Stratifying for risk factors in three categories according to Creasman GOG study (grading and depth of myometrial invasion), 75% of patients avoid postoperative radiotherapy [4]. Very often pelvic radiotherapy is performed in intermediate risk cases where lymphadenectomy has been omitted or incompletely performed, because of the presumed higher risk of pelvic sidewall recurrence from occult pelvic nodal disease. Sharma et al. in a SEER data analysis on 58,776 women with endometrioid adenocarcinoma stage I-II concluded that lymphadenectomy plays an important role in the allocation of adjuvant treatment; women who undergo lymphadenectomy are less likely to receive whole pelvic radiation therapy. Moreover, they found that the effects of lymphadenectomy are most pronounced in women with high/intermediate-risk tumors and greatest for patients who have 10 or more nodes removed [14].

PORTEC-1 randomized study on adjuvant radiotherapy on stage I endometrial cancer found no survival difference, but the radiotherapy arm reported more frequent and severe toxicities [15]. The effectiveness of adjuvant brachytherapy is also high, PORTEC-2 showing a 0.9% vaginal recurrence rate with low morbidity, compared with 19% for a similar cohort without adjuvant treatment in PORTEC [16]. In another randomized study (GOG99, external beam radiotherapy without brachytherapy for intermediate-risk node-negative lymphadenectomy patients) the major difference was the number of vaginal vault recurrences; local recurrence 1.6% for radiotherapy vs. 7.4% for no adjuvant therapy at 2 years. Perhaps, lymphadenectomy in intermediate-risk cases plus adjuvant brachytherapy for node-negative patients may achieve pelvic disease control with minimal morbidity.

Pelvic radiotherapy does not improve survival in endometrial cancer. Therefore, it is not surprising that a surgical procedure confined to the pelvis does not affect the prognosis. Ideal treatment should identify patients with extra-uterine disease outside of the radiotherapy field. While the presence of extra uterine sites of disease may change treatment approaches; the impact of those changes on survival is much less clear. Because the use of lymphadenectomy did not statistically significantly change the rate of patients who did not receive adjuvant therapy, we assume that lymph node status was not generally used to spare patients from unnecessary treatment whenever appropriate. The use of pelvic radiotherapy in high-risk patients in both treatment groups may have resulted in similar treatments in the pelvis and, consequently, similar recurrence and survival outcomes [17].

Is Lymphadenectomy Therapeutic?

Recently two randomized studies have been published and both did not confirmed a therapeutic role of the systematic lymphadenectomy. Benedetti Panici et al. designed a study on preoperative stage I disease randomized to systematic vs. no lymphadenectomy (n=537). The trial was designed to detect an improvement difference of 8% in 5-year overall survival, from 80% to 88%. No difference in survival was detected between the two arms. However this study present a few pitfalls such as the inclusion of low-risk patients, the lack of systematic para-aortic lymphadenectomy, the lack of strict criteria for adjuvant therapy. The lymphadenectomy did not change the rate of patients who did not receive adjuvant therapy and, above all, only 13.3% of the overall population have lymph node metastases [18]. The second randomized trial (ASTEC) were planned to randomize 1,400 women to detect an improvement in 5-yrs OS from 80% in the standard surgery group to 90% in the lymphadenectomy group (HR=0.47). The results of ASTEC trial show no evidence of benefit in terms of overall or recurrence-free survival for pelvic lymphadenectomy in women with early endometrial cancer. Therefore, pelvic lymphadenectomy cannot be recommended as routine procedure for therapeutic purposes outside of clinical trials. But even this study presents important pitfalls: inclusion of patients with stage IA-IB G1-2 (44.7% of cases), low number of nodes positive cases, median node count 12, para-aortic lymphadenectomy not included, surgical staging not used to modulate postsurgical treatment, 49% of Pfannenstiel incision, no central pathology review, 20% of non-endometriod histology [19]. On the basis of the study of Crossman 70 to 80 of the patients should have had positive para-aortic nodes, yet only in 4 patients (0.3%) were the para-aortic nodes positive. Whilst Chan et al. analyzing the SEER data on 12,333 patients found that the survival increase with the increase of lymph node removed. In details, SEER data demonstrated that intermediate-risk and high-risk patients (stage IB, grade 3; stages IC-IV, all grades) and patients with nodal disease (stages IIIC-IV) benefit from lymphadenectomy [5]. As well, Cragun reported that patients underwent lymphadenectomy with tumor grade 3 and at least 11 lymph node removed had an improvement on OS and DFS. In addition, Cragun stated that when controlling for administration of adjuvant radiotherapy in the multivariate analysis, the association between extent of lymphadenectomy and improved survival remained in high-risk patients (poorly differentiated, outer-half myometrial invasion, papillary serous or clear-cell histologic type) [20]. Recently, Hiura et al. in a series of 284 endometrial cancers treated with systematic pelvic and aortic lymphadenectomy plus adjuvant chemotherapy, concluded that this approach could improve long-term survival in patients with aortic metastasis [21]. A Japanese retrospective cohort analysis on survival effect of paraortic lymphadenectomy in endometrial cancer (SEPAL study) comparing 325 patients submitted to pelvic lymphadenectomy vs. 346 patients submitted to pelvic plus para-aortic lymphadenectomy, reported a survival advantage for patients fully staged (pelvic and aortic). The authors reported a significant survival benefit for intermediate and high-risk patients and also concluded that pelvic lymphadenectomy alone might be insufficient in patients at risk of nodes metastasis advocating a centralization of surgical advanced procedures in specialized centers [14].

Are There Some Patients Who Are at Such Low-Risk That Lymphadenectomy Can Be Safely Omitted?

Cahn et al reported the data on analysis 12,333 low-risk patients (well to moderately-differentiated, inner-half myometrial invasion, and endometrioid or mucinous histologic type) and no improvement associated with lymphadenectomy in low-risk patients [5]. Cragun, in a study published in 2005, stated that in low-risk patients the lymphadenectomy can be omitted [20].

Sentinel Lymph Node (SLN) Technique

Intraoperative lymphatic mapping and SLN biopsy have generated much interest to reduce the invasiveness of lymphatic nodal dissection. SLN technique is widely employed in the management of breast cancer and melanoma patients, and is under investigation in vulvar cervical cancer and endometrial cancer (Figure 1).

No definitive data are mature on that interesting topic. Debate starts form the way of tracer injection, pericervical versus hystereoscopic and the role (diagnostic ± therapeutic) of such a procedure which still remain in the field of experimental therapy. Literature data on identification rate of sentinel node varies largely and it depends on the type of tracer used and on the site of injection of tracer (Table 1). The SLN detection rate was 69% and 81% for pericervical versus hysteroscopic way of tracer injection, respectively. In the hysteroscopic group the false negative rate is significantly lower and it is significantly higher (about 46%) the paraortic sentinel node detection. This could be an indirect confirmation that hysteroscopic injection allows to the tracer to follow the same anatomic routes involved in the lymphatic spread of the endometrial cancer.

In our feasibility study published in 2004 eighteen patients with endometrial adenocarcinoma were submitted to hysteroscopic injection of technetium sub-endometrially and around the lesion. At the time 0 the patient underwent office operative hysteroscopy without anesthesia. Uterine distension was obtained by means of saline solution. The fluid bag was placed 50 cm above the patient's plane so that the intracavitary pressure did not exceed 40 mm of mercury.

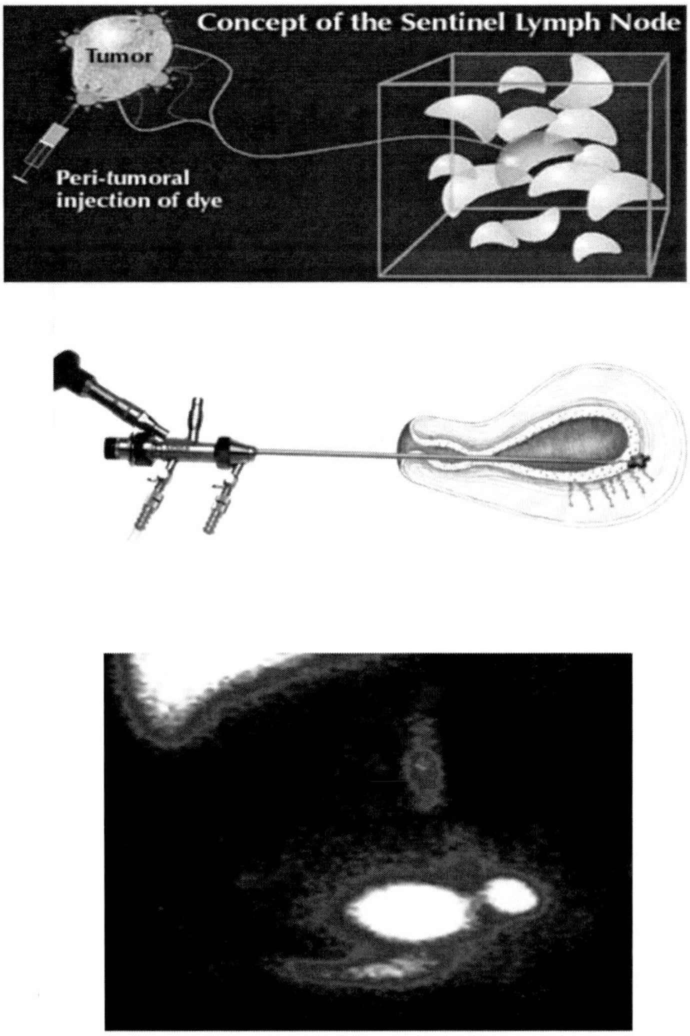

Figure 1. Concept and technique of sentinel node in endometrial cancer.

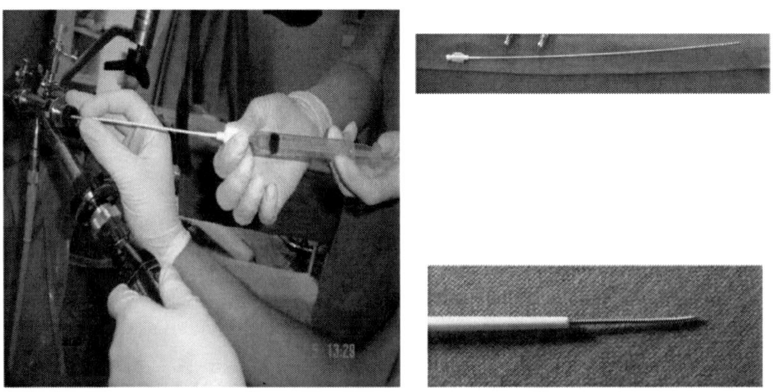

Figure 2. Hysteroscopic injection of technetium for sentinel node in endometrial cancer.

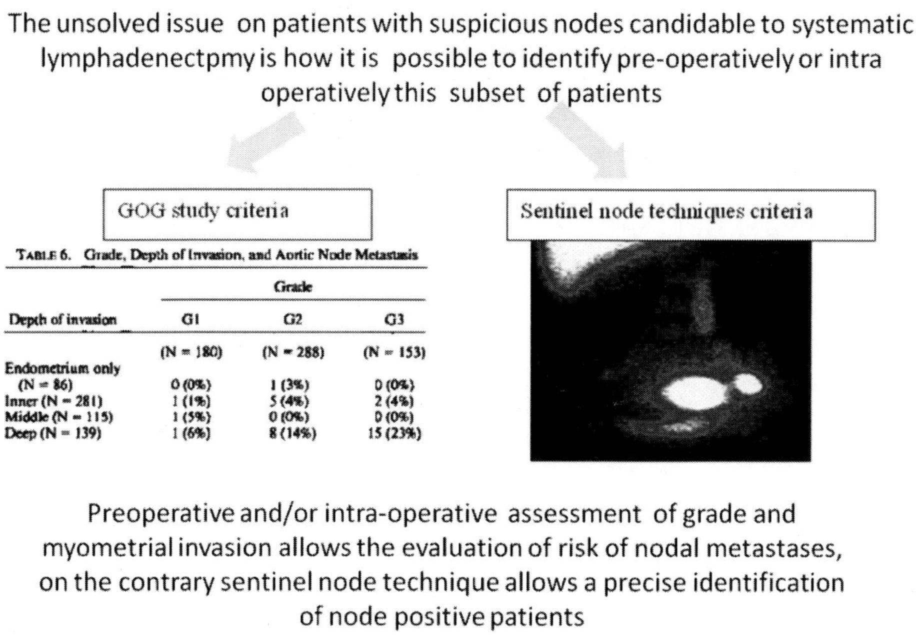

TABLE 6. Grade, Depth of Invasion, and Aortic Node Metastasis

	Grade		
Depth of invasion	G1	G2	G3
	(N = 180)	(N = 288)	(N = 153)
Endometrium only (N = 86)	0 (0%)	1 (3%)	0 (0%)
Inner (N = 281)	1 (1%)	5 (4%)	2 (4%)
Middle (N = 115)	1 (5%)	0 (0%)	0 (0%)
Deep (N = 139)	1 (6%)	8 (14%)	15 (23%)

Figure 3. Sentinel node criteria in endometrial cancer.

After localization of the tumor, we injected, through a 23-gauge needle 30 cm in length, 111 MBq of 99Tc. The injection was performed around the lesion, or, if the uterine cavity was totally involved by disease, at 3, 6, 9, and 12 o’clock. (Figure 2).

Published series report that SLN biopsy could be a trade-off between systematic lymphadenectomy and no dissection at all in patients with endometrial cancer of low or intermediate risk.

The unsolved issue on patients with suspicious nodes eligible for systematic lymphadenectomy is how it is possible to identify pre-operatively or intra operatively this subset of patients. Preoperative and/or intra-operative assessment of grade and myometrial invasion, according to GOG study, allows the evaluation of risk of nodal metastases, on the contrary sentinel node technique allows a precise identification of node positive patients (Figure 3). Moreover adding SLN mapping to current surgical staging procedures may increase the likelihood of detecting metastatic cancer cells in regional lymph nodes and could provide important data to tailor adjuvant therapy [22-33].

Conclusion

In endometrial cancer literature, the acquisition of lymphatic tissue for surgical staging has been referred to as: biopsies, lymph node sampling, selective lymphadenectomy, complete or systematic lymphadenectomy. While nodes count is used as surrogates for assessing the completeness of lymphadenectomy, it is subjected not only to anatomic variations between patients, but also inter-institutional and inter pathologist variations. Certainly, the true incidence of positive nodes is often underestimated because of the limited number of nodes removed and the intrinsic limitations of the pathologic analysis of samples.

Surgical staging was not used to modulate postsurgical treatment. In fact, the lymphadenectomy did not change the rate of patients who did not receive adjuvant therapy.

In the ASTEC study high and/or intermediate-risk cases underwent second randomization to avoid differences in postsurgical treatment on the basis of nodal histology, any differences being attributed to lymphadenectomy. The frustrating consequence is that we cannot assess the clinically relevant comparison between high and/or intermediate-risk node-negative lymphadenectomy without adjuvant therapy and conventional surgery with adjuvant radiotherapy. In addition, very often pelvic radiotherapy is performed for intermediate-risk histological cases where lymphadenectomy has been omitted or incompletely performed, because of the presumed higher risk of pelvic sidewall recurrence from occult pelvic nodal disease.

Table 1. Literature review on sentinel node detection in endometrial cancer

Author	Year	N° PTS	Inj Site	treacer	Identification %
Burke et al	1996	15	M	B	67
Echt et al	1999	8	M	B	0
Holub	2002	13	M	B	62
		12	M + C	B	83
Pelosi et al	2003	16	C	B+T	94
Niikura	2003	28	H	T	82
Barranger et al.	2004	17	C	B+T	94
Maccauro et al.	2004	26	H	B+T	100
Fersis et al	2004	10	H	T	70
Raspagliesi et al.	2004	18	H	B+T	100
Holub et al	2004	25	M + C	B	84
Bats et al	2005	26	C	B+T	81
Gien et al	2005	16	H + M	B	44
Frumovitz et al	2006	10	M	T	0
		8	M	B+T	100
Deloye JF	2007	60	H	B+T	82
Lopes LAF	2007	40	M	B	77
Ballester M	2008	39	C	T	57
		7	C	B + T	91
Perrone et al	2008	23	C	T	74
		17	H	T	35
Bats AS	2008	43	C	B +T	70
Abu-rustum N	2009	21	C	B+T	
		21	C +M	B+T	92
INT 2010	2010	66	H	T	97

Legend. B: blu dye; C: cervical; M: myometrial; H: hysteroscopic injection, T: technetium.

The phase III trials have documented no evidence of benefit in terms of overall or recurrence-free survival for pelvic lymphadenectomy in a population including 87-91% of node negative patients. Lymphadenectomy is not indicated in low-risk / negative-nodes endometrial cancer. Lymphadenectomy seems to show therapeutic effects only in high-risk / positive-nodes patients and could be used to tailor adjuvant therapies.

In this subset of patients, considering the significant para-aortic nodes involvement, para-aortic lymphadenectomy could identify patients with extrauterine disease outside of the radiotherapy field.

The unsolved issue is how it is possible to identify pre-operatively or intra operatively this subset of patients eligible for systematic lymphadenectomy. SLN detection will compete with emerging technologies such as new MRI, PET-TC, and molecular markers in the identification of subset of patients addressable to lymph node dissection.

References

[1] Pecorelli, S. Revised FIGO staging for carcinoma of the vulva, cervix, and endometrium. *Int. J. Gynaecol. Obstet.* 2009;105:103-4.

[2] Morrow, CP; Bundy, BN; Kurman, RJ; Creasman, WT; Heller, P; Homesley, HD; et al. Relationship between surgical-pathological risk factors and outcome in clinical stage I and II carcinoma of the endometrium: a Gynecologic Oncology Group study. *Gynecol. Oncol.* 1991;40:55-65.

[3] Lurain, JR; Rice, BL; Rademaker, AW; Poggensee, LE; Schink, JC; Miller, DS Prognostic factors associated with recurrence in clinical stage I adenocarcinoma of the endometrium. *Obstet. Gynecol.* 1991;78:63-9.

[4] Creasman, WT; Morrow, CP; Bundy, BN; Homesley, HD; Graham, JE; Heller, PB. Surgical pathologic spread patterns of endometrial cancer. A Gynecologic Oncology Group Study. *Cancer* 1987;60(Suppl):2035-41.

[5] Chan, JK; Cheung, MK; Huh, WK; Osann, K; Husain, A; Teng, NN; et al. Therapeutic role of lymph node resection in endometrioid corpus cancer: a study of 12;333 patients. *Cancer* 2006;107:1823-30.

[6] Soliman, PT; Frumovitz, M; Spannuth, W; Greer, MJ; Sharma, S; Schmeler, KM; et al. Lymphadenectomy during endometrial cancer staging: practice patterns among gynecologic oncologists. *Gynecol. Oncol.* 2010;119:291-4.

[7] Belinson, JL; Lee, KK; Badger, GJ; Pretorius, RG; Jarrell, MA. Clinical stage I adenocarcinoma of the endometrium analysis of recurrences and the potential benefit of staging lymphadenectomy. *Gynecol. Oncol.* 1992;44:17-23.

[8] Benedetti Panici, PL; Scambia, G; Baiocchi, G; Greggi, S; Mancuso, S. Technique and feasibility of radical para-aortic and pelvic lymphadenectomy for gynecologic malignancies: a prospective study. *Int. J. Gynecol. Cancer* 1991;1:133-40.

[9] McMeekin, DS; Lashbrook, D; Gold, M; Scribner, DR; Kamelle, S; Tillmanns, TD; et al. Nodal distribution and its significance in FIGO stage IIIc endometrial cancer. *Gynecol. Oncol.* 2001;82:375-9.

[10] Mariani, A; Dowdy, SC; Cliby, WA; Haddock, MG; Keeney, GL; Lesnick, TG; et al. Efficacy of systematic lymphadenectomy and adjuvant radiotherapy in node-positive endometrial cancer patients. *Gynecol. Oncol.* 2006;101:200-8.
[11] Mariani, A; Dowdy, SC; Cliby, WA; Gostout, BS; Jones, MB; Wilson, TO; et al. Prospective assessment of lymphatic dissemination in endometrial cancer: a paradigm shift in surgical staging. *Gynecol. Oncol.* 2008;109:11-8.
[12] Klopp, AH; Jhingran, A; Ramondetta, L; Lu, K; Gershenson, DM; Eifel, PJ. Node-positive adenocarcinoma of the endometrium: outcome and patterns of recurrence with and without external beam irradiation. *Gynecol. Oncol.* 2009;115:6-11.
[13] Hoekstra, AV; Kim, RJ; Small, W Jr; Rademaker, AW; Helenowski, IB; Singh, DK; et al. FIGO stage IIIC endometrial carcinoma: prognostic factors and outcomes. *Gynecol. Oncol.* 2009;114:273-8.
[14] Sharma, C; Deutsch, I; Lewin, SN; Burke, WM; Qiao, Y; Sun, X; et al. Lymphadenectomy influences the utilization of adjuvant radiation treatment for endometrial cancer. *Am. J. Obstet. Gynecol.* 2011;205:562.e1-9Todo, Y; Kato, H; Kaneuchi, M; Watari, H; Takeda, M; Sakuragi, N. Survival effect of para-aortic lymphadenectomy in endometrial cancer (SEPAL study): a retrospective cohort analysis. *Lancet* 2010;375:1165-72.
[15] Creutzberg, CL; van Putten, WL; Koper, PC; Lybeert, ML; Jobsen, JJ; Wárlám-Rodenhuis, CC; et al. Surgery and postoperative radiotherapy versus surgery alone for patients with stage-1 endometrial carcinoma: multicentre randomised trial. PORTEC Study Group. Post Operative Radiation Therapy in Endometrial Carcinoma. *Lancet* 2000;355:1404-11.
[16] Nout, RA; Smit, VT; Putter, H; Jürgenliemk-Schulz, IM; Jobsen, JJ; Lutgens, LC; et al; PORTEC Study Group. Vaginal brachytherapy versus pelvic external beam radiotherapy for patients with endometrial cancer of high-intermediate risk (PORTEC-2): an open-label, non-inferiority, randomised trial. *Lancet* 2010;375:816-23.
[17] Keys, HM; Roberts, JA; Brunetto, VL; Zaino, RJ; Spirtos, NM; Bloss, JD; et al; Gynecologic Oncology Group. A phase III trial of surgery with or without adjunctive external pelvic radiation therapy in intermediate risk endometrial adenocarcinoma: a Gynecologic Oncology Group study. *Gynecol. Oncol.* 2004;92:744-51.
[18] Benedetti Panici, P; Basile, S; Maneschi, F; Lissoni, A; Signorelli, M; Scambia, G; et al. Systematic pelvic lymphadenectomy vs. no lymphadenectomy in early-stage endometrial carcinoma: randomized clinical trial. *J. Natl. Cancer Inst.* 2008;100: 1707-16.
[19] ASTEC study group; Kitchener, H; Swart, AM; Qian, Q; Amos, C; Parmar, MK. Efficacy of systematic pelvic lymphadenectomy in endometrial cancer (MRC ASTEC trial): a randomised study. *Lancet* 2009;373:125-36.
[20] Cragun, JM; Havrilesky, LJ; Calingaert, B; Synan, I; Secord, AA; Soper, JT; et al. Retrospective analysis of selective lymphadenectomy in apparent early-stage endometrial cancer. *J. Clin. Oncol.* 2005;23:3668-75.
[21] Hiura, M; Nogawa, T; Matsumoto, T; Yokoyama, T; Shiroyama, Y; Wroblewski, J. Long-term survival in patients with para-aortic lymph node metastasis with systematic retroperitoneal lymphadenectomy followed by adjuvant chemotherapy in endometrial carcinoma. *Int. J. Gynecol. Cancer* 2010;20:1000-5.

[22] Veronesi, U; Paganelli, G; Viale, G; Luini, A; Zurrida, S; Galimberti, V; et al. A randomized comparison of sentinel-node biopsy with routine axillary dissection in breast cancer. *N. Engl. J. Med.* 2003;349:546-53.

[23] Estourgie, SH; Nieweg, OE; Valdes Olmos, RA; Hoefnagel, CA; Kroon, BB. Review and evaluation of sentinel node procedures in 250 melanoma patients with a median follow-up of 6 years. *Ann. Surg. Oncol.* 2003;10:681-8.

[24] Makar, AP; Scheistroen, M; van den Weyngaert, D; Trope, CG. Surgical management of stage I and II vulvar cancer: the role of the sentinel node biopsy. Review of literature. *Int. J. Gynecol. Cancer* 2001;11:255-62.

[25] Van der Zee, AG; Oonk, MH; De Hullu, JA; Ansink, AC; Vergote, I; Verheijen, RH; et al. Sentinel node dissection is safe in the treatment of early-stage vulvar cancer. *J. Clin. Oncol.* 2008;26:884-9.

[26] Dargent, D; Martin, X; Mathevet, P. Laparoscopic assessment of the sentinel lymph node in early stage cervical cancer. *Gynecol. Oncol.* 2000;79:411-5.

[27] Burke, TW; Levenback, C; Tornos, C; Morris, M; Wharton, JT; Gershenson, DM. Intraabdominal lymphatic mapping to direct selective pelvic and paraaortic lymphadenectomy in women with high-risk endometrial cancer: results of a pilot study. *Gynecol. Oncol.* 1996;62:169-73.

[28] FIGO news. Corpus cancer staging. *Int J Gynecol Obstet* 1989;28: 190.

[29] Raspagliesi, F; Ditto, A; Kusamura, S; Fontanelli, R; Vecchione, F; Maccauro, M; et al. Hysteroscopic injection of tracers in sentinel node detection of endometrial cancer: a feasibility study. *Am. J. Obstet. Gynecol.* 2004;191:435-9.

[30] Khoury-Collado, F; Murray, MP; Hensley, ML; Sonoda, Y; Alektiar, KM; Levine, DA; et al. Sentinel lymph node mapping for endometrial cancer improves the detection of metastatic disease to regional lymph nodes. *Gynecol. Oncol.* 2011;122:251-4.

[31] Ballester, M; Dubernard, G; Lécuru, F; Heitz, D; Mathevet, P; Marret, H; et al. Detection rate and diagnostic accuracy of sentinel-node biopsy in early stage endometrial cancer: a prospective multicentre study (SENTI-ENDO). *Lancet Oncol.* 2011;12:469-76.

[32] Selvaggi, L; Cormio, G; Ceci, O; Loverro, G; Cazzolla, A; Bettocchi, S. Hysteroscopy does not increase the risk of microscopic extrauterine spread in endometrial carcinoma. *Int. J. Gynecol. Cancer* 2003;13:223-7.

[33] Kasamatsu, T; Onda, T; Katsumata, N; Sawada, M; Yamada, T; Tsunematsu, R; et al. Prognostic significance of positive peritoneal cytology in endometrial carcinoma confined to the uterus. *Br. J. Cancer* 2003;88:245-50.

In: Endometrial Cancer: Prevention, Diagnosis and Treatment ISBN: 978-1-62257-740-8
Editor: Stefano Greggi

Chapter VIIIb

The Problem of Lymphadenectomy: Contra

Pierluigi Benedetti Panici[1,*], Violante Di Donato[1], Stefano Basile[2], Filippo Bellati[1], Angela Musella[1], Assunta Casorelli[1], Giorgia Perniola[1], Innocenza Palaia[1], Claudia Marchetti[1], Giovanna Salerno[2]

[1]Gynecology and Obstetrics, "Sapienza" University, Rome, Italy
[2]Obstetrics and Gynecology, "Santa Chiara" Hospital, Pisa, Italy

Abstract

Endometrial cancer treatment includes peritoneal cytology, total hysterectomy, bilateral salpingo-oophorectomy. However, there is no general consensus on the surgical approach to endometrial cancer and therefore surgical practice varies widely around the world. Lymph node status still remains difficult to be assessed pre-operatively and intra-operatively with the highest level of accuracy. Currently, the role of lymphadenectomy is completely recognized with a staging aim, but its possible therapeutic role remains a particularly debated issue. For this reason, performing lymphadenectomy in all women affected by endometrial cancer seems to burden complications rate, without a substantial survival benefit. Clinical evidence takes us to recommend lymphadenectomy in high risk patients only when the real risk of nodal spread justifies the morbidity of the procedure (particular histotypes, suspected advanced disease), but its therapeutic role has not been demonstrated. In the future the oncologic community may develop the use of accurate molecular markers to preoperatively select patients to undergo complete lymphadenectomy. However, to better define all the unsolved questions, high quality scientific evidence in endometrial cancer clinico-surgical management is mandatory.

[*] E-mail address: pierluigi.benedettipanici@uniroma1.it

Endometrial cancer (EC) is surgically staged since the International Federation of Gynecologic and Obstetrics (FIGO) established it in 1988 [1]. This decision was supported by the findings of a large prospective surgical-pathologic study of patients with clinical stage I and II EC performed by the Gynecologic Oncology Group (GOG) [2]. The International Federation of Gynecology and Obstetrics (FIGO) published in May 2009 the new staging system for EC [3]. Compared to the 1988 criteria, the new classification introduces the following changes: 1) former stage IA and IB have been combined; 2) past stage IIA has been eliminated, so that only cervical stroma involvement is considered stage II disease; 3) positive peritoneal cytology for EC is no longer considered a condition for disease upstaging (although FIGO still recommends the collection of peritoneal washings, recognizing the predictive value of positive cytological findings when combined with other poor-prognosis factors); 4) stage IIIC has been divided into IIIC1 and IIIC2 in accordance with the absence or presence of positive para-aortic nodes respectively. Therefore histotype, depth of myometrial invasion, site and extent of extra-uterine spread of disease were all fundamental criteria for staging according to the FIGO system.

Surgical treatment for EC includes peritoneal cytology, total hysterectomy, bilateral salpingo-oophorectomy.

Traditional indication to pelvic lymphadenectomy associated or not with aortic node dissection is related to some parameters: non-endometrioid histotype, poorly differentiated carcinoma, more than half myometrial involvement, extra-uterine spread of disease. In patients with non-endometrioid cancer, omentectomy, appendectomy and peritoneal biopsies are indicated.

Concerning pelvic lymphadenectomy, lymph nodal assessment in all cases leads to a low rate of patients with positive lymph nodes (about 9%). Conversely, selection of high-risk patients and performance of systematic nodal dissection in both pelvic and para-aortic areas allow the identification of nodal metastases in 22% of cases, thus sparing unnecessary surgical procedures in 27% of cases. Overall, 67% of patients with lymphatic dissemination have para-aortic lymph node metastases, with 16% having isolated nodal disease confined to the para-aortic area [4].

Lymphatic involvement represents the main way of endometrial cancer spread and it is associated with tumor histotype, myometrial invasion, cancer grading, extra-uterine spread of disease (in particular adnexal involvement), and therefore stage of disease. Traditional staging for EC requires the assessment of pelvic and aortic lymph nodes. Lymphadenectomy provides for an accurate staging and prognosis, therefore may indicate postoperative treatments in high risk patients [4].

In 1987 GOG 33 study [2] reported the rate of pelvic and aortic nodal metastases among patients at clinical early stage disease. Patients with no myometrial invasion and/or any grade of disease or grade 1 tumors involving less than the outer third of the myometrium had the lowest rate of pelvic nodal metastases (0-3%). Nodal dissection in these patients is, therefore, extremely unlikely to produce any benefit, while it increases the risk of surgical complications. More recently, some investigators reported that patients with endometrioid grade 1 or 2 disease and superficial myometrial invasion have no risk of lymphatic metastases if tumor diameter is 2 cm or less [4]. On the other hand, patients demonstrating myometrial invasion to the outer third had the highest rate of pelvic node metastases (11-34%). The reported risk of lymph nodal metastases in early stage disease ranges from 5% for low risk patients (grade IA or IB tumors) to 20% for high risk patients. According to some authors, high risk patients would constitute about 20% of patients with apparent early stage of disease.

The extent of lymphadenectomy in order to perform an accurate surgical staging remains a debated topic, with unsolved questions about nodal stations most frequently involved and the optimal number of nodes to resect. Concerning aortic lymphadenectomy, a topic particularly debated is the level of aortic nodal resection: aortic bifurcation, inferior mesenteric artery or up to renal vessels. Lymphadenectomy is accomplished by several risks. Median operative time is significantly higher when lymphadenectomy is performed in addition to the standard total hysterectomy and bilateral salpingo-oophorectomy, with intra-operative and post-operative complications occurring more frequently [5,6]. Moreover, patients with EC are often elderly, obese and medically unfit, making wise limiting surgical risks as possible. As most women present low risk early stage disease, the probability of lymph node involvement in these cases is generally considered quite low (5-10%), making ten to twenty full staging procedures necessary to diagnose a single case of nodal metastasis. On this background many authors recommend systematic lymphadenectomy only in selected high risk patients, when the significant risks of positive lymph nodes justifies the morbidity associated with the procedure.

To date, the role of lymphadenectomy is completely recognized with a staging aim, but its possible therapeutic role remains a particularly debated issue.

In fact, even though nodal status is considered an important prognostic factor [4], there is no evidence from randomized clinical trials (RCTs) that lymph nodal dissection increases survival in patients affected by clinical early stage disease [5,6].

However, an apparent therapeutic role of lymphadenectomy is suggested for high risk patients by some retrospective analyses [5-8].

In 2008 a multicenter Italian group investigated in a large randomized trial the role of pelvic lymphadenectomy in clinical early stage EC. The study took in consideration all clinical stage I EC with the exception of patients at lowest risk (intraoperative pathological assessment showing a well differentiated tumor with concomitant depth of myometrial invasion less than 50%). Five hundred and fourteen patients were randomized: 264 patients were assigned to systematic pelvic lymphadenectomy arm and 250 to no lymphadenectomy (or removal of grossly bulky nodes) arm. The median number of pelvic lymph nodes removed was 26 (range 21-35) in the pelvic lymphadenectomy arm. Pelvic systematic lymphadenectomy improved surgical staging: patients with lymph node metastases resulted statistically higher in lymphadenectomy arm than in no-lymphadenectomy one (13.3% vs. 3.2% $p<0.001$). However, no significant differences were found in terms of overall survival and disease-free survival between lymphadenectomy (OS: 81%, DFS: 85.9%) and no lymphadenectomy (OS: 81.7%, DFS: 90%) arm. Moreover, operative time was significantly higher among women undergoing lymphadenectomy and both early and late post-operative complications occurred significantly more frequently in patients submitted to systematic pelvic lymphadenectomy (12.1% vs. 4.8% for early complications and 18.6% vs. 8.8% for late complications) [5]. Most of the difference in morbidity was due to lymphocysts and lymphedema that occurred in 35 (13.3%) patients in the lymphadenectomy arm and four (1.6%) patients in the no-lymphadenectomy arm. Deep venous thrombosis occurred in four patients (1.6%) (two in each arm), and pulmonary embolism occurred in two patients (0.8%) undergoing lymphadenectomy. Two cases (0.8%) of bladder-vaginal fistula occurred in the lymphadenectomy arm, and bowel obstruction occurred in four patients (1.6%) in each arm. No surgical procedure-related deaths occurred.

Similar results in terms of survival were successively obtained also in ASTEC trial, conducted on 1408 women affected by clinical stage I endometrial carcinoma [6]. Also in this trial no significant differences were found in terms of overall survival and disease free survival between lymphadenectomy (OS: 80%, DFS: 73%) and standard surgical procedure (OS: 81%, DFS: 79%) arm. The median length of operation was 50% longer when lymphadenectomy was performed. The risk of developing short-term major surgical complications was generally low in both groups but more women in the lymphadenectomy group than in standard surgery group suffered from some specific complications, such as ileus (3% vs. 1%), deep vein thrombosis (1% vs. 0.1%), lymphocyst (1% vs. 0.3%) and the major wound dehiscence (1% vs. 0.3%).

There were no statistically significant differences in the use of adjuvant treatment, with no further treatment administered to 69% in the lymphadenectomy arm and 65% in the no lymphadenectomy arm. Although not statistically significantly different, type of adjuvant treatment differed slightly between the two arms, with more chemotherapy and less radiation therapy being used in the surgically staged patients. Lymphadenectomy seems to maintain its importance in determining patient's prognosis and tailoring adjuvant therapy [9].

Moreover, a more recent Cochrane meta-analysis resuming the results of these two multicenter trials has confirmed the lack of benefits in survival by pelvic lymphadenectomy in patients with preoperative stage I EC [10].

The major criticism moved to these RCTs was the lack of systematic para-aortic lymphadenectomy and the inclusion of low-intermediate risk patients in the trials. The rate of nodal metastases reported by lymphadenectomy (9-13%) in the RCTs [5,6] was substantially similar to that found in retrospective series [4,11]. In the Italian trial, after complete pelvic lymphadenectomy surgeons selected the patients (majority of whom had grade 3 tumor or bulky or suspected/positive pelvic or aortic lymph nodes) who should receive aortic lymphadenectomy (26%) [5]. Also the rate of isolated aortic and pelvic plus aortic metastases (2.8% and 7.2%) was in keeping with literature data (2.8% and 6.7%, respectively) [4].

After the publication of the two RCTs a large retrospective study (SEPAL) was reported [11]. This study compared a series of patients affected by endometrial cancer from a Japanese hospital, where para-aortic lymph node dissection was routinely performed, with a series of patients from another nearby hospital where it was not performed. This study reported the limitations and the intrinsic bias related to a retrospective analyses: demography of para-aortic group appeared to be younger than expected, para-aortic lymphadenectomy series had a higher proportion of women who received adjuvant chemotherapy compared to other series, who in turn where more likely to receive adjuvant radiotherapy. SEPAL study reported that overall survival was significantly longer in patients who received both pelvic and para-aortic lymphadenectomy. This difference was confirmed in the sub analysis including intermediate/high risk patients, whereas the type of lymphadenectomy was not related to survival in low risk patients. Although retrospective, the SEPAL study suggests that high-risk patients may benefit from a more aggressive surgery, including systematic lymphadenectomy extended to the para-aortic area.

According to GOG 33 study [2] patients with aortic lymph nodal involvement had at least one of the following characteristics: bulky pelvic lymph nodes, macroscopic adnexal metastases or a grade 3 tumor with outer myometrial involvement. As already stated, in our opinion all this features could be assessed intraoperatively and para-ortic lymphadenectomy avoided when these features are absent.

Furthermore lymphadenectomy failed in reducing nodal recurrence (lymphadenectomy arm: 1.5% vs. no lymphadenectomy arm: 1.6%), as well as to impact the natural history of disease: similar hematogenous (5.2% vs. 5.6%) and peritoneal recurrences by implants (5.6% vs. 5.2%) [5].

For all the above mentioned reasons, performing lymphadenectomy in all women affected by EC seems to burden complications rate, without a substantial survival benefit.

Since lymph nodal status represents an adverse prognostic factor while nodal dissection does not improve survival, we can speculate that the prognosis in patients with nodal involvement is unfavorable whatever lymphadenectomy is performed or not.

Clinical evidence takes us to recommend lymphadenectomy in high risk patients only when the real risk of nodal spread justifies the morbidity of the procedure (particular histotypes, suspected advanced disease), but its therapeutic role has not been demonstrated.

To date, lymphadenectomy can be performed with the aim of an accurate retroperitoneal staging. So, where are we now? Is it worth to allow the complications associated with the procedure only for staging purpose ?

Does the very low rate of skip aortic metastases (1-2%) justify systematic pelvic and aortic lymphadenectomy in all patients?

Nodal status is scarcely assessed in a pre-operative setting, also considering that about 40% of nodal metastases are < 2 mm in diameter.

Unfortunately we still lack of preoperative imaging techniques having an optimal accuracy in assessing nodal status, therefore allowing surgeons to remove only supposed positive nodes [12]. Several studies have been performed in order to investigate the sensitivity and specificity of magnetic resonance imaging (MRI), computed tomography (CT) and positron emission tomography (PET)/CT in nodal involvement detection in oncologic patients, however a gold standard imaging technique is not available yet.

Concerning MRI, in literature is reported a sensitivity rate of 30-64.3%, and a specificity rate of 69-93%. On the other side for CT scan is reported a sensitivity of 35-43% and a specificity rate of 65-97%, but above all for PET/CT scan are reported rates of sensitivity and specificity of 30-100% and 83-99%, respectively in assessing nodal metastasis.

Some studies have analyzed the use of sentinel lymph node procedure in breast and vulvar cancer. Similarly in endometrial cancer some authors reported that the sentinel node detection rate ranges from 77% to 94%, depending on user skills, with false negative rate decreasing with higher user experience [13]. Nowadays, sentinel node (SN) procedure in EC is still debated and further studies are needed to define its role and efficacy in endometrial carcinoma [14].

In the future the oncologic community may develop the use of accurate molecular markers to predict the metastatic potential of endometrial cancer, with the aim of preoperatively select patients to undergo complete lymphadenectomy. Several biomolecular factors have been investigated in basic research assays in last decades. However, further studies are needed to better define their role in predicting nodal metastases accurately and making possible to identify new tailored therapies. There are established risks associated with lymphadenectomy, but these risks seem to decrease in skilled hands. In future postoperative targeted treatments could improve patients survival without unnecessary exposure to radiation and/or chemotherapy.

In conclusion, there is no general consensus on the surgical approach to EC and therefore surgical practice varies widely around the world. Lymph node status still remains difficult to be assessed pre-operatively and intra-operatively with the highest level of accuracy. The goal would be to detect preoperatively lymph node metastases but, to date, we can do it only by intraoperative histological assessment, with a limited level of accuracy. To better define all the unsolved questions, high quality scientific evidence in EC clinico-surgical management is mandatory.

References

[1] Kichener, H; Jones, HW III; Bertelsen, K; et al. Cancer of the corpus uteri. In: Pecorelli, S; at al. *Staging Classification and Clinical Practice Guidelines for Gynecological Cancers*. Amsterdam: Elsevier; 2000.

[2] Creasman, WT; Morrow, CP; Bundy, BN; et al. Surgical pathologic spread patterns of endometrial cancer. A Gynecologic Oncology Group Study. *Cancer* 1987;60(8 Suppl):2035-41.

[3] Lewin, SN. Revised FIGO staging system for endometrial cancer. *Clin Obstet Gynecol* 2011;54:215-8.

[4] Mariani, A; Dowdy, SC; Cliby, WA. Prospective assessment of lymphatic dissemination in endometrial cancer: a paradigm shift in surgical staging. *Gynecol Oncol* 2008;109:11-8.

[5] Benedetti Panici, P; Basile, S; Maneschi, F; et al. Systematic lymphadenectomy vs. no lymphadenectomy in early-stage endometrial carcinoma: randomized clinical trial. *J Natl Cancer Inst* 2008;100:11707-16.

[6] Kichener, H; Swart, AM; Qian, Q; et al. Efficacy of systematic pelvic lymphadenectomy in endometrial cancer (MRC ASTEC trail): a randomised study. *Lancet* 2009;373:125-36.

[7] Chan, JK; Cheung, MK; Huh, WK; et al. Therapeuthic role of lymph node resection in endometrioid corpus cancer:a study of 12;333 patients. *Cancer* 2006;107:1823-30.

[8] Smith, DC; Macdonald, OK; Lee, CM; et al. Survival impact of lymph node dissection in endometrial adenocarcinoma: a surveillance; epidemiology; and end results analysis. *Int J Gynecol Cancer* 2008;18:255-61.

[9] Walsh, CS; Karlan, BY. Lymphadenectomy's role in early endometrial cancer: prognostic or therapeutic? *J Natl Cancer Inst* 2008;100:1660-1.

[10] May, K; Bryant, A; Dickinson, HO; et al. Lymphadenectomy for the management of endometrial cancer (review). *Cochrane Database Syst Rev* 2010;1:CD007585.

[11] Todo, Y; Kato, H; Kaneuchi, M. Survival effect of para-aortic lymphadenectomy in endometrial cancer (SEPAL study): a retrospective cohort analysis. *Lancet* 2010;375:1165-72.

[12] Kitchener, HC. Sentinel node biopsy in endometrial cancer: a win scenario? *Lancet Oncology* 2011;12:413-4.

[13] Ballester, M; Dubernard, G; Rouzier, R; et al. Use of the sentinel node procedure to stage endometrial cancer. *Ann Surg Oncol* 2008;15:1523-9.

[14] Ballester, M; Dubernard, G; Lecuru F; al. Detection rate and diagnostic accuracy of sentinel-node biopsy in early stage endometrial cancer: a prospective multicentre study (SENTI-ENDO). *Lancet Oncology* 2011;12:469-76.

In: Endometrial Cancer: Prevention, Diagnosis and Treatment ISBN: 978-1-62257-740-8
Editor: Stefano Greggi

Chapter IX

Surgical Staging and Disease-Based Postoperative Treatment: The Mayo Clinic Experience

Shikha Sarangi and Andrea Mariani*
Gynecologic Oncology,
Mayo Clinic, Rochester,
MN, US

Abstract

Endometrial cancer is the sixth most common malignancy among females worldwide and the most common cancer of the female genital tract.

Although surgical staging with hysterectomy and bilateral salpingo-oophorectomy is considered the main treatment of endometrial cancer, there is controversy regarding the need of performing lymphadenectomy.

In this chapter we discuss the need and extent of lymphadenectomy, based on the Mayo Clinic experience.

Also, in contrast to the traditional modality-based approach for postoperative treatment, we discuss our Mayo Clinic approach, characterized by disease-based individualized treatment.

Introduction

In this chapter we will discuss our experience at the Mayo Clinic, Rochester, Minnesota, in treating endometrial carcinoma (EC), with special emphasis on the role of surgical staging and postoperative disease-based adjuvant therapy.

---

* E-mail address: sarangi.shikha@mayo.edu.

Pathways of Spread

Endometrial carcinoma has 4 pathways of spread which can be present alone or in combination: (1) contiguous (mainly to the vagina); (2) lymphatic; (3) hematogenous; and (4) peritoneal.

In an unselected population of 915 patients (without history of other malignancies) who received treatment of EC at Mayo Clinic, Rochester, Minnesota, over a 13-year period, the rate of relapse was 5%, 9%, 6%, and 6% through these four dissemination pathways, respectively.

Vaginal

Histologic grade 3 and lymphovascular space invasion are proven predictors of vaginal relapse in stage I EC [1]. The addition of vaginal brachytherapy to the initial surgical treatment can significantly reduce the risk of such recurrence [2].

Hematogenous

Deep myometrial invasion (> 50% for all stages and > 66% for stage I) is the strongest predictor of hematogenous recurrence [3].

Table 1. Rates of recurrence at 5 years according to the different risk categories for 915 patients (Mariani A. et al.) [3]

Risk Category	Recurrence rate at 5 years
Hematogenous	
All stages	
Myometrial invasion ≤ 50%	4%
Myometrial invasion > 50%	28%
Stage I (negative lymph nodes)	
Myometrial invasion < 66%	2%
Myometrial invasion ≥ 66%	34%
Lymphatic	
No risk factors	2%
Cervical stromal invasion and/or positive lymph nodes	31%
Peritoneal	
Stage IV disease	63%
Stage II-III disease and ≥ 2 risk factors [a]	21%
Stage I-III disease and ≤ 1 risk factor [a]	1%
Overall [b]	
Not at risk [c]	2%
At risk [c]	46%

a: cervical stromal invasion, nonendometrioid histologic subtype, positive lymph nodes, positive result on peritoneal cytologic evaluation;

b: excluding vaginal recurrences;

c: for at least 1 of the 3 categories of recurrence (i.e., hematogenous, lymphatic, or peritoneal).

Lymphatic

Lymphatic spread is more likely to occur when cervical stromal involvement and positive lymph nodes are present [3].

Peritoneal

Predictors of peritoneal relapse are: 1) stage IV disease, or 2) stage II-III disease with 2 or more of the following risk factors: cervical invasion, peritoneal cytologic results positive for EC, positive lymph nodes, and non endometrioid histologic findings (Table 1) [3].

Patterns of Lymphatic Spread

Systematic pelvic and para-aortic lymphadenectomy is not only one of the most important steps to assess the presence of extra-uterine spread of disease, but also for guiding targeted postoperative treatment. Patients with endometrioid grade 1 or 2 disease and superficial myometrial invasion have a probability close to 0% of lymphatic metastases when tumor diameter is 2 cm or less (Table 2) [4].

Therefore, it is possible to identify a group of patients in which lymphadenectomy is likely to increase the risk of surgical complications without producing any benefit.

Table 2. Patients at low risk for lymph node metastasis (i.e., myometrial invasion < 50%, grade 1-2, endometrioid histologic subtype, or no macroscopic tumor outside the uterine corpus) - Stratification in accordance with tumor diameter and pelvic lymph node metastases (Mariani et al.) [4]

Pelvic Lymph Node Metastases			
Tumor Diameter (cm)	Patients (No.)	Pelvic Lymphadenectomy (No.)	Positive Pelvic Lymph Nodes (No.)
≤ 2	123	59	0
> 2	169	107	8

Overall, 67% of patients with lymphatic dissemination have para-aortic lymph node metastases, with 16% having isolated nodal disease confined to the para-aortic area (Table 3). Moreover, 60% of patients with nodal involvement above the inferior mesenteric artery have negative homolateral infra-mesenteric para-aortic nodes [5].

Table 3. The frequency of observed endometrial cancer metastases to the pelvic or para-aortic node bearing region, or both, in patients with lymphatic dissemination who have had a systematic pelvic and para-aortic lymphadenectomy (Mariani A et al.) [5]

Node Site Positive for Metastasis	Nodes (N=57)	
	Positive (No.)	Positive (%)
Pelvic region only	19	33%
Pelvic plus para-aortic regions	29	51%
Para-aortic region only	9	16%

These above findings suggest that when nodal dissection is considered necessary in the treatment of an EC patient, it should involve the para-aortic area up to the level of the renal vessels. Selection of at-risk patients, with use of the criteria given in Table 4, and performance of systematic nodal dissection in both pelvic and para-aortic areas allow the identification of nodal metastases in 22% of cases, sparing unnecessary surgical procedures in 27% of cases [5].

Treatment

Surgical staging has been recommended since 1988. But performing pelvic and para-aortic lymphadenectomy in all patients has not been universally accepted. Our current protocol for surgical management of endometrial cancer at Mayo Clinic includes surgical staging peritoneal cytology, hysterectomy and bilateral salpingo-oophorectomy. Whether to perform lymphadenectomy or not is decided by tumor diameter, myometrial invasion and histologic grade and subtype (determined by frozen section) and the evidence of extrauterine disease (Table 4) [6].

Table 4. Surgical guidelines for the treatment of endometrial cancer at Mayo Clinic, Rochester, Minnesota (2004-2008) (Mariani et al.) [6]

Treatment: Hysterectomy, Bilateral Salpingo-oophorectomy, Peritoneal Cytologic Evaluation, and Bilateral Pelvic and Para-aortic Lymphadenectomy up to the Renal Vessels
1. Can omit lymphadenectomy if: (A) all of the following: no myometrial invasion, endometrioid, and no evidence of tumor outside the corpus (independent of grade or tumor diameter) (B) all of the following: endometrioid, grade 1 or 2 tumor, myometrial invasion $< 50\%$, tumor diameter ≤ 2 cm, and no evidence of tumor outside the corpus
2. If no endometrioid (serous, clear cells), add complete omentectomy, appendectomy, and peritoneal biopsies (i.e., 11 pairs of cul-de-sac, bladder peritoneum, R diaphragm, R/L colic gutters, R/L pelvic sidewall, small-/large-bowel serosa and mesentery, and any suspicious area)

Disease-Based Adjuvant Therapy

Adjuvant therapy has traditionally been modality based, which is external radiotherapy supplemented with vaginal brachytherapy. The optimal treatment approach should minimize overtreatment by identifying patients not requiring lymphadenectomy, radiotherapy or chemotherapy and minimize undertreatment by identifying those patients who will benefit from lymphadenectomy or radiation or chemotherapy or a combination of these modalities. At Mayo Clinic, we have introduced the concept of disease-based individualized treatment.

In patients with adequate surgical staging, in general, we suggest:

- external beam radiotherapy for preventing lymphatic recurrences in the pelvic and para-aortic areas, in patients with documented lymphatic dissemination;
- vaginal brachytherapy in patients at risk of vaginal recurrence (Table 1) [1];

- chemotherapy in presence of risk factors for hematogenous recurrences (Table 1);
- the administration of chemotherapy for the prevention of abdominal recurrences based on the results of the GOG 122 study [7] and on our finding of extra-abdominal recurrences in 43% of patients with abdominal failure (Table 1) [8].

Considering the 1988 FIGO staging classification, patients with stage IIIA and with one or more risk factors (Table 5) are at risk for distant extra-abdominal recurrence and may benefit from systemic chemotherapy.

Table 5. Prognostic subgroups in patients with stage IIIA endometrial cancer (Mariani et al.) [9]

	Stage IIIA1 Low Risk	Stage IIIA1 High Risk	Stage IIIA2
Characteristics	Positive peritoneal cytology (as the only sign of extra-uterine disease)	Positive peritoneal cytology (as the only sign of extra-uterine disease)	Positive adnexae, Uterine serosal invasion (± Positive peritoneal cytology)
Histo-pathologic Characteristics	No Risk Factors *	At least one risk factor *	

* lympho-vascular invasion, myometrial invasion ≥ 50%, non-endometrioid histologic subtype, histologic grade 3, cervical invasion.

Moreover, in stage IIIC, we can identify subsets of patients. Those who have lymphatic metastasis as the only site of extrauterine disease are at risk of lymphatic failure, whereas those with other associated sites of extrauterine disease (i.e., adnexal, vaginal or cervical invasion, positive peritoneal cytology, uterine serosal involvement) are more likely to recur in extra-nodal sites (Table 6) [10].

Table 6. Recurrences according to stage IIIC subsets (Mariani et al.) [10]

Stage Subset	N	Recurrences Total Extranodal
$IIIC^{0}$	22	7 (32%) 1 (5%) [a] *p=0.04 p<0.01*
$IIIC^{ab}$	24	16 (67%) 9 (41%) [b]
Totals	46	23 (50%) 10 (23%) [b]

$IIIC^{0}$: lymph node metastases only.

$IIIC^{ab}$: lymph node metastases plus peritoneal cytologic and/or vaginal and/or uterine serosa and/or adnexal involvement.

Therefore, the subset of patients in stage IIIC with extrauterine disease limited to the lymph nodes will potentially benefit from external radiotherapy only, whereas the subset with other sites of extrauterine disease will potentially benefit from the addition of systemic chemotherapy.

Conclusion

Due to the recognized limitations of the prospective randomized trials on lymphadenectomy in endometrial cancer [18,19], at this point, there is no widely accepted evidence in literature about whether to avoid lymphadenectomy and treat patients based on uterine risk factors only [20], or to perform lymphadenectomy and offer targeted postoperative treatment [3]. A new randomized controlled trial is needed to reach a consensus. In our opinion, the trial should include only patients at high risk of lymphatic metastasis; it should also have an in-built quality control of lymph node dissection and extent of surgery.

Finally, it should analyze (as primary or secondary outcomes) the overall and cancer-specific survival, healthcare cost, quality of life, sites of recurrence and treatment related morbidity. Sentinel lymph node procedure may be an ancillary part of the prospective trial as well [21].

References

[1] Mariani, A; Dowdy, SC; Keeney, GL; Haddock, MG; Lesnick, TG; Podratz, KC. Predictors of vaginal relapse in stage I endometrial cancer. *Gynecol. Oncol.* 2005;97:820-7.

[2] Elliott, P; Green, D; Coates, A; Krieger, M; Russell, P; Coppleson, M; et al. The efficacy of postoperative irradiation in preventing vaginal recurrence in endometrial cancer. *Int. J. Gynecol. Cancer* 1994;4:84-93.

[3] Mariani, A; Dowdy, SC; Keeney, GL; Long, HJ; Lesnick, TG; Podratz, KC. High-risk endometrial cancer subgroups: candidates for target-based adjuvant therapy. *Gynecol. Oncol.* 2004;95:120-6.

[4] Mariani, A; Webb, MJ; Keeney, GL; Haddock, MG; Calori, G; Podratz, KC. Low-risk corpus cancer: is lymphadenectomy or radiotherapy necessary? *Am. J. Obstet. Gynecol.* 2000;182:1506-19.

[5] Mariani, A; Dowdy, SC; Cliby, WA; Gostout, BS; Jones, MB; Wilson, TO; et al. Prospective assessment of lymphatic dissemination in endometrial cancer: a paradigm shift in surgical staging. *Gynecol. Oncol.* 2008;109:11-8.

[6] Mariani, A; Keeney, GL; Aletti, G; Webb, MJ; Haddock, MG; Podratz, KC. Endometrial carcinoma: paraaortic dissemination. *Gynecol. Oncol.* 2004;92:833-8.

[7] Randall, ME; Filiaci, VL; Muss, H; Spirtos, NM; Mannel, RS; Fowler, J; et al; Gynecologic Oncology Group Study. Randomized phase III trial of whole-abdominal irradiation versus doxorubicin and cisplatin chemotherapy in advanced endometrial carcinoma: a Gynecologic Oncology Group Study. *J. Clin. Oncol.* 2006;24:36-44.

[8] Mariani, A; Webb, MJ; Keeney, GL; Aletti, G; Podratz, KC. Endometrial cancer: predictors of peritoneal failure. *Gynecol. Oncol.* 2003;89:236-42.

[9] Mariani, A; Webb, MJ; Keeney, GL; Aletti, G; Podratz, KC. Assessment of prognostic factors in stage IIIA endometrial cancer. *Gynecol. Oncol.* 2002;86:38-44.

[10] Mariani, A; Webb, MJ; Keeney, GL; Lesnick, TG; Podratz, KC. Surgical stage I endometrial cancer: predictors of distant failure and death. *Gynecol. Oncol.* 2002;87:274-80.

[11] Mariani, A; Dowdy, SC; Keeney, GL; Long, HJ; Lesnick, TG; Podratz, KC. High-risk endometrial cancer subgroups: candidates for target-based adjuvant therapy. *Gynecol. Oncol.* 2004;95:120-6.

[12] Mariani, A; Dowdy, SC; Cliby, WA; Haddock, MG; Keeney, GL; Lesnick, TG; et al. Efficacy of systematic lymphadenectomy and adjuvant radiotherapy in node-positive endometrial cancer patients. *Gynecol. Oncol.* 2006;101:200-8.

[13] Mariani, A; Webb, MJ; Keeney, GL; Aletti, G; Podratz, KC. Predictors of lymphatic failure in endometrial cancer. *Gynecol. Oncol.* 2002;84:437-42.

[14] Mariani, A; Webb, MJ; Galli, L; Podratz, KC. Potential therapeutic role of para-aortic lymphadenectomy in node-positive endometrial cancer. *Gynecol. Oncol.* 2000;76: 348-56.

[15] Mariani, A; Webb, MJ; Keeney, GL; Calori, G; Podratz, KC. Hematogenous dissemination in corpus cancer. *Gynecol. Oncol.* 2001;80:233-8.

[16] Podratz, KC; Mariani, A; Webb, MJ. Staging and therapeutic value of lymphadenectomy in endometrial cancer. *Gynecol .Oncol.* 1998;70:163-4.

[17] Creutzberg, CL; van Putten, WL; Wárlám-Rodenhuis, CC; van den Bergh, AC; de Winter, KA; Koper, PC; et al. Outcome of high-risk stage IC, grade 3, compared with stage I endometrial carcinoma patients: the Postoperative Radiation Therapy in Endometrial Carcinoma Trial. *J. Clin. Oncol.* 2004;22:1234-41.

[18] Uccella, S; Podratz, KC; Aletti, GD; Mariani, A. Lymphadenectomy in endometrial cancer. *Lancet* 2009;373:1170-1.

[19] Uccella, S; Podratz, KC; Aletti, GD; Mariani, A. Re: Systematic pelvic lymphadenectomy vs no lymphadenectomy in early-stage endometrial carcinoma: randomized clinical trial. *J .Natl. Cancer Inst.* 2009;101:897-8.

[20] Creutzberg, CL; van Putten, WL; Koper, PC; Lybeert, ML; Jobsen, JJ; Warlam-Rodenhuis, CC; et al; PORTEC Study Group. Surgery and postoperative radiotherapy versus surgery alone for patients with stage-1 endometrial carcinoma: multicentre randomised trial. *Lancet* 2000;355:1404-11.

[21] Kitchener, HC. Sentinel-node biopsy in endometrial cancer: a win-win scenario? *Lancet Oncol.* 2011;12:413-4.

In: Endometrial Cancer: Prevention, Diagnosis and Treatment ISBN: 978-1-62257-740-8
Editor: Stefano Greggi

Chapter X

Conservative Treatment of Early Disease: A Literature Review

Stefano Greggi*[*]*, Giuseppe Laurelli and Cono Scaffa
Gynecologic Oncology, National Cancer Institute "G. Pascale,"
Naples, Italy

Abstract

Approximately one fourth **of** women with endometrial cancer are diagnosed in fertile age. Nevertheless, the current standard of surgical approach is preclusive of fertility. Primary progestin therapy, sometimes combined with local surgical excision, has been used as conservative treatment in early well differentiated tumors. The worldwide experience and data, however, are still limited due to the small number of cases, potential methodological bias, and the use of different therapeutic regimes. In our experience, we have tested the feasibility and efficacy of combined operative hysteroscopy and hormone therapy as fertility-preserving treatment in a cohort of selected young women with FIGO stage IA (intramucous) well differentiated endometrial cancer (n=14). Treatment consisted of hysteroscopic ablation of the lesion and the myometrial tissue below, followed by oral megestrol acetate for 6 months or levonorgestrel-medicated intrauterine device for 12 months. With a median follow-up of 46 months, one patient recurred after 5 months from operative hysteroscopy and underwent definitive surgery, one patient showed an endometrial hyperplasia without atypia at the 3 and 6 month hysteroscopy control, with negative controls thereafter; three patients have attempted to conceive and one of them conceived and term delivered a healthy baby. A systematic review of the literature data published in the last twenty years on patients with endometrial cancer conservatively treated with fertility-sparing aims is reported. Twenty-eight papers on clinical series (n=347) and 7 unfavorable case reports are shown. By means of different strategies (hormonal therapy ± hysteroscopic resection) and using different drugs, a mean of 72% complete response was obtained, with a 23% relapse rate (only 4 disease-related deaths due to recurrence in the abdomen or distance site). So far, combined approach of operative hysteroscopy and hormonal therapy has been used only in very limited group of

[*] E-mail address: s.greggi@istitutotumori.na.it.

patients: of 20 cases treated, only one has relapsed (5%), compared to a mean of 24% following exclusive medical treatment reported in our review; although limited by a comparison not methodologically correct, it may be argued that operative hysteroscopy is of benefit in terms of cure. Twenty-eight percent of complete responders subsequently conceived with or without assisted reproduction technology, while the pregnancy rates ranging from 32% to 100% in patients attempting to conceive.

Introduction

Endometrial cancer is the most frequent gynecological malignancy. Twenty-five percent of endometrial cancer are diagnosed in premenopausal women and almost 5% in women up to 40 years aged with a history of estrogen- or hormone-related disorders, such as ovarian dysfunction, chronic anovulation, infertility, obesity, and polycystic ovary syndrome [1-6].

When arising in young women, endometrial cancer usually presents with favorable prognostic features, that is, as a focal, well differentiated lesion, with minimal or absent myometrial invasion [3,7]. This profile corresponds to the type 1 endometrial cancer, which correlates with the estrogen/progesterone receptor positive (ER+/PR+) pattern [8]. Primary progestin therapy has been demonstrated to be effective in early well differentiated tumors and in poor operative candidates with response rates ranging from 58-100% [9].

Currently, the therapeutic approach to an early stage endometrial cancer consists of a staging laparotomy/laparoscopy, including a total abdominal hysterectomy and bilateral salpingo-oophorectomy (TAH-BSO), peritoneal washings, and lymphadenectomy (pelvic and aortic), depending on the pathological risk profile pre- and intraoperatively determined [10,11]. Therefore, the current standard of surgical approach is preclusive of fertility. So far, conservative management has been experimented anedoctically or in very small series of selected young patients with early endometrial cancer [12-20]. Progestin therapies, mostly medroxyprogesterone acetate (MPA) and megestrol acetate (MA) [7], sometimes combined with local surgical excision by hysteroscopy or repeated dilation and curettage, have been used as conservative treatments.

Data on conservative treatment are, therefore, still limited due to the small numbers of cases, potential methodological bias, and the use of different therapeutic regimes. This chapter reports our experience and a systematic review of the literature data. Such a review may be of help for better understanding the critical issues of conservative approach in endometrial cancer.

Our Experience

Subjects and Methods

We evaluated the outcome of a cohort of young women with clinically diagnosed early endometrial cancer who were selected for fertility preservation, and treated by combined hysteroscopic resection and oral MA or levonorgestrel-medicated intrauterine device (LNG-IUD). Fourteen endometrial cancer patients aged up to 40 years who desired childbearing and/or retaining their fertility were enrolled into a prospective pilot study to assess the outcome of investigational fertility-preserving treatment at the Gynecological Oncology Department, National Cancer Institute in Naples.

Selection criteria were considered in a two-step procedure: a) screening phase: age up to 40 years; histologically proven well differentiated endometrioid endometrial cancer; absence of radiologic evidence of myometrial/cervical invasion, pelvic/aortic lymph node involvement, and/or ovarian tumors; normal (< 35 IU/ml) CA125 serum levels; strong desire to preserve fertility and complete the follow-up program; (oncology and fertility) counseling and informed consent; b) enrollment phase: histological confirmation of well differentiated endometrioid ER+/PR+ (by either ligand binding or immunohistochemistry) endometrial cancer; absence of hysteroscopic evidence of myometrial/cervical invasion. Further exclusion criteria were: history of previous/concomitant cancer (except for adequately treated skin basal cell or in situ cervical cancer); patient belonging to a family with hereditary non-polyposis colorectal cancer (HNPCC, Lynch II syndrome); multifocal endometrial cancer; synchronous ovarian cancer at magnetic resonance imaging (MRI) or laparoscopy; contraindications for progestin treatment or IUD insertion.

The screening clinical workup consisted of: general and gynecological examinations; diagnostic hysteroscopy with endometrial biopsy (if not yet performed or in case of unclear findings) (4-mm telescope with a 30° forward oblique lens and 5-mm diagnostic sheath; illumination by a high-intensity cold light source via a fiber-optic cable, and all procedures monitored by a video camera; hysteroscope inserted under direct vision with no cervical dilation; uterine cavity distended with carbon dioxide (CO_2) using a hystero-insufflator: 35 ml/min flow rate, pressure < 90 mmHg); chest-X-ray; transvaginal ultrasound (TVUS); abdomen-pelvis MRI; serum CA125.

Those patients fitting all the screening criteria, underwent the subsequent procedures: operative hysteroscopy under general anesthesia (cervix dilated to 10-mm with Hegar's dilator, introduction of a 10-mm resectoscope with 0° lens; uterine distension with 1.5% glycine solution under gravity inflow of 70 mmHg pressure; irrigant fluid collection in 3 liters graduated cylinders and monitored carefully; a 5-mm cutting loop electrode and 100 W of pure cutting output power were used to resect the endometrial lesion and a small layer of the myometrium below) [21, 22]. Patients were enrolled only in case of pathologically confirmed no evidence of myometrial invasion. Due to a higher incidence of synchronous ovarian tumors in endometrial cancer patients under 45 year old compared to older patients (10-29% vs. 2-5%) [23, 24], a diagnostic laparoscopy was incorporated (following the hysteroscopy) in the enrollment workup [25, 26] of the last 8 patients.

One week after operative hysteroscopy, the first 6 patients received oral MA (160 mg/day) for 6 months, while to the subsequent 8 patients a 52 mg LNG-IUD was inserted, and removed after 12 months. Three months after starting oral MA medication or LNG-IUD insertion, patients entered the follow-up phase undergoing gynecological examination, serum CA125, and hysteroscopy with multiple endometrial biopsies three-monthly for one year; an abdomen-pelvis computerized tomography (CT) scan was performed after the first 6 months. After 12 months, patients still in complete remission wishing pregnancy are encouraged to conceive (with or without assisted reproduction technology, ART). In the second year of the follow-up program, the non-pregnant patients were submitted to gynecological examination, TVUS, serum CA125 every 3 months, hysteroscopy with endometrial biopsies and abdomen-pelvis CT scan every 6 months. In the following 3-5 years, the patients underwent gynecological examination, TVUS, serum CA125 every 6 months. In case of conception, pregnant patients were followed through a routine obstetrical schedule, with a follow-up visit three months after term of pregnancy. Patients showing no response to progestin therapy underwent standard surgery (TAH-BSO, peritoneal washings). Women who failed in their attempt to conceive or who successfully completed childbearing, were encouraged to undergo definitive surgery.

Median follow-up time is 46 months (range 19-85).

Results

Fourteen patients with FIGO Stage IA (intramucous) well differentiated endometrioid ER+/PR+ endometrial cancer (median age 38 years, range 26-40; median body mass index, BMI, 26 Kg/m^2, range 23-53) were enrolled into the study. Three patients (21%) showed a BMI > 30 (Table 1). In particular, the endometrial tumor diameter was ≤ 2 cm in 12 cases (86%) and about 3 cm in the remaining two. The tumor site was the corpus in all cases, of which 3 (21%) close to the tubaric angle. Most patients (11, 79%) were nulligravidae, with a history of infertility in two (14%). Three (31%) have had one baby, wishing further pregnancies and/or to preserve their fertility. While all patients underwent oncologic counseling, only 7 (50%), although referred to, underwent fertility counseling.

The first 6 patients (43%) received oral MA (160 mg/day) for 6 months, while to the subsequent 8 patients (57%) a 52 mg LNG-IUD was inserted, and removed after 12 months.

No perioperative complications occurred. The first 6 patients were treated on a day-surgery basis, while the last 8 (additional laparoscopy) with a median hospital stay of 2 days (range 2-3). Hormonal therapies were well tolerated with no cases of treatment interruption. The patients compliance to follow-up was good with the hysteroscopy missed in only 3 out of the total 56 (5%) planned controls.

After a minimum 19 month follow-up (median 46, range 19-85), local recurrence has been detected in one patient (7%) (LNG-IUD group) 5 months from hysteroscopic treatment. The patient underwent definitive surgery (TAH-BSO, peritoneal washings) with evidence of a FIGO Stage IA (intramucous). Further, endometrial hyperplasia without atypia was diagnosed in one patient (7%) (MA group) at the 3 and 6-month hysteroscopy, with negative controls thereafter following 2 further months of therapy. Endometrial cancer relapse (BMI 53 Kg/m^2) and hyperplasia (BMI 31 Kg/m^2) were only seen in two of the three obese patients (Table 1). Three patients (two from MA group, one from LNG-IUD group) have attempted to conceive without ART. One of them conceived and term delivered an healthy baby 14 month from the end of follow-up. All patients, including those showing local recurrence and undergoing definitive surgery, have no evidence of disease (NED) at the moment (Table 1).

Review of the Literature

During the last years, conservative management has been more frequently proposed, based on the excellent prognosis of early stage well differentiated endometrioid endometrial cancer and the high response of type 1 endometrial cancer to progestin therapies.

Table 1. Conservative treatment of early endometrial cancer: clinical findings and follow-up of 14 patients with endometrial cancer (FIGO stage IA, intramucous; ER+/PR+) treated with combined hysteroscopic resection and hormone therapy

Case	Age *years*	BMI Kg/m^2	Histotype/ Grade	Hormone Therapy	Relapse (Months)	Pregnancy	Follow-up *months*	Current Status
1	40	24	E / G1	MA	No	No	85	NED
2	39	25	E / G1	MA	No	No	83	NED
3	38	26	E / G1	MA	No	No	74	NED
4	36	27	E / G1	MA	No	NFTD	68	NED
5	37	31	E / G1	MA	No $_a$	No	62	NED
6	38	25	E / G1	MA	No	No	56	NED
7	37	23	E / G1	LNG-IUD	No	No	49	NED
8	39	28	E / G1	LNG-IUD	No	No	43	NED
9	39	26	E / G1	LNG-IUD	No	No	36	NED
10	39	48	E / G1	LNG-IUD	No	No	34	NED
11	37	23	E / G1	LNG-IUD	No	No	32	NED
12	40	24	E / G1	LNG-IUD	No	No	25	NED
13	28	53	E / G1	LNG-IUD	Yes (5)	No $_b$	23	NED
14	26	27	E / G1	LNG-IUD	No	No	19	NED

Legend. BMI: body mass index; E: endometrioid; ER+/PR+: estrogen/progesterone receptor positive; G1: well differentiated; LNG-IUD: 52mg levonorgestrel-intrauterine device for 12 months; MA: megestrol acetate 160 mg/day for 6 months; NED: no evidence of disease; NFTD: normal full time delivery.

Notes. a: endometrial hyperplasia without atypia; b: submitted to definitive surgery.

Based on literature reviews published in the early 2000s, the outcomes of such management in early stage patients seem to be similar to that of conventional therapy with no impact on survival [17,27].

A systematic literature review has been performed using MEDLINE to identify all clinical series (prospective and retrospective) published over the last two decades (between January 1992 and December 2011) involving endometrial cancer patients conservatively treated with fertility-sparing aims. Case reports and studies not having the specific aim of preservation of fertility were excluded. Some case reports, however, have been included because of reporting unfavorable outcomes not otherwise described (including one case report on conservative treatment of atypical endometrial hyperplasia).

Therefore, 28 papers on clinical series (n=347) are shown in Table 2 [4,12-14,16, 17,22,28-49] and 7 case reports are shown in Table 3 [50-56]. By means of different strategies (hormonal therapy ± hysteroscopic resection) and using different drugs (bromocriptine, gonadotropin-releasing hormone, levonorgestrel, megestrol, medroxyprogesterone, norethisterone, oral contraceptive, hydroxyprogesterone, progesterone, tamoxifen), on average, a 72% complete response was obtained (18-100). Among complete responders, a relapse developed in 23% of cases (0-67) and a pregnancy was achieved in 28% (0-100) (Tables 2,3).

Our study [43,44] includes the largest series of invasive endometrial cancer treated by combined hysteroscopy and progestin therapy published thus far in the English literature. Moreover, the long median follow-up period (46 months) makes our results reliable. Only one patient (7%) recurred 5 months from the endoscopic treatment and was submitted to definitive surgery without evidence of disease progression. One further patient showed endometrial hyperplasia without atypia, at 3 and 6 months, likely persistent after hysteroscopy, which was reverted to a normal histology by oral progestin therapy at the 9-month control. There were no high-grade and/or non-endometrioid tumors missed on the screening endometrial biopsies compared with the final pathology (hysteroscopic specimens). Such accuracy of pathological assessment can be explained by the selection of cases both in terms of hormone-receptor status (100% ER+/PR+), and tumor dimension (86% < 2 cm). Moreover, clinical staging based on pelvic MRI was accurate in terms of myometrial involvement, with no cases of myoinvasion detected by hysteroscopy. Transvaginal ultrasound, when in expert hands, shows comparable results to those of MRI in detecting myometrial infiltration [57], and the combined use of it with MRI has been suggested. Regardless of MRI / TVUS diagnostic accuracy, however, the presence of a well differentiated tumor significantly predicts an intramucous stage of disease [23]. Therefore, in the light of the considerations above, the hysteroscopic resection including the myometrium under lesion may be considered redundant, but, it is, however, the most accurate procedure to define histology and myometrial involvement; thus, we believe reasonable to incorporate it into such an experimental treatment protocol.

Operative hysteroscopy can be considered not only diagnostic but also therapeutic in treating an endometrial lesion, compared to the conventional approach consisting of blunt endometrial curettage only followed by hormonal therapy. So far, results from a combined approach of operative hysteroscopy and hormone-therapy have been published only by Mazzon et al. [22] and by our group [43]. Of 20 patients treated, only one patient has relapsed (5%), compared to a mean of 24% following exclusive medical treatment reported in our

Table 2. Conservative treatment of early endometrial cancer: 1992-2011 clinical series with fertility-sparing aims (n=347)

Author, Year [Ref.]	**n**	**Study Type**	**Age** *years*	**Histotype /Grade**	**Hysteroscopic Resection**	**Hormone Therapy**	**Complete Response** *n*	**Relapse** *n*	**DOD** *n*	**Patients who conceived** *n*	**Mean Follow-up** *months*
Kim, 1997 [12]	7	Retro	19-41	E / G1	no	MA	4 (57%)	2 (50%)	-	-	13
Randall, 1997 [13]	14	Retro	20-33	E / G1	no	MA ± TAM / MAP / OC / B	9 (64%)	1 (11%)	-	2 (22%)	40
Sardi, 1998 [28]	4	Retro	29-35	E / G1	no	MPA	3 (75%)	-	-	2 (67%)	36
Imai, 2001 [29]	15	Retro	< 40	vv / G1-2	no	MPA	8 (53%)	3 (38%)	-	2 (25%)	59
Kaku, 2001 [14]	12	Retro	21-40	E / G1	no	MPA	9 (75%)	2 (22%)	-	2 (22%)	31
Wang, 2002 [16]	9	Pro	30-39	E / G1	no	MA ± TAM	8 (89%)	4 (50%)	-	4 (50%)	69
Gotlieb, 2003 [17]	13	Retro	23-40	vv / G1-2	no	MA / MPA / HOPC / NETA	13 (100%)	5 (38%)	-	4 (31%)	82
Lowe, 2003 [30]	2	Retro	27-38	E / G1	no	MA	2 (100%)	-	-	2 (100%)	40-96 (range)
Niwa, 2005 [31]	12	Retro	23-34	E / G1	no	MPA	12 (100%)	8 (67%)	-	7 (58%)	56
Ota, 2005 [4]	12	Retro	22-40	E / G1	no	MPA	5 (42%)	2 (40%)	1	4 (80%)	53
Yang, 2005 [32]	6	Pro	27-39	E / G1	no	MA	4 (67%)	2 (50%)	-	2 (50%)	49
Minaguchi, 2007 [33]	19	Retro	19-37	E / G1	no	MPA	15 (79%)	3 (20%)	-	3 (20%)	41
Ushijima, 2007 [34]	22	Pro	32 (mean)	n/r / G1	no	MPA	14 (64%)	8 (57%)	-	4 (34%)	48
Yamazawa, 2007 [35]	9	Pro	28-40	E / G1	no	MPA	7 (78%)	2 (29%)	-	4 (57%)	39

Table 2. (Continued)

Author, Year [Ref.]	n	Study Type	Age years	Histotype /Grade	Hysteroscopic Resection	Hormone Therapy	Complete Response n	Relapse n	DOD n	Patients who conceived n	Mean Follow-up months
Eftekhar, 2009 [36]	21	Pro	21-45	E / G1	no	MA	18 (86%)	3 (17%)	-	5 (28%)	48
Hahn, 2009 [37]	35	Retro	21-43	E / G1	no	MA / MPA	22 (63%)	9 (41%)	-	10 (45%)	39
Han, 2009 [38]	7	Retro	27-35	E / G1-2	no	MA / MPA	6 (86%)	-	-	6 (100%)	38-75 (range)
Signorelli, 2009 [39]	11	Pro	< 40	n/r / G1	no	P	2 [a] (18%)	-	-	4 [a] (36%)	≥ 36
Yu, 2009 [40]	8	Retro	25 (mean)	E / G1	no	MA / MPA / HOPC	5 (63%)	1 (20%)	-	-	32
Cade, 2010 [41]	16	Retro	23-53	n/r / n/r	no	MA and/or LNG-IUD	10 (63%)	-	-	3 (30%)	27
Mao, 2010 [42]	6	Retro	26-31	E / G1-3	no	MA / MPA	4 (67%)	-	-	3 (75%)	51
Mazzon, 2010 [22]	6	Pro	26-38	E / G1	yes	MA	6 (100%)	-	-	4 (67%)	51
Laurelli, 2011 [43,44]	14	Pro	26-40	E / G1	yes	MA / LNG-IUD	14 (100%)	1 (7%)	-	1 (7%)	46
Kim, 2011 [45]	5	Pro	33-41	n/r / G1	no	MPA plus LNG-IUD	4 (80%)	-	-	-	10
Minig, 2011 [46]	14	Pro	22-40 [b]	E / G1	no	GnRH plus LNG-IUD	8 (57%)	2 (25%)	-	1 (13%)	29 [b]
Park, 2011 [47]	14	Retro	21-38	E / G1	no	MA / MPA	13 (93%)	4 (31%)	-	4 (31%)	47
Perri, 2011 [48]	27	Retro	24-43	E / G1	no	MA / MPA / HOPC / NETA ± LNG-IUD	24 (89%)	15 (62%)	-	14 (58%)	57
Shirali, 2011 [49] [c]	16	Pro	24-42	E / G1	no	MA	10 (63%)	-	-	4 (40%)	n/r

Legend. B: bromocriptine; E: endometrioid; G1: well differentiated; GnRH: gonadotropin-releasing hormone; LNG-IUD: levonorgestrel-intrauterine device; MA: megestrol acetate; MPA: medroxyprogesterone acetate; NETA: norethisterone acetate; n/r: not reported; OC: oral contraceptive; OHPC: hydroxyprogesterone caproate; P: progesteron; Pro: prospective; Retro: retrospective; TAM: tamoxifen; vv: various.

Notes. a: patients were encouraged to attempt to conceive immediately after start of treatment, regardless of response; b: including cases with atypical endometrial hyperplasia; c: 9 patients already included in the Eftekhar series

Table 3. Conservative treatment of early endometrial cancer: 1992-2011 case reports about unfavorable outcomes

Author, Year [Ref.]	Age *years*	Histotype / Grade	Hysteroscopic Resection	Hormone Therapy	Initial Complete Response	Relapse Months	Site of Relapse	Status
Yasuda, 2004 [50]	31	AEH	no	MPA	yes	36	Peritoneal carcinomatosis	DOD
Ferrandina, 2005 [51]	38	E / G1	no	DHD	yes	20	Endometrium, cervix, ovaries peritoneum, omentum, liver, lungs, lymph nodes, bones	DOD
Huang, 2005 [52]	36	E / G1	no	1. MA; 2. TAM + LA	no	5	1. Endometrium; 2. Ovary	n/r
Cormio, 2006 [53]	31	E / G1	no	MA	yes	24	1. Endometrium; 2. Pelvis; 3. Brain, choroid, lung	DOD
Hurst, 2008 [54]	31	E / G1	no	MA	yes	48	Endometrium	NED
Kothari, 2008 [55]	24	E / G2	no	MA + LNG-IUD	yes	27	1. Endometrium; 2. Peritoneum	NED
Vandenput, 2009 [56]	25	E / G1	no	LNG-IUD	yes	19	Endometrium	NED

Legend. AEH: atypical endometrial hyperplasia; DHD: dihydrogesterone; DOD: died of disease; E: endometrioid; G1: well differentiated; LA: leuprolide acetate; LNG-IUD: levonorgestrel-intrauterine device; MA: megestrol acetate; MPA: medroxyprogesterone acetate; NED: no evidence of disease; n/r: not reported; TAM: tamoxifen.

review (Tables 2,3). Although such a comparison is not methodologically correct, it may be argued that operative hysteroscopy is of benefit in terms of cure.

In the our series, the only recurrent endometrial cancer occurred in one of the three obese patients enrolled. Patients with endometrial cancer are obese in a remarkable proportion of cases, particularly in a subset of young patients. Duska et al. reported a 48% obese among 95 < 40 year old endometrial cancer patients retrospectively collected [23]. When reported, overweight (≥ 25 or ≥ 30 BMI) is in fact present in about one third of cases enrolled into conservative management protocols (43/136, 32%) [4,14,22,23,31,32,36,42,45-47,58]. This is consistent with the disease pattern usually seen in younger patients with a more favorable prognostic profile (type 1 endometrial cancer). Nevertheless, obesity, which is part of the endometrial cancer-related metabolic syndrome, remains a significant risk factor of endometrial transformation even after primary treatment. Based on those series in which relapse and BMI are analyzed, approximately 50% of obese patients recur [14,22,23,31,32,43,44].

Only four disease-related deaths have been so far reported following conservative treatment [4,50,51,53]. In spite of initial response, these fatal relapses occurred in the abdomen or distance site (Tables 2,3). A critical analysis of the case reports reveals, however, that PR status was negative or not assessed in two patients while in a third p53 was highly expressed despite PR positive status. Moreover, it is to be noticed that extrauterine relapses (adnexal, peritoneal) have been reported in further three cases [36,52,55], even without a fatal outcome (Tables 2,3): one case presenting with PR negative status [52] and two cases with moderately-poorly differentiated tumor, besides refusing definitive surgery in the presence of disease persistence / relapse [36,55].

Delayed definitive surgery is usually suggested at childbearing completion further than in non-responding and recurrent patients. In this respect, it is noticeable three cases of residual carcinoma was found in the surgical specimens of three patients undergoing definitive surgery 6, 8 and 22 months after delivery [19].

In the first cases of our series, we administered a MA-based hormonal therapy, while more recently LNG-IUD was adopted. Based on our review, MA with MPA represent the drugs mainly used showing an overall complete response rate of 42-100% and recurrence rates of 0-67% (Table 2). LNG-IUD showed higher concentrations of progestin to the uterine mucosa compared to oral MA, and superior results in endometrial hyperplasia compared with oral MA [59,60]. Moreover, LNG-IUD proved to be effective in early endometrial cancer with complete histological remission in 33-100% of cases [15,41,43,44]. The optimal hormonal therapy, however, is not yet defined both in terms of progestin used and dosage, and treatment duration.

In our series, 3 patients attempted to conceive and one (33%) successfully conceived without ART use and term delivered an healthy baby. The low pregnancy rate is explained first by the low proportion of conception attempt among our patients. This seems to be related to the strong desire to preserve their fertility rather than to childbearing, and this is why only 50% of them underwent a proper fertility counseling. In our literature review, a mean of 28% of complete responders (0-100%) subsequently conceived with or without ART (Table 2), while the pregnancy rates ranging from 32% to 100% in patients attempting to conceive [4,7,15,22,31,34,35,42].

In conclusion, in young patients, the evaluation of the fertility-sparing options should always be extensively discussed in the light of a standard definitive procedure. A fertility-sparing approach is still to be considered experimental and offered in the framework of scientific protocols conducted in cancer centers. The gynecological oncologist and gynecological pathologist expertise is, in fact, crucial to ensure the correct decision making process within a complex algorithm for fertility preservation.

In our experience, conservative combined operative hysteroscopy and progestin therapy showed to have a role for the safe and effective management of early endometrial cancer in selected patients wishing to preserve fertility.

References

[1] Gallup, DG; Stock, RJ. Adenocarcinoma of the endometrium in women 40 years of age and younger. *Obstet Gynecol* 1984;64:417.

[2] Sherman, ME. Theories of endometrial carcinogenesis: a multidisciplinary approach. *Mod Pathol* 2001;13:295-308.

[3] Benshushan, A. Endometrial adenocarcinoma in young patients: evaluation and fertility-preserving treatment. *Eur J Obstet Gynecol Reprod Biol* 2004;117:132-7.

[4] Ota, T; Yoshida, M; Kimura, M; Kinoshita, K. Clinicopathologic study of uterine endometrial carcinoma in young women aged 40 years and younger. *Int J Gynecol Cancer* 2005;15:657-62.

[5] Rackow, BW; Arici, A. Endometrial cancer and fertility. *Curr Opin Obstet Gynecol* 2006;18:245-52.

[6] Creasman, WT; Odicino, F; Maisonneuve, P; Quinn, MA; Beller, U; Benedet, JL; et al. Carcinoma of the corpus uteri. *Int J Gynaecol. Obstet* 2006;95(Suppl1):S105-43.

[7] Ramirez, PT; Frumovitz, M; Bodurka, DC; Sun, CC; Levenback, C. Hormonal therapy for the management of grade 1 endometrial adenocarcinoma: a literature review. *Gynecol Oncol* 2004;95:133-8.

[8] Ehrlich, CE; Young, PC; Stehman, FB; Sutton, GP; Alford, WM. Steroid receptors and clinical outcome in patients with adenocarcinoma of the endometrium. *Am J Obstet Gynecol* 1988;158:796-807.

[9] American College of Obstetricians and Gynecologists. ACOG practice bulletin, clinical management guidelines for obstetrician-gynecologists: management of endometrial cancer. *Obstet Gynecol* 2005;106:413-25.

[10] Gadducci, A; Cosio, S; Genazzani, AR. Treatment planning in endometrial cancer. *Cancer Therapy* 2003;1:373-91.

[11] Leitao, MM. Current and future surgical approaches in the management of endometrial carcinoma. *Future Oncol* 2008;4:389-401.

[12] Kim, YB; Holschneider, CH; Ghosh, K; Nieberg, RK; Montz, FJ. Progestin alone as primary treatment of endometrial carcinoma in premenopausal women. Report of seven cases and review of the literature. *Cancer* 1997;79:320-7.

[13] Randall, TC; Kurman, RJ. Progestin treatment of atypical hyperplasia and well-differentiated carcinoma of the endometrium in women under age 40. *Obstet Gynecol* 1997;90:434-40.

[14] Kaku, T; Yoshikawa, H; Tsuda, H; Sakamoto, A; Fukunaga, M; Kuwabara, Y; et al. Conservative therapy for adenocarcinoma and atypical endometrial hyperplasia of the

endometrium in young women: central pathologic review and treatment outcome. *Cancer Lett* 2001;167:39-48.

[15] Montz, FJ; Bristow, RE; Bovicelli, A; Tomacruz, R; Kurman, RJ. Intrauterine progesterone treatment of early endometrial cancer. *Am J Obstet Gynecol* 2002;186:651-7.

[16] Wang, CB; Wang, CJ; Huang, HJ; Hsueh, S; Chou, HH; Soong, YK; et al. Fertility-preserving treatment in young patients with endometrial adenocarcinoma. *Cancer* 2002;94:2192-8.

[17] Gotlieb, WH; Beiner, ME; Shalmon, B; Korach, Y; Segal, Y; Zmira, N; et al. Outcome of fertility-sparing treatment with progestins in young patients with endometrial cancer. *Obstet Gynecol* 2003;102:718-25.

[18] Yahata, T; Fujita, K; Aoki, Y; Tanaka, K. Long-term conservative therapy for endometrial adenocarcinoma in young women. *Hum Reprod* 2006;21:1070-5.

[19] Chiva, L; Lapuente, F; González-Cortijo, L; Carballo, N; García, JF; Rojo, A; et al. Sparing fertility in young patients with endometrial cancer. *Gynecol Oncol* 2008;111(Suppl2):S101-4.

[20] Wu, HM; Lai, CH; Huang, HY; Soong, YK. A successful live twin birth by in vitro fertilization after conservative treatment of recurrent endometrial cancer. *Chang Gung Med J* 2008;31:102-6.

[21] Mazzon, I; Corrado, G; Morricone, D; Scambia, G. Reproductive preservation for treatment of stage IA endometrial cancer in a young woman: hysteroscopic resection. *Int J Gynecol Cancer* 2005;15:974-8.

[22] Mazzon, I; Corrado, G; Masciullo, V; Morricone, D; Ferrandina, G; Scambia, G. Conservative surgical management of stage IA endometrial carcinoma for fertility preservation. *Fertil Steril* 2010;93:1286-9.

[23] Duska, LR; Garrett, A; Rueda, BR; Haas, J; Chang, Y; Fuller, AF. Endometrial cancer in women 40 years old or younger. *Gynecol Oncol* 2001;83:388-93.

[24] Walsh, C; Holschneider, C; Hoang, Y; Tieu, K; Karlan, B; Cass, I. Coexisting ovarian malignancy in young women with endometrial cancer. *Obstet Gynecol* 2005;106:693-9.

[25] Morice, P; Fourchotte, V; Sideris, L; Gariel, C; Duvillard, P; Castaigne, D. A need for laparoscopic evaluation of patients with endometrial carcinoma selected for conservative treatment. *Gynecol Oncol* 2005;96:245-8.

[26] Shamshirsaz, AA; Withiam-Leitch, M; Odunsi, K; Baker, T; Frederick, PJ; Lele, S. Young patients with endometrial carcinoma selected for conservative treatment: a need for vigilance for synchronous ovarian carcinomas, case report and literature review. *Gynecol Oncol* 2007;104:757-60.

[27] Jadoul, P; Donnez, J. Conservative treatment may be beneficial for young women with atypical hyperplasia or endometrial adenocarcinoma. *Fertil Steril* 2003;80:1315-24.

[28] Sardi, J; Anchezar Henry, JP; Paniceres, G; Gomez Rueda, N; Vighi, S. Primary hormonal treatment for early endometrial carcinoma. *Eur J Gynaecol Oncol* 1998;19:565-8.

[29] Imai, M; Jobo, T; Sato, R; Kawaguchi, M; Kuramoto, H. Medroxyprogesterone acetate therapy for patients with adenocarcinoma of the endometrium who wish to preserve the uterus-usefulness and limitations. *Eur J Gynaecol Oncol* 2001;22:217-20.

[30] Lowe, MP; Cooper, BC; Sood, AK; Davis, WA; Syrop, CH; Sorosky, JI. Implementation of assisted reproductive technologies following conservative

management of FIGO grade I endometrial adenocarcinoma and/or complex hyperplasia with atypia. *Gynecol Oncol* 2003;91:569-72.

[31] Niwa, K; Tagami, K; Lian, Z; Onogi, K; Mori, H; Tamaya, T. Outcome of fertility-preserving treatment in young women with endometrial carcinomas. *BJOG* 2005;112:317-20.

[32] Yang, YC; Wu, CC; Chen, CP; Chang, CL; Wang, KL. Reevaluating the safety of fertility-sparing hormonal therapy for early endometrial cancer. *Gynecol Oncol* 2005;99:287-93.

[33] Minaguchi, T; Nakagawa, S; Takazawa, Y; Nei, T; Horie, K; Fujiwara, T; et al.Combined phospho-Akt and PTEN expressions associated with post-treatment hysterectomy after conservative progestin therapy in complex atypical hyperplasia and stage Ia, G1 adenocarcinoma of the endometrium. *Cancer Lett* 2007;248:112-22.

[34] Ushijima, K; Yahata, H; Yoshikawa, H; Konishi, I; Yasugi, T; Saito, T; et al. Multicenter phase II study of fertility-sparing treatment with medroxyprogesterone acetate for endometrial carcinoma and atypical hyperplasia in young women. *J Clin Oncol* 2007;25:2798-803.

[35] Yamazawa, K; Hirai, M; Fujito, A; Nishi, H; Terauchi, F; Ishikura, H; et al. Fertility-preserving treatment with progestin, and pathological criteria to predict responses, in young women with endometrial cancer. *Hum Reprod* 2007;22:1953-8.

[36] Eftekhar, Z; Izadi-Mood, N; Yarandi, F; Shojaei, H; Rezaei, Z; Mohagheghi, S. Efficacy of megestrol acetate (megace) in the treatment of patients with early endometrial adenocarcinoma: our experiences with 21 patients. *Int J Gynecol Cancer* 2009;19:249-52.

[37] Hahn, HS; Yoon, SG; Hong, JS; Hong, SR; Park, SJ; Lim, JY; et al. Conservative treatment with progestin and pregnancy outcomes in endometrial cancer. *Int J Gynecol Cancer* 2009;19:1068-73.

[38] Han AR; Kwon YS; Kim DY; Kim JH; Kim YM; Kim YT; et al. Pregnancy outcomes using assisted reproductive technology after fertility-preserving therapy in patients with endometrial adenocarcinoma or atypical complex hyperplasia. *Int J Gynecol Cancer* 2009;19:147-51.

[39] Signorelli M; Caspani G; Bonazzi C; Chiappa V; Perego P; Mangioni C. Fertility-sparing treatment in young women with endometrial cancer or atypical complex hyperplasia: a prospective single-institution experience of 21 cases. *BJOG* 2009;116:114-8.

[40] Yu M; Yang JX; Wu M; Lang JH; Huo Z; Shen K. Fertility-preserving treatment in young women with well-differentiated endometrial carcinoma and severe atypical hyperplasia of endometrium. *Fertil Steril* 2009;92:2122-4.

[41] Cade, TJ; Quinn, MA; Rome, RM; Neesham, D. Progestogen treatment options for early endometrial cancer. *BJOG* 2010;117:879-84

[42] Mao, Y; Wan, X; Chen, Y; Lv, W; Xie, X. Outcomes of conservative therapy for young women with early endometrial adenocarcinoma. *Fertil Steril* 2010;93:283-5.

[43] Laurelli, G; Di Vagno, G; Scaffa, C; Losito, S; Del Giudice, M; Greggi, S. Conservative treatment of early endometrial cancer: preliminary results of a pilot study. *Gynecol Oncol* 2011;120:43-6.

[44] Laurelli, G; Scaffa, C; Scala, F; Losito, NS; Del Giudice, M; Greggi, S. Conservative treatment of early endometrial cancer (EC). *Int J Gynecol Cancer* 2011;21:Suppl3.

[45] Kim, MK; Yoon, BS; Park, H; Seong, SJ; Chung, HH; Kim, JW; et al. Conservative treatment with medroxyprogesterone acetate plus levonorgestrel intrauterine system for early-stage endometrial cancer in young women: pilot study. *Int J Gynecol Cancer* 2011;21:673-7.

[46] Minig, L; Franchi, D; Boveri, S; Casadio, C; Bocciolone, L; Sideri, M. Progestin intrauterine device and GnRH analogue for uterus-sparing treatment of endometrial precancers and well-differentiated early endometrial carcinoma in young women. *Ann Oncol* 2011;22:643-9.

[47] Park, H; Seok, JM; Yoon, BS; Seong, SJ; Kim, JY; Shim, JY; et al. Effectiveness of high-dose progestin and long-term outcomes in young women with early-stage, well-differentiated endometrioid adenocarcinoma of uterine endometrium. *Arch Gynecol Obstet* 2011 Jun 25. [Epub ahead of print]

[48] Perri, T; Korach, J; Gotlieb, WH; Beiner, M; Meirow, D; Friedman, E; et al. Prolonged conservative treatment of endometrial cancer patients: more than 1 pregnancy can be achieved. *Int J Gynecol Cancer* 2011;21:72-8.

[49] Shirali, E; Yarandi, F; Eftekhar, Z; Shojaei, H; Khazaeipour, Z. Pregnancy outcome in patients with stage 1a endometrial adenocarcinoma, who conservatively treated with megestrol acetate. *Arch Gynecol Obstet* 2011 Jul 30. [Epub ahead of print]

[50] Yasuda, M; Matsui, N; Kajiwara, H; Yoshiyuki Osamura, R; Miyamoto, T; Murakami, M; et al. Malignant transformation of atypical endometrial hyperplasia after progesterone therapy showing germ-cell tumor-like differentiation. *Pathol Int* 2004;54:451-6.

[51] Ferrandina, G; Zannoni, GF; Gallotta, V; Fotia, E; Mancuso, S; Scambia, G. Progression of conservatively treated endometrial carcinoma after full term pregnancy: a case report. *Gynecol Oncol* 2005;99:215-7.

[52] Huang, SY; Jung, SM; Ng, KK; Chang, YC; Lai, CH. Ovarian metastasis in a nulliparous woman with endometrial adenocarcinoma failing conservative hormonal treatment. *Gynecol Oncol* 2005;97:652-5.

[53] Cormio, G; Martino, R; Loizzi, V; Resta, L; Selvaggi, L. A rare case of choroidal metastasis presented after conservative management of endometrial cancer. *Int J Gynecol Cancer* 2006;16:2044-8.

[54] Hurst, SA; Hartzfeld, KM; Del Priore, G. Occult myometrial recurrence after progesterone therapy to preserve fertility in a young patient with endometrial cancer. *Fertil Steril* 2008;89:724.e1-3.

[55] Kothari, R; Seamon, L; Cohn, D; Fowler, J; O'Malley, DM. Stage IV endometrial cancer after failed conservative management: a case report. *Gynecol Oncol* 2008;111:579-82.

[56] Vandenput, I; Van Eygen, K; Moerman, P; Vergote, I; Amant, F. Ineffective attempt to preserve fertility with a levonorgestrel-releasing intrauterine device in a young woman with endometrioid endometrial carcinoma: a case report and review of the literature. *Eur J Gynaecol Oncol* 2009;30:313-6.

[57] Savelli, L; Ceccarini, M; Ludovisi, M; Fruscella, E; De Iaco, PA; Salizzoni, E; et al. Preoperative local staging of endometrial cancer: transvaginal sonography vs magnetic resonance imaging. *Ultrasound Obstet Gynecol* 2008;31:560-6.

[58] Zivanovic, O; Carter, J; Kauff, ND; Barakat, RR. A review of the challenges faced in the conservative treatment of young women with endometrial carcinoma and risk of ovarian cancer. *Gynecol Oncol* 2009;115:504-9.

[59] Vereide, AB; Arnes, M; Straume, B; Maltau, JM; Ørbo, A. Nuclear morphometric changes and therapy monitoring in patients with endometrial hyperplasia: a study comparing effects of intrauterine levonorgestrel and systemic medroxyprogesterone. *Gynecol Oncol* 2003;91:526-33.

[60] Ørbo, A; Arnes, M; Hancke, C; Vereide, AB; Pettersen, I; Larsen, K. Treatment results of endometrial hyperplasia after prospective D-score classification A follow-up study comparing effect of LNG-IUD and oral progestins versus observation only. *Gynecol Oncol* 2008;111:68-73.

In: Endometrial Cancer: Prevention, Diagnosis and Treatment ISBN: 978-1-62257-740-8
Editor: Stefano Greggi

Chapter XI

The Role of Levonorgestrel-Releasing Intra-Uterine System in the Treatment of Endometrial Hyperplasia and Carcinoma: High Quality Evidence Is Still Lacking

***Fadi Alfhaily*[1*] *and Ayman A. Ewies*[2]**
[1]Obstetrics and Gynecology,
Colchester Hospital University NHS Foundation Trust, UK
[2]Gynecology, Sandwell and West Birmingham Hospitals NHS Trust, UK

Abstract

Endometrial hyperplasia is a commonly seen gynaecological condition that affects women of all age groups. Endometrial cancer is the most frequent gynaecological malignancy in Europe and North America with almost 75% of cases present in the early stage.

Currently, there are no professional body guidelines for the management of endometrial hyperplasia. Whereas, hysterectomy is the most preferred treatment option for atypical endometrial hyperplasia and carcinoma, there is no consensus regarding the first line management of women with hyperplasia without cytological atypia. Some recent reports documented that levonorgestrel-releasing intra-uterine system (LNG-IUS) has been successfully used to treat endometrial hyperplasia without cytological atypia, and selected cases of atypical endometrial hyperplasia and well-differentiated early stage endometrial carcinoma.

This chapter provides an up to date review of the studies that evaluated the use of LNG-IUS (Mirena®; Schering Health Care, Burgess Hill, UK), releasing 20 μg of LNG per day, in treating endometrial hyperplasia and carcinoma. We found that the published

* E-mail address: fadi.alfhaily@nhs.net.

literature is scarce of high quality evidence to reliably inform clinical practice in this area. Further, there is no evidence from randomized controlled trials that LNG-IUS prevents the development of endometrial hyperplasia or carcinoma in tamoxifen-treated women.

Introduction

Endometrial hyperplasia is diagnosed in 5-10% of women of all age groups presenting with abnormal uterine bleeding [1]. It was found that approximately 1-3% of simple and complex endometrial hyperplasia progress to carcinoma over 10 years and 8-29% of atypical hyperplasia progress to carcinoma over 4 years [2].Endometrial cancer is the most common gynaecological malignancy in Europe and North America, and is the seventh cause of death from cancer in women [3,4]. There were around 40,000 cases diagnosed in 2007 with almost 75% of them presenting with FIGO stage I disease [4].

Management options for endometrial hyperplasia depend on patient's age, desire for maintaining fertility, the histological type and surgical risks [5]. While hysterectomy is the preferred treatment option for atypical endometrial hyperplasia, there is no consensus regarding the initial management of women with endometrial hyperplasia without cytological atypia [6]. Non-surgical therapeutic strategies in endometrial hyperplasia aim to induce disease regression and prevent progression to cancer. These strategies, if successful, could reduce the number of hysterectomies performed for this condition and hence reduce morbidity and health care costs [7]. Currently, there are no professional body guidelines for the management of endometrial hyperplasia.

Endometrial hyperplasia and carcinoma often develop when the endometrium is continuously exposed to unopposed endogenous or exogenous estrogen, and it can be reversed by progestogen therapy. Progestogen has both indirect anti-estrogenic and direct anti-proliferative effects on the endometrium [8,9]. The main progestational agents used to treat endometrial hyperplasia were oral progestogens; norethisterone acetate, megestrol acetate, and medroxyprogesterone acetate [7]. More recently, the levonorgestrel-releasing intra-uterine system (LNG-IUS), developed primarily as a contraceptive device, has also been used to treat selected cases of endometrial hyperplasia and early stage endometrial carcinoma. This system has the advantage, over the conventional progestogen therapy, of the steady release of levonorgestrel (LNG), high endometrial concentration of the hormone and guaranteed patient's compliance [7]. LNG-IUS releases constant continuous dose of progestogen with endometrial concentrations up to 100 times higher than that of oral tablet containing 30 μg of LNG [10,11].

Pharmacokinetics of Levonorgestrel

LNG is a synthetic steroid (gestagen) that has potent progestational and androgenic effects but lacks estrogen-like activity [12]. Plasma LNG is bound mainly (64%) to sex hormone binding globulin (SHBG) to form a stable long-lived complex from which it dissociates slowly, whereas 35% is bound to albumin and 1.3% only is the free fraction [13]. There is a significant positive correlation between the concentrations of LNG and SHBG irrespective of the mode of administration, although marked inter-individual variations of SHBG levels exist [13-15]. Moreover, there are wide inter and intra-individual variations in serum concentrations and pharmacokinetic parameters of LNG, irrespective of the route of administration [16].

Following the insertion of LNG-IUS, LNG is initially released at a rate of 20 μg/day. Subsequently, this rate decreases progressively to half that value after 5 years. A stable serum concentration, without peaks and troughs, occurs after the first few weeks following insertion [17]. The reported steady-state LNG serum levels in LNG-IUS users ranged in different studies between 455-1601 pmol/l compared to 800 pmol/l after oral administration of 30 μg LNG [18]. However, Nilsson et al. found that the concentrations of LNG in the endometrial tissue were 2586 pmol/g and 11.2 pmol/g of wet tissue weight in the users of a LNG-releasing IUS that releases 30 μg daily and in those taking oral contraceptive pill containing 250 μg LNG, respectively [10].

LNG is completely metabolised by the common pathways of steroid metabolism with clearance rate from serum of approximately 1 ml/min/kg. However, metabolic clearance rates vary among individuals by several-fold, which partially explains the wide variations in serum concentrations in individuals using LNG-containing contraceptive products [16].

The serum levels decline biphasically with half-lives of 12-24 min and 20h, respectively. About 45% of LNG and its metabolites are excreted in the urine and 32% are excreted in faeces, mostly as glucuronide conjugates [17]. The half-life of metabolite excretion is about 1 day; however, some studies reported values as short as 9h and others as long as 80h [19]. This means that women with slow metabolic clearance rates could have, at any one point, up to three times higher serum levels of LNG than average [11].

The Relevant LNG-IUS Effects on Endometrial Morphology

Histological Effects

The high local levels of LNG lead to changes in the endometrial features which are characteristic and relatively constant, and are in keeping with the effects of both a progestogenic compound and a mechanical device [20]. These include dilated thin-walled vesicles associated with a thinning of the surface epithelium which shows complex intercellular junctions, lateral interdigitating microvilli and continuous prominent basal laminae.

It also induces extensive stromal pseudodecidualization; endometrial glandular atrophy, leukocytic infiltration, and decrease in glandular and stromal mitoses. The glandular epithelial cells become thinner within 6 months of LNG-IUS insertion, and remain so throughout insertion period. [21-23]. Further, the extracellular matrix becomes compact rather than oedematous, and the epithelial cell projections through the basal lamina get fewer in number and less complex in shape [24]. Other histological features were reported including the presence of foci of stromal myxoid change and stromal haemosiderin pigment. Reactive atypia of surface glands, glandular metaplastic changes, stromal necrosis and calcifications were also found in some cases [20].

Immunohistochemical Effects

Immunohistochemical studies found a significant increase in granulocyte-macrophage colony stimulating factor expression in the endometrial stroma after insertion of LNG-IUS [21]. Further, there was significant increase in glandular and stromal prolactin receptor expression, an infiltrate of CD56+ large granular lymphocytes and CD68+ macrophages, insulin-like growth factor binding protein-1 [21,25], vascular endothelial growth factor [26], and reduced expression of the proliferative marker Ki67 [27]. All these changes are consistent with decidualization and are evident for at least up to 12 months post insertion. LNG-IUS therapy also led to significant reduction in endometrial progesterone receptor expression, and this appears to be a marker for the strong endometrial anti-proliferative effect of the LNG at a cellular level resulting in an inhibition of estrogen bioactivity and endometrial suppression [25,28-29].

Effects on Endometrial Vasculature and Uterine Artery Blood Flow

Some Doppler studies found an increase in the mean uterine artery Pulsatility Index (PI) in the mid-luteal phase within 3-6 months of insertion of LNG-IUS, and this increase correlated with the serum levels of LNG [30,31]. Other studies revealed significant increase in Resistance Index (RI) and reduction in the subendometrial flow in the spiral arteries and uterine volume up to one year after the insertion of the LNG-IUS [32-34]. These changes could be the progestogenic effects that abolish the vasodilatory effect of estrogen.

The Role of LNG-IUS in the Protection of Endometrium

As an Adjunct to Estrogen Replacement Therapy

There is strong evidence that LNG-IUS prevents the endometrial proliferation associated with estrogen replacement therapy (ERT) leading to predominantly inactive endometrium, which is characterized by pseudodecidualization of the stroma and glandular atrophy [21,23,35]. Seven randomized controlled trials (RCTs) [36-42], five cohort studies [43-47] and three observational studies [48-50] have described the use of LNG-IUS to protect the endometrium from endometrial hyperplasia or malignant transformation during exogenous ERT in perimenopausal and postmenopausal women. Endometrial suppression (inactive or atrophic) was achieved in all studies.

Further, a recent case-control study showed that the use of LNG-IUS alongside estradiol in hormone replacement therapy (HRT) regimens was associated with reduced risk of endometrial cancer; the odds ratio for sequential estradiol-progestogen therapy was 0.67 (95%CI: 0.52-0.86), for continuous estradiol-progestogen therapy was 0.45 (95%CI: 0.27-0.73), and for estradiol plus LNG-IUS was 0.39 (95%CI: 0.17-0.88). This reduced risk persisted for up to 10 years while using continuous estradiol-progesterone therapy and estradiol plus LNG-IUS [51].

As an Adjunct to Tamoxifen in Breast Cancer Survivors

Tamoxifen is a selective estrogen receptor modulator that has been used successfully as an adjuvant therapy in the treatment of advanced breast cancer in postmenopausal patients with positive estrogen receptors. However, it was shown to be associated with various endometrial pathologies such as endometrial polyps, hyperplasia and carcinoma [52,53]. The reported relative risk of developing endometrial carcinoma in these women ranged from 1.3 to 7.5 compared to the age-matched controls not using tamoxifen [54]. The management of the asymptomatic postmenopausal patient on tamoxifen is controversial, and the use of LNG-IUS was suggested to help reducing endometrial pathology.

Two RCTs [55,56], one cohort study [57] and one observational study of six cases [58] have examined the effectiveness of the LNG-IUS in preventing the development of endometrial polyps, hyperplasia and carcinoma in women taking tamoxifen following breast cancer. A Cochrane review of the two RCTs documented that the LNG-IUS in tamoxifen users led to a significant reduction inthe incidence of endometrial polyps (Peto odds ratio 0.14, 95%CI: 0.03-0.61); however neither trial was sufficiently powered to detect whether the device leads to significant changes in the incidence of endometrial hyperplasia or carcinoma, nor whether it leads to any increased risk of breast cancer recurrence [59]. A cohort study of postmenopausal breast cancer women on tamoxifen showed significant difference ($p<0.05$) between those who had LNG-IUS inserted for 36 months ($n=70$) and controls ($n=72$). No cases of hyperplasia and four cases of polyps were diagnosed in the former group, while four cases of hyperplasia and 14 cases of polyps were diagnosed in the second group [57]. Gardner et al [60] found that the endometrial benign changes (histological decidual or atrophic response) and the protective effect against polyp formation occur only during the use of LNG-IUS.

Given the unproven safety of the LNG-IUS in breast cancer survivors, there is a need for longer term randomized studies to determine the benefit to risk balance, and the probability recurrence in these women. The World Health Organization medical eligibility criteria for contraceptive use recommended that LNG-IUS usage by women with current breast cancer presents an unacceptable risk and for those with a past history of breast cancer (no disease for 5 years) the risks outweigh the benefits [61]. The reluctance to use LNG-IUS may be based on the concerns that the high stable systemic levels of LNG may be sufficient through its progestogenic effect to promote tumourigenesis or to blunt the anti-tumor effect of tamoxifen on the breast [62]. A retrospective cohort study assessed the recurrence rate among 79 breast cancer Belgian survivors who used LNG-IUS in comparison with 120 non-users who were closely matched for age at diagnosis, tumor stage, tumor grade, and treatment modalities. It found no increased risk of breast cancer recurrence associated with use of the LNG-IUS after the diagnosis. However, in a subgroup analysis of women who developed breast cancer while using an LNG IUS and who continued to use it, a statistically significant higher risk of recurrence was found [63]. On the other hand, a large population-based study of 17360 Finnish LNG-IUS users showed no difference in the incidence of breast cancer when they were compared with the average Finnish female population (data derived from the Finnish Cancer Registry) aged between 30 and 54 years [64].

The Role of LNG-IUS in the Treatment of Endometrial Hyperplasia

To date, there are no RCTs to assess the role of LNG-IUS in the management of endometrial hyperplasia. In the literature, seven prospective observational non-comparative studies and two case reports showed that using LNG-IUS in the treatment of peri- and postmenopausal women with endometrial hyperplasia without atypia has caused regression in the majority of reported cases. However, mixed results were obtained on using it to treat atypical endometrial hyperplasia.

The largest prospective observation study, included 105 women with endometrial hyperplasia (96 without atypia and 9 with atypia) who were unfit for surgery and treated with LNG-IUS, revealed endometrial regression in 90% (94/105) of women by two years; the majority of them (96%) achieved this within the first year of use. Regression occurred in 88 (92%) women without atypia and 6 (67%) with atypia as well as in all 22 women with endometrial hyperplasia associated with HRT. All 13 women with failed treatment underwent hysterectomy and one case of endometrial carcinoma was identified [65]. The other 6 prospective studies, collectively included a mixture of peri- and postmenopausal women with endometrial hyperplasia without atypia (n=85) and atypical endometrial hyperplasia (n=19), reported that LNG-IUS induced regression on biopsy in all cases in the former group and 16/19 (84.2%) in the second group. The follow up period varied between 12-90 months [28,66-70]. Interestingly, Lee et al. noticed that as long as LNG-IUS was kept in situ, the endometrial hyperplasia did not recur [66].

Two case reports showed the progression of atypical endometrial hyperplasia to carcinoma despite treatment with LNG-IUS, suggesting that caution should be exercised before offering it to these women, and close monitoring should be practised [71,72].

LNG-IUS Versus Oral Progestogen in the Treatment of Endometrial Hyperplasia

Oral progestogen was used to treat endometrial hyperplasia with some success; [9,73,74] however, there are wide variations amongst investigators as regards the optimal type, regimen (dose and route) and duration of oral therapy [75]. It is plausible to argue that women with endometrial hyperplasia need continuous treatment and high level of compliance in order to ensure complete regression which may not be guaranteed with oral progestogen therapy. In addition, the endometrial progestogen concentrations when delivered through an intrauterine device were found to exceed that of the oral therapy by several folds [10].

The comparative studies in the literature that compared oral progestogen therapy versus LNG-IUS in women with endometrial hyperplasia revealed that the histological regression with LNG-IUS therapy was more robust and more reliable, and the recurrence of the disease was less frequent. This may be due to the uniform suppression of the endometrium throughout the whole thickness caused by the high tissue concentrations. A recent meta-analysis of 24 observational studies (1001 women), evaluating the regression rate of endometrial hyperplasia in LNG-IUS users versus oral progestogens users, showed that oral therapy achieved a lower pooled regression rate compared with LNG-IUS for complex hyperplasia (66% *vs.* 92%; p<0.01) and atypical hyperplasia (69% *vs.* 90%; p=0.03). However, there was no statistical difference in simple hyperplasia (89% *vs.* 96%; p=0.41) [7]. The encouraging findings of these studies should be interpreted with cautions given the observational design, and small sample, poor quality and the lack of direct comparison between LNG-IUS and oral progestogen therapy in most of them.

Two other studies were published and not included in the previously mentioned meta-analysis. In a cohort study (published as an abstract) with a mean follow up duration of 25 months, 209 women with endometrial hyperplasia were treated with LNG-IUS and 96 with oral progestogens. Gallos et al. found a regression rate of 92% and 74% in LNG-IUS and oral therapy groups, respectively (OR 4.25; 95%CI: 2.14-8.42), and the duration from diagnosis to regression was shorter in the LNG-IUS group (8.4±6.9 *vs.* 10±12.6 months). In addition, the relapse of hyperplasia during follow-up was less common in LNG-IUS (8.4%) when compared to oral therapy (28.6%) (OR 4.38; 95%CI: 2.11-9.07) [76]. Another prospective long-term follow up trial done in eight different hospitals in North Norway, evaluated three different treatment options for 258 women with endometrial hyperplasia; 66 had LNG-IUS inserted for 3-108 months, 85 had medroxyprogesterone acetate 10 mg for 10 days per cycle for 3-6 months and 107 had no treatment. At 6 months of follow-up, the regression rate was 100%, 54% and 50% in the three groups, respectively. Long-term follow-up for 56-108 months showed a regression rate of 100%, 60% and 49%, respectively. Also, the regression rate was 100% for those who retained the LNG-IUS (n=44) and 63% for those who had it removed (n=22). The response to LNG-IUS was significantly higher than the other two groups, and there was no statistically significant difference between oral progestogen and observation groups. Nevertheless, it is not possible from the study to quantify the response according to the presence or absence of cytological atypia since the authors used a unique morphometric scoring system [77].

The Role of LNG-IUS in the Treatment of Early Endometrial Cancer

It may be possible to extrapolate the endometrial suppression data observed in LNG-IUS users as an adjunct to ERT and tamoxifen, and in treating endometrial hyperplasia and hypothesize that the risk of endometrial cancer may be reduced in long-term users of LNG-IUS. However, there is no data relating its use to an increased or decreased risk of endometrial cancer. The absence of publications showing association does not necessarily indicate lack of association between LNG-IUS and endometrial cancer. In the literature, there are only two case reports and a case series which showed that endometrial carcinoma has developed in four premenopausal women despite having LNG-IUS inserted as a contraceptive or to treat heavy periods [78-80].

Hysterectomy is the preferred primary treatment for well-differentiated early stage endometrial carcinoma. Although the majority of endometrial cancer cases occur in postmenopausal women, 2-14% of cases occur in those <40 years of age. Therefore, in selected cases when preserving fertility is a priority, a uterine-sparing treatment may be the option [9,81,82] Further, there is a room for an alternative to surgical treatment for women who are at high risk for surgery [83].

A literature review of the available limited sized case series and cohort studies (in total 81 cases, 27 articles) has shown an overall 76% cure rate on using oral progestogen therapy in women with well-differentiated stage 1 endometrial carcinoma [83]. This evidence, although limited in quality, suggests a plausible role for LNG-IUS in early stage disease. There are three prospective observational studies in the literature that assessed the outcome of treatment of early stage endometrial carcinoma with LNG-IUS [84-86]. In addition, there are 2 case reports and 2 case series that showed cure in 3 out of 7 cases and no data available for one patient who died of pneumonia [87-90]. Another 2 case reports [91,92] described successful reversion of the cancer on endometrial biopsies on using a combination of oral progestogens and LNG-IUS.

Recently, Bifulco et al.suggested that hysteroscopic resection of the focal endometrial atypical lesion preserving the basal endometrial layer followed by insertion of LNG-IUS may be an alternative option in young women desiring to preserve fertility. In a prospective study, of 14 women with mean age 32.6±3.5 years who had a diagnosis of atypical polypoid adenomyoma (*n*=4), atypical endometrial hyperplasia (*n*=6) and well differentiated grade 1 endometrial carcinoma (*n*=4) and underwent that intervention, no patient had a progression of the endometrial disease at 24 months of follow-up. Ten women had a complete remission with normal functional endometrium; four of them conceived following removal of the device. The other two women had a partial response i.e. regression of endometrial carcinoma to atypical hyperplasia; however, no recurrence was detected at the end of follow up period [84]. Wheeler et al. [85] treated 16 women diagnosed with well-differentiated endometrioid carcinoma with oral progestogen and another 10 with LNG-IUS. Eleven women (42.3%) showed complete remission (6 from the LNG-IUS group), 10 (38.5%) had persistent disease over a median follow-up period of 12 months (4 from the LNG-IUS group) and 5 (19.2%) regressed to complex atypical hyperplasia (all from the oral therapy group). Montz et al. [86] reported one year follow up data of 12 women with FIGO stage IA grade 1 endometrioid endometrial carcinoma who were considered to be high risk for surgery and treated with LNG-IUS. There was no residual disease in 6 out of 12 women at 3 months, 7 out of 11 women at 6 months, 7 out of 9 women at 9 months, and 6 out of 8 women at 12 months.

Clearly, it is impossible to obtain valid conclusions from these small observational studies, and these women should be informed that the option of conservative management is not the standard treatment for their disease and close observation is mandatory to diagnose possible recurrence or progression [93,94].

Pregnancy after Treatment of Endometrial Hyperplasia and Endometrial Carcinoma with LNG-IUS

There are two prospective studies [84,93], a case series [95] and a case report [96] in the literature which documented the outcome regarding conception following LNG-IUS treatment. Out of the 29 women with either atypical endometrial hyperplasia or carcinoma included in all studies, 10 managed to conceive. Five of them were treated only with LNG-IUS [93,95]; four underwent resection of the focal endometrial lesion prior to LNG-IUS insertion [84] and one received combined therapy of LNG-IUS and oral medroxyprogesterone acetate [96].

Given the fear of recurrence of endometrial hyperplasia or carcinoma after removal of the device or delivery, some investigators suggested that LNG-IUS should be re-inserted in the postpartum [95].

Conclusion

Although the current data on using LNG-IUS in endometrial hyperplasia without atypia may be encouraging, but there is no enough evidence to recommend LNG-IUS as a standard management in women with atypical endometrial hyperplasia and well-differentiated early stage endometrial carcinoma. The strength of the findings is limited by the dearth of primary literature, unreliability of the data because of the small numbers and the risk of bias in most of the studies because of their poor quality. Further, the interpretation of the positive findings should also take into account publication bias, which is likely to result in preferential reporting of cases with good outcome, leading to possible overestimation of the effect.

The scarcity of high quality evidence to reliably inform the clinicians in this area makes the efficacy of LNG-IUS still in doubt. It may be considered in young women wishing to spare their fertility or when there are considerable surgical risks. Nonetheless, to overcome the pitfalls of observational studies, a well-designed, adequately powered, prospective, controlled trial is required to establish the short and long-term efficacy and safety, and to better define the selection criteria, optimum duration of treatment, follow up protocols and outcome.Similarly, there is no evidence from RCTs that LNG-IUS prevents endometrial hyperplasia or carcinoma in breast cancer women taking tamoxifen, and the impact on the risk of breast cancer recurrence is unclear.

References

[1] Kurman, RJ; Kaminski, PF; Norris, HJ. The behavior of endometrial hyperplasia. A long-term study of "untreated" hyperplasia in 170 patients. *Cancer* 1985;56:403-12.

[2] Trimble, CL; Kauderer, J; Zaino, R; Silverberg, S; Lim, PC; Burke, JJ 2nd; et al. Concurrent endometrial carcinoma in women with a biopsy diagnosis of atypical endometrial hyperplasia: a Gynecologic Oncology Group study. *Cancer* 2006;106: 812-9.

[3] Plataniotis, G; Castiglione, M. Endometrial cancer: ESMO Clinical Practice Guidelines for diagnosis; treatment and follow-up. *Ann. Oncol.* 2010;Suppl 5:v41-5.

[4] Jemal, A; Siegel, R; Ward, E; Murray, T; Xu, J; Thun, MJ. Cancer statistics, 2007. *CA Cancer J. Clin.* 2007;57:43-66.

[5] Montgomery, BE; Daum, GS; Dunton, CJ. Endometrial hyperplasia: a review. *Obstet. Gynecol. Surv.* 2004;59:368-78.

[6] Clark, TJ; Neelakantan, D; Gupta, JK. The management of endometrial hyperplasia: an evaluation of current practice. *Eur. J. Obstet. Gynecol. Reprod.Biol.* 2006;125:259-64.

[7] Gallos, ID; Shehmar, M; Thangaratinam, S; Papapostolou, TK; Coomarasamy, A; Gupta, JK. Oral progestogens vs levonorgestrel-releasing intrauterine system for endometrial hyperplasia: a systematic review and metaanalysis. *Am. J. Obstet. Gynecol.* 2010;203:547 e1-10.

[8] Ferenczy, A; Gelfand, M. The biologic significance of cytologic atypia in progestogen-treated endometrial hyperplasia. *Am. J. Obstet. Gynecol.* 1989;160:126-31.

[9] Randall, TC; Kurman, RJ. Progestin treatment of atypical hyperplasia and well-differentiated carcinoma of the endometrium in women under age 40. *Obstet. Gynecol.* 1997;90:434-40.

[10] Nilsson, CG; Haukkamaa, M; Vierola, H; Luukkainen, T. Tissue concentrations of levonorgestrel in women using a levonorgestrel-releasing IUD. *Clin. Endocrinol. (Oxf)* 1982;17:529-36.

[11] Ewies AA. Levonorgestrel-releasing intrauterine system--the discontinuing story. *Gynecol. Endocrinol.* 2009;25:668-73.

[12] Lemus, AE; Vilchis, F; Damsky, R; Chavez, BA; Garcia, GA; Grillasca, I; et al. Mechanism of action of levonorgestrel: in vitro metabolism and specific interactions with steroid receptors in target organs. *J. Steroid Biochem. Mol. Biol.* 1992;41:881-90.

[13] Kuhnz, W; al-Yacoub, G; Fuhrmeister, A. Pharmacokinetics of levonorgestrel and ethinylestradiol in 9 women who received a low-dose oral contraceptive over a treatment period of 3 months and; after a wash-out phase; a single oral administration of the same contraceptive formulation. *Contraception* 1992;46:455-69.

[14] Xiao, BL; Zhou, LY; Zhang, XL; Jia, MC; Luukkainen, T; Allonen, H. Pharmacokinetic and pharmacodynamic studies of levonorgestrel-releasing intrauterine device. *Contraception* 1990;41:353-62.

[15] Jia, MC; Zhou, LY; Ren, S; Dong, L; Xiao, B. Serum SHBG levels during normal menstrual cycle and after insertion of levonorgestrel-releasing IUD. *Adv. Contracept* 1992;8:33-40.

[16] Fotherby, K. Levonorgestrel. Clinical pharmacokinetics. *Clin. Pharmacokinet* 1995;28:203-15.

[17] RxList: the Internet Drug Index. Mirena (levonorgestrel-releasing) Intrauterine System; http://www.rxlist.com/mirena-drug.htm

[18] Weiner, E; Victor, A; Johansson, ED. Plasma levels of d-norgestrel after oral administration. *Contraception* 1976;14:563-70.

[19] The electronic Medicines Compendium (eMC). http://www.medicines.org.uk/EMC/medicine/1829/SPC/Mirena/

[20] Phillips, V; Graham, CT; Manek, S; McCluggage, WG. The effects of the levonorgestrel intrauterine system (Mirena coil) on endometrial morphology. *J. Clin. Pathol.* 2003;56:305-7.

[21] Critchley, HO; Wang, H; Jones, RL; Kelly, RW; Drudy, TA; Gebbie, AE; et al. Morphological and functional features of endometrial decidualization following long-term intrauterine levonorgestrel delivery. *Hum. Reprod.* 1998;13:1218-24.

[22] Sheppard, BL. Endometrial morphological changes in IUD users: a review. *Contraception* 1987;36:1-10.

[23] Silverberg, SG; Haukkamaa, M; Arko, H; Nilsson, CG; Luukkainen, T. Endometrial morphology during long-term use of levonorgestrel-releasing intrauterine devices. *Int. J. Gynecol. Pathol.* 1986;5:235-41.

[24] Pakarinen, PI; Lahteenmaki, P; Lehtonen, E; Reima, I. The ultrastructure of human endometrium is altered by administration of intrauterine levonorgestrel. *Hum. Reprod.* 1998;13:1846-53.

[25] Jones, RL; Critchley, HO. Morphological and functional changes in human endometrium following intrauterine levonorgestrel delivery. *Hum. Reprod.* 2000;15 Suppl 3:162-72.

[26] Roopa, BA; Loganath, A; Singh, K. The effect of a levonorgestrel-releasing intrauterine system on angiogenic growth factors in the endometrium. *Hum. Reprod.* 2003;18: 1809-19.

[27] Salmi, A; Pakarinen, P; Peltola, AM; Rutanen, EM. The effect of intrauterine levonorgestrel use on the expression of c-JUN; oestrogen receptors; progesterone receptors and Ki-67 in human endometrium. *Mol. Hum. Reprod.* 1998;4:1110-5.

[28] Wildemeersch, D; Janssens, D; Pylyser, K; De Wever, N; Verbeeck, G; Dhont, M; et al. Management of patients with non-atypical and atypical endometrial hyperplasia with a levonorgestrel-releasing intrauterine system: Long-term follow-up. *Maturitas* 2007;57:210-3.

[29] Guttinger, A; Critchley, HO. Endometrial effects of intrauterine levonorgestrel. *Contraception* 2007;75:S93-8.

[30] Jarvela, I; Raudaskoski, T; Tekay, A; Jouppila, P. Effect of the levonorgestrel-releasing intrauterine system on the uterine artery pulsatility index in postmenopausal hormone replacement therapy. *Ultrasound Obstet. Gynecol.* 1997;10:350-5.

[31] Jarvela, I; Tekay, A; Jouppila, P. The effect of a levonorgestrel-releasing intrauterine system on uterine artery blood flow; hormone concentrations and ovarian cyst formation in fertile women. *Hum. Reprod.* 1998;13:3379-83.

[32] Zalel, Y; Gamzu, R; Shulman, A; Achiron, R; Schiff, G; Lidor, A. The effect of the levonorgestrel-releasing intrauterine system--when does it manifest? *Contraception* 2003;67:473-6.

[33] Zalel, Y; Shulman, A; Lidor, A; Achiron, R; Mashiach, S; Gamzu, R. The local progestational effect of the levonorgestrel-releasing intrauterine system: a sonographic and Doppler flow study. *Hum. Reprod.* 2002;17:2878-80.

[34] Haberal, A; Kayikcioglu, F; Gunes, M; Kaplan, M; Ozdegirmenci, O. The effect of the levonorgestrel intrauterine system on uterine artery blood flow 1 year after insertion. *Ultrasound Obstet. Gynecol.* 2006;27:316-9.

[35] Andersson, K; Odlind, V; Rybo, G. Levonorgestrel-releasing and copper-releasing (Nova T) IUDs during five years of use: a randomized comparative trial. *Contraception* 1994;49:56-72.

[36] Boon, J; Scholten, PC; Oldenhave, A; Heintz, AP. Continuous intrauterine compared with cyclic oral progestin administration in perimenopausal HRT. *Maturitas* 2003;46:69-77.

[37] Raudaskoski, T; Tapanainen, J; Tomas, E; Luotola, H; Pekonen, F; Ronni-Sivula, H; et al. Intrauterine 10 microg and 20 microg levonorgestrel systems in postmenopausal women receiving oral oestrogen replacement therapy: clinical; endometrial and metabolic response. *BJOG* 2002;109:136-44.

[38] Raudaskoski, TH; Lahti, EI; Kauppila, AJ; Apaja-Sarkkinen, MA; Laatikainen, TJ. Transdermal estrogen with a levonorgestrel-releasing intrauterine device for climacteric complaints: clinical and endometrial responses. *Am. J. Obstet. Gynecol.* 1995;172: 114-9.

[39] Andersson, K; Stadberg, E; Mattsson, LA; Rybo, G; Samsioe, G. Intrauterine or oral administration of levonorgestrel in combination with estradiol to perimenopausal women--effects on lipid metabolism during 12 months of treatment. *Int. J. Fertil. Menopausal. Stud.* 1996;41:476-83.

[40] Suhonen, SP; Allonen, HO; Lahteenmaki, P. Sustained-release estradiol implants and a levonorgestrel-releasing intrauterine device in hormone replacement therapy. *Am. J. Obstet. Gynecol.* 1995;172:562-7.

[41] Suhonen, SP; Holmstrom, T; Allonen, HO; Lahteenmaki, P. Intrauterine and subdermal progestin administration in postmenopausal hormone replacement therapy. *Fertil. Steril.* 1995;63:336-42.

[42] Andersson, K; Mattsson, LA; Rybo, G; Stadberg, E. Intrauterine release of levonorgestrel--a new way of adding progestogen in hormone replacement therapy. *Obstet. Gynecol.* 1992;79:963-7.
[43] Suvanto-Luukkonen, E; Kauppila, A. The levonorgestrel intrauterine system in menopausal hormone replacement therapy: five-year experience. *Fertil. Steril.* 1999;72:161-3.
[44] Suvanto-Luukkonen, E; Malinen, H; Sundstrom, H; Penttinen, J; Kauppila, A. Endometrial morphology during hormone replacement therapy with estradiol gel combined to levonorgestrel-releasing intrauterine device or natural progesterone. *Acta Obstet. Gynecol. Scand.* 1998;77:758-63.
[45] Suvanto-Luukkonen, E; Sundstrom, H; Penttinen, J; Laara, E; Pramila, S; Kauppila, A. Percutaneous estradiol gel with an intrauterine levonorgestrel releasing device or natural progesterone in hormone replacement therapy. *Maturitas* 1997;26:211-7.
[46] Antoniou, G; Kalogirou, D; Karakitsos, P; Antoniou, D; Kalogirou, O; Giannikos, L. Transdermal estrogen with a levonorgestrel-releasing intrauterine device for climacteric complaints versus estradiol-releasing vaginal ring with a vaginal progesterone suppository: clinical and endometrial responses. *Maturitas* 1997;26:103-11.
[47] Kalogirou, D; Antoniou, G; Karakitsos, P; Kalogirou, O; Antoniou, D; Giannikos, L. A comparative study of the effects of an estradiol-releasing vaginal ring combined with an oral gestagen versus transdermal estrogen combined with a levonorgestrel-releasing IUD: clinical findings and endometrial response. *Int. J. Fertil. Menopausal Stud.* 1996;41:522-7.
[48] Hampton, NR; Rees, MC; Lowe, DG; Rauramo, I; Barlow, D; Guillebaud, J. Levonorgestrel intrauterine system (LNG-IUS) with conjugated oral equine estrogen: a successful regimen for HRT in perimenopausal women. *Hum. Reprod.* 2005;20: 2653-60.
[49] Varila, E; Wahlstrom, T; Rauramo, I. A 5-year follow-up study on the use of a levonorgestrel intrauterine system in women receiving hormone replacement therapy. *Fertil. Steril.* 2001;76:969-73.
[50] Suhonen, S; Holmstrom, T; Lahteenmaki, P. Three-year follow-up of the use of a levonorgestrel-releasing intrauterine system in hormone replacement therapy. *Acta Obstet. Gynecol. Scand.* 1997;76:145-50.
[51] Jaakkola, S; Lyytinen, HK; Dyba, T; Ylikorkala, O; Pukkala, E. Endometrial cancer associated with various forms of postmenopausal hormone therapy: a case control study. *Int. J. Cancer* 128:1644-51.
[52] Cohen, I; Perel, E; Flex, D; Tepper, R; Altaras, MM; Cordoba, M; et al. Endometrial pathology in postmenopausal tamoxifen treatment: comparison between gynaecologically symptomatic and asymptomatic breast cancer patients. *J. Clin. Pathol.* 1999;52:278-82.
[53] De Muylder, X; Neven, P; De Somer, M; Van Belle, Y; Vanderick, G; De Muylder, E. Endometrial lesions in patients undergoing tamoxifen therapy. *Int. J. Gynaecol. Obstet.* 1991;36:127-30.
[54] Daniel, Y; Inbar, M; Bar-Am, A; Peyser, MR; Lessing, JB. The effects of tamoxifen treatment on the endometrium. *Fertil. Steril.* 1996;65:1083-9.

[55] Chan, SSC; Tam, WH; Yeo, W; Yu, MMY; Ng, DPS; Wong, AWY; et al. A randomised controlled trial of prophylactic levonorgestrel intrauterine system in tamoxifen-treated women. *BJOG* 2007; 114:1510-5.

[56] Gardner, FJE; Konje, JC; Abrams, KR; Brown, LJR; Khanna, S; Al-Azzawi, F; et al. Endometrial protection from tamoxifen-stimulated changes by a levonorgestrel-releasing intrauterine system: A randomised controlled trial. *Lancet* 2000;356:1711-7.

[57] Kesim, MD; Aydin, Y; Atis, A; Mandiraci, G. Long-term effects of the levonorgestrel-releasing intrauterine system on serum lipids and the endometrium in breast cancer patients taking tamoxifen. *Climacteric* 2008;11:252-7.

[58] Turnbull, LW tr; Manton, DJ; Purdie, DW. The effects of progestogen on the endometrium of long-term users of tamoxifen treated breast cancer patiens using transvaginal scanning and MRI. *Br. J. Radiol.* 1998;71:45(S).

[59] Chin, J; Konje, JC; Hickey, M. Levonorgestrel intrauterine system for endometrial protection in women with breast cancer on adjuvant tamoxifen. *Cochrane database of systematic reviews* 2009:CD007245.

[60] Gardner, FJ; Konje, JC; Bell, SC; Abrams, KR; Brown, LJ; Taylor, DJ; et al. Prevention of tamoxifen induced endometrial polyps using a levonorgestrel releasing intrauterine system long-term follow-up of a randomised control trial. *Gynecol. Oncol.* 2009;114:452-6.

[61] World-Health-Organization-(WHO). Medical Eligibility Criteria for Contraceptive Use. 2000. Geneva; Switzerland.

[62] Varma R; Sinha D; Gupta JK. Non-contraceptive uses of levonorgestrel-releasing hormone system (LNG-IUS)--a systematic enquiry and overview. *Eur. J. Obstet. Gynecol. Reprod.Biol.* 2006;125:9-28.

[63] Trinh, XB; Tjalma, WA; Makar, AP; Buytaert, G; Weyler, J; van Dam, PA. Use of the levonorgestrel-releasing intrauterine system in breast cancer patients. *Fertil. Steril.* 2008;90:17-22.

[64] Backman, T; Rauramo, I; Jaakkola, K; Inki, P; Vaahtera, K; Launonen, A; et al. Use of the levonorgestrel-releasing intrauterine system and breast cancer. *Obstet. Gynecol.* 2005;106:813-7.

[65] Varma, R; Soneja, H; Bhatia, K; Ganesan, R; Rollason, T; Clark, TJ; et al. The effectiveness of a levonorgestrel-releasing intrauterine system (LNG-IUS) in the treatment of endometrial hyperplasia--a long-term follow-up study. *Eur. J. Obstet. Gynecol. Reprod.Biol.* 2008;139:169-75.

[66] Lee, SY; Kim, MK; Park, H; Yoon, BS; Seong, SJ; Kang, JH; J et al. The effectiveness of levonorgestrel releasing intrauterine system in the treatment of endometrial hyperplasia in Korean women. *J. Gynecol. Oncol.* 2010;21:102-5.

[67] Haimovich, S; Checa, MA; Mancebo, G; Fuste, P; Carreras, R. Treatment of endometrial hyperplasia without atypia in peri- and postmenopausal women with a levonorgestrel intrauterine device. *Menopause* 2008;15:1002-4.

[68] Wildemeersch, D; Dhont, M. Treatment of nonatypical and atypical endometrial hyperplasia with a levonorgestrel-releasing intrauterine system. *Am. J. Obstet. Gynecol.* 2003;188:1297-8.

[69] Perino, A; Quartararo, P; Catinella, E; Genova, G; Cittadini, E. Treatment of endometrial hyperplasia with levonorgestrel releasing intrauterine devices. *Acta Eur. Fertil.* 1987;18:137-40.

[70] Scarselli, G; Tantini, C; Colafranceschi, M; Taddei, GL; Bargelli, G; Venturini, N; et al. Levo-norgestrel-nova-T and precancerous lesions of the endometrium. *Eur. J. Gynaecol. Oncol.* 1988;9:284-6.

[71] Corrado, G; Baiocco, E; Carosi, M; Vizza, E. Progression of conservatively treated endometrial complex atypical hyperplasia in a young woman: a case report. *Fertil. Steril.* 2008;90:2006 e5-8.

[72] Kresowik, J; Ryan, GL; Van Voorhis, BJ. Progression of atypical endometrial hyperplasia to adenocarcinoma despite intrauterine progesterone treatment with the levonorgestrel-releasing intrauterine system. *Obstet. Gynecol.* 2008;111:547-9.

[73] Gotlieb, WH; Beiner, ME; Shalmon, B; Korach, Y; Segal, Y; Zmira, N; et al. Outcome of fertility-sparing treatment with progestins in young patients with endometrial cancer. *Obstet. Gynecol.* 2003;102:718-25.

[74] Chiva, L; Lapuente, F; Gonzalez-Cortijo, L; Carballo, N; Garcia, JF; Rojo A; et al. Sparing fertility in young patients with endometrial cancer. *Gynecol. Oncol.* 2008;111:S101-4.

[75] Marsden, DE; Hacker, NF. Optimal management of endometrial hyperplasia. *Best Pract Res Clin Obstet Gynaecol* 2001;15:393-405.

[76] Gallos, ID; Krishan, P; Shehmar, M; Gupta, JK. LNG-IUS vs. oral progestogens for endometrial hyperplasia. A comparative cohort study with long term follow-up. *Gynecol. Surg.* 2009;6.

[77] Orbo, A; Arnes, M; Hancke, C; Vereide, AB; Pettersen, I; Larsen, K. Treatment results of endometrial hyperplasia after prospective D-score classification: a follow-up study comparing effect of LNG-IUD and oral progestins versus observation only. *Gynecol. Oncol.* 2008;111:68-73.

[78] Abu, J; Brown, L; Ireland, D. Endometrial adenocarcinoma following insertion of the levonorgestrel- releasing intrauterine system (mirena) in a 36-year-old woman. *Int. J. Gynecol. Cancer* 2006;16:1445-7.

[79] Flemming, R; Sathiyathasan, S; Jackson, A. Endometrioid adenocarcinoma after insertion of a levonorgestrel-releasing intrauterine system. *J. Minim. Invasive Gynecol.* 2008;15:771-3.

[80] Jones, K; Georgiou, M; Hyatt, D; Spencer, T; Thomas, H. Endometrial adenocarcinoma following the insertion of a Mirena IUCD. *Gynecol. Oncol.* 2002;87:216-8.

[81] Crissman, JD; Azoury, RS; Barnes, AE; Schellhas, HF. Endometrial carcinoma in women 40 years of age or younger. *Obstet. Gynecol.* 1981;57:699-704.

[82] Garrett, A; Quinn, MA. Hormonal therapies and gynaecological cancers. *Best Pract. Res. Clin. Obstet. Gynaecol.* 2008;22:407-21.

[83] Ramirez, PT; Frumovitz, M; Bodurka, DC; Sun, CC; Levenback, C. Hormonal therapy for the management of grade 1 endometrial adenocarcinoma: a literature review. *Gynecol. Oncol.* 2004;95:133-8.

[84] Bifulco, G; Di Spiezio Sardo, A; De Rosa, N; Bertrando, A; Lavitola, G; Spinelli, ML; et al. Fertility-sparing combined hysteroscopic and medical treatment of atypical endometrial lesions in young women. *Gynecological Surgery;* 7(Suppl1): ESGE Barcellona, 1-3 ottobre 2010.

[85] Wheeler, DT; Bristow, RE; Kurman, RJ. Histologic alterations in endometrial hyperplasia and well-differentiated carcinoma treated with progestins. *Am. J. Surg. Pathol.* 2007;31:988-98.

[86] Montz, FJ; Bristow, RE; Bovicelli, A; Tomacruz, R; Kurman, RJ. Intrauterine progesterone treatment of early endometrial cancer. *Am. J. Obstet. Gynecol.* 2002;186:651-7.

[87] Wildemeersch, D; Anderson, E; Lambein, K; Pauwels, P; Dhont, M. Successful treatment of early endometrial carcinoma by local delivery of levonorgestrel: a case report. *Obstet. Gynecol. Int.* 2010;2010:431950.

[88] Fambrini, M; Bargelli, G; Peruzzi, E; Buccoliero, AM; Pieralli, A; Andersson, KL; et al. Levonorgestrel-releasing intrauterine system alone as primary treatment in young women with early endometrial cancer: case report. *J. Minim. Invasive Gynecol.* 2009;16:630-3.

[89] Dhar, KK; Needhi Rajan, T; Koslowski, M; Woolas, RP. Is levonorgestrel intrauterine system effective for treatment of early endometrial cancer? Report of four cases and review of the literature. *Gynecol. Oncol.* 2005;97:924-7.

[90] Bahamondes, L; Ribeiro-Huguet, P; De Andrade, KC; Leon-Martins, O; Petta, CA. Levonorgestrel-releasing intrauterine system (Mirena) as a therapy for endometrial hyperplasia and carcinoma. *Acta Obstet. Gynecol. Scand.* 2003;82:580-2.

[91] Tanmahasamut, P; Wongwananuruk, T. Challenging regimen for long-term conservative treatment of endometrial adenocarcinoma in young women: A case report and review of the literature. *Case Rep. Oncol.* 2010;3:380-5.

[92] Giannopoulos, T; Butler-Manuel, S; Tailor, A. Levonorgestrel-releasing intrauterine system (LNG-IUS) as a therapy for endometrial carcinoma. *Gynecol. Oncol.* 2004;95:762-4.

[93] Cade, T; Quinn, M; Rome, R; Neesham, D. Progestogen treatment options for early endometrial cancer. *BJOG* 2010;117:879-83.

[94] Scarselli, G; Bargelli, G; Taddei, GL; Marchionni, M; Peruzzi, E; Pieralli, A; et al. Levonorgestrel-releasing intrauterine system (LNG-IUS) as an effective treatment option for endometrial hyperplasia: A 15-year follow-up study. *Fertil. Steril.* 2011;95:420-2.

[95] Qi, X; Zhao, W; Duan, Y; Li, Y. Successful pregnancy following insertion of a levonorgestrel-releasing intrauterine system in two infertile patients with complex atypical endometrial hyperplasia. *Gynecol. Obstet. Invest* 2008;65:266-8.

[96] Ercan, CM; Duru, NK; Sakinci, M; Alanbay, B; Karasahin, KE; Baser, I. Successful twin pregnancy achieved by assisted reproductive technology in a patient with polycystic ovary syndrome with complex atypical endometrial hyperplasia treated with levonorgestrel-releasing intrauterine system. *Gynecol. Endocrinol.* 2010;26:125-8.

In: Endometrial Cancer: Prevention, Diagnosis and Treatment ISBN: 978-1-62257-740-8
Editor: Stefano Greggi

Chapter XII

Rare Uterine Cancer: Serous Papillary Cancer and Its Molecular Genetics

***Grazia Artioli*[1*] *and Jacopo Wabersich*[2]**
[1]Oncology - Haematology, Mirano Hospital, Venice, Italy
[2]Obstetrics and Gynecology, Mirano Hospital, Venice, Italy

Abstract

Endometrial cancer is the most common malignant tumor of the female genital tract. Uterine papillary serous carcinoma (UPSC) is a rare but aggressive subtype of endometrial cancer, although it represents only 10% of all endometrial cancer cases. Some studies described BRCA mutation associated with UPSC but definitive recommendation for hysterectomy to prevent primary uterine cancer as part of BRCA-associate cancer spectrum does not seem warranted.

Several studies have suggested that endometrioid endometrial cancer (UEC) and UPSC are distinct neoplasms with different molecular basis. UPSC shows often estrogen and progesterone receptors negative, tendency to deep myometrial invasion and grade and high frequency to spread to lymph node. UPSC and UEC have different molecular genetics which distinct two different type of tumors in the same organ.

K-Ras mutation is present in UEC and it is a sign of good prognosis. Tashiro et. al described a high number of p53 positivity for mutation in UPSC and that atrophic uterine epithelium in which these tumors arise may be and early acquisition of p53 mutations. Even in intraepithelial cancer, p53 is already mutated and this mutation arise advantage for metastasis. p53 mutation is an early steps in the endometrial carcinogenesis because it is present in the intraepithelial carcinomas, instead in UEC p53 inactivation is a late step.

UPSC is a different type of endometrial cancer and has to be considered a high risk subtype to be treated with chemotherapy/radiotherapy even in early stage.

[*] E-mail address: grazia.artioli@yahoo.it.

Introduction

Endometrial cancer is the most common malignant tumor of the female genital tract. Uterine papillary serous carcinoma (UPSC) is a rare but aggressive subtype of endometrial cancer, although it represents only 10% of all endometrial cancer cases [1].

Several studies have suggested that endometrioid endometrial cancer (UEC) and UPSC are distinct neoplasms with different molecular basis. UPSC was established as a distinct type of endometrial cancer by Lauchlan and Hendrickson et al. in 1982 [2]. Later Bokhman described two different types of endometrial carcinoma: Type I with endometrioid histology that arises in young women with obesity, hyperlipidemia and hyperestrogenism and Type II that is a poorly differentiated endometrioid, clear cell and serous histology in older women with non hormonal risk factors [3]. The purpose of this chapter is to describe UPSC as a different uterus carcinoma. We will first address the question of which kind of molecular basis may have UPSC and which treatment is the best option.

Histopathology

UPSC is described as a different endometrial cancer that often develops in the setting of endometrial atrophy and has poor prognostic factors as: estrogen and progesterone negative receptors, tendency to deep myometrial invasion, high grade, high frequency to spread to lymph node and higher stages at diagnosis.

Hendrickson et al. described a papillary architecture supported by a fibrovascular framework identical to that seen in serous ovarian carcinoma [2,4-5].

Christopherson et al. examined 46 cases of papillary endometrial adenocarcinoma and emphasized other features including multiple papillary arborizations, cellular stratification, cell desquamation, and variations in the nuclear morphology [6].

Chen et al. in 1985 reviewed all the papillary tumors of the endometrium and divided in UPSC as defined by Hendrickson et al., and in well-differentiated adenocarcinoma of the endometrium with papillary features characterized by thin papillae covered by relatively uniform neoplastic epithelial cells [7].

Type II tumors represent 10% to 20% of the sporadic endometrial carcinomas and usually arise in a background of atrofic endometrium through a mechanism unrelated to estrogen.

The stroma presented edematous papillae and was covered by highly pleomorphic cells containing hyperchromatic nuclei. The majority of cases showed marked anaplasia and very enlarged nuclei and psammoma-bodies are found in about 30% of cases.

Endometrial Intraepithelial Carcinoma (EIC)

Sherman et al. were the first to describe EIC as a precursor lesion of UPSC. EIC is defined morphologically as the replacement of endometrial surface epithelium and glands by frankly malignant cells that resemble the cells of the invasive high grade endometrial carcinoma. EIC can be considered a form of cancer rather than a precursor. Dysplastic lesions have never been described in the process of UPSC development or between benign endometrium lesions and serous EIC. The classical microscopic features are constituted of smaller, cuboidal cells with a papillary architecture consisting of fibrous stalks, tufted stratification of epithelial lining with associated stromal support [8]. Sharon et al. showed that endometrial glandular dysplasia (EmGD) may be a newly defined precursos lesion of UPSC by morphology. They conclude that EmGD frequently shows loss of heterozygosity (LOH) of multiple chromosomal loci, particulary 17p and 1p, similar to those found in UPSC, suggesting a similar pathogenesis for these two lesions. In the study, they found that LOH at 2p16 region was 17% in EmGD, 31% in EIC and 23% in UPSC. The role of those finding has to be clarified.

Today, therefore, gynecologists must learn to recognize and handle this type of lesions because they can hide the presence of a concomitant UPSC [9].

Molecular Basis

Lax S. et al. show that 17% of UEC have p53 mutation and 25% and K-RAS cod 12 mutations. The K-RAS mutation is frequent in UEC (26%) grade 1 and rare in UPSC (2%), and occur early in carcinogenesis steps. The K-RAS mutation occurs more frequently in microsatellite instability (MSI) negative UEC tumors compared with MSI positive.

MSI is about 9-23% in UEC (0% in UPSC), while p53 mutation is very common and is described c-herb2 amplification in UPSC (16-62%)

Those results showed that inside the endometrial tumors there are two distinct kind of tumors with distinct genotypes.

p53

p53 mutation is an early step in the endometrial carcinogenesis, because it is present in the intraepithelial carcinomas, while in UEC p53 inactivation is a late step (10-20%).

The presence of p53 mutation can provide cells with a selective growth advantage leading to tumor progression and its inactivation is an intragenic mutation followed by loss of the remaining wild-type allele. Although the p53 gene consists of a total of 11 exons and 905 mutations, it often occurs in exons 5 to 8.

Tashiro et al. describe a high number of p53 positivity for mutation in UPSC and show that atrophic uterine epithelium in which these tumors arise may be an early acquisition of p53 mutations. Aneuploidy is commonly found in USCP and may reflect the fact that p53 gene mutation is part of an early step of carcinogenesis and can cause a poor outcome of patients affected by the disease. p53 mutation is an early event and is present in 100% of EIC.

PTEN

PTEN: gene encodes a 55 kDa protein, which has been shown to play a role in cell growth and survival. PTEN is a tumor suppressor gene and its loss of heterozygosity and decrease in protein expression is described in endometrial cancer but not in UPSC.

C-erbB2

C-erbB2 is a member of the human epithelial growth factor receptor family. Satin showed that c-erb2 amplification is present in 80% of UPSC cases [10-11].

Hereditary Syndromes and Serous Papillary Adenocarcinoma of Uterus

BRCA1 and BRCA2 Mutations Syndrome

It is unclear whether endometrial cancer is a part of BRCA syndrome and whether BRCA positive women affected by endometrial cancer have better prognosis than sporadic cases. All studies showing a BRCA mutation in UPSC are done among Askenazi Jewish population screened only for their 3 more frequent mutations.

In those studies, all women had a personal or familial cases of breast/ ovarian cancer.

Lavie described a population of 51 Ashkenazi women, of them 8/13 affected by UPSC with a previous diagnosis of breast cancer and 1 ovarian cancer were BRCA mutated. The median age at diagnosis was 71. At present, this study is the richest in literature, showing a high number of UPSC in BRCA population [12]. In Biron-Shental study in a group of women with personal history of breast and ovarian cancer, 6 out of 22 had BRCA1-2 mutations. Other cases were described as case reports [13].

Goshen et al. study did not find BRCA1-2 mutations among 56 women with UPSC. Based on those relative low numbers of women, as showed in table 1, definitive recommendation for hysterectomy to prevent primary uterine cancer as part of BRCA-associate cancer spectrum does not seem warranted. A relevant bias is that the disease has been studied only in Jewish population and studies in a larger population are needed [14].

The rare presence of UPSC in BRCA carrier women, as shown in table 1, does not allow the screening for the disease right now, because UPSC is an unusual endometrial type of cancer and BRCA mutation is rare, as well.

No cases of clear cell uterus carcinoma are described in literature as associated to BRCA syndrome [19].

Hereditary Non-Polyposis Colorectal Cancer (HNPCC) Syndrome

Endometrial carcinoma is one of the most common cancer in the HNPCC syndrome. MSI has been reported to be more common in endometrioid (MSI has been reported in 25-45% of all endometrial carcinoma) than non-endometrioid cancers. Microsatellite instability is characterized by the accumulation of mutations during DNA replication. An HJ. et al. studied the clinicopathological phenotype of endometrial cancer associated with MSI. There is a relationship between PTEN and MSI given the higher rates of PTEN mutations in tumors with MSI 60-80% compared with those without MSI 24-35% [20,21,22,23].

Table 1. Studies on association between BRCA mutation and UPSC

Author, Year	n	Race	BRCA1	BRCA2	UPSC
Lavie O, 2010 [12]	51	Jewish	7	1	n/a
Kwon JS, 2008 [15]	3	Jewish	3	0	2
Biron-Shental T, 2006 [13]	22	Jewish	3	3	6
Lavie O, 2005 [16]	Case report	-	0	1	1
Levine DA, 2001 [17]	199	Jewish	1	2	3
Goshen R, 2000 [14]	56	-	0	0	0
Honreich G, 1999 [18]	Case report	Jewish	2	0	1

Surgical Treatment

The Society of Gynecologic Oncology (SGO) recommends to perform peritoneal washing, total hysterectomy with bilateral salpingoophorectomy, pelvic and para-aortic lymphadenectomy [24]. Lymphadenectomy may also provide a therapeutic benefit in patients with high-grade endometrial cancer [25]. Thomas et al, to confirm the importance of optimal stage and cytoreduction, considered two groups of patients in stage IIIC and IV, the first with residual of disease < 1 cm (optimal cyitoreduction) and the second with suboptimal reduction; he observed that the optimal group presents a significant improved median time to recurrence, and that median survival was 9 months vs. 6 (p=0.04) and 20 months vs. 12 (p=0.02), respectively [26]. The absence of visible residual disease is considered as an independent predictor of overall survival. At present, the International Federation of Gynecology and Obstetrics (FIGO) staging of endometrial cancer does not include the study of omentum. UPSC is described by the presence of psammomatous bodies with histological characteristics similar to ovarian papillary serous adenocarcinoma with a tendency to spread to the peritoneum surface [27].

Chan and Geisler considered omentectomy and peritoneal biopsies as a part of the surgical staging [28,29]. On the other hand, in a study of 18 patients with omental positive disease, Gehrig at al. showed that 16 of them had macroscopic disease of omentum and only two cases had macroscopic and microscopic omental disease as well, Gehrig concluded that routine omentectomy may not be necessary [30]. The limits of this study are that the cases are small in number and retrospective.

Lymph-vascular space invasion (LVSI) and myometrial deep invasion are not predictive of spread of disease and therefore it should consider to perform omentectomy and peritoneal biopsies.

Adjuvant Chemotherapy

Due to its aggressive phenotype, UPSC treated with radiotherapy and chemotherapy seems to improve survival even in the early stage. UPSC has a significant risk to develop extrapelvic recurrence and has poor survival.

In the experience of Kelly et al. for staged I UPSC, platinum-based chemotherapy showed to improve disease-free survival (p<0.01) and overall survival (p<0.05) after a median follow-up of 38 months [4]. In 2009, Fader published a retrospective study about early stage UPSC well staged at surgery and treated with platinum-taxane based chemotherapy ± pelvic radiation therapy or observation alone. The risk of recurrence was lower for patients receiving chemotherapy (11.2%) compared with patient receiving RT alone (25%) and observation (30.3%). PFS was 81.5% in CTRT, 64.1% in RT alone and 64.7% in observation alone. In stage IB and IC, patients receiving CT ± RT experienced a similar recurrence to that of non-treated patients. Even though data have showed improved survival for patient treated with chemotherapy, at present there are no randomized studies in stage I UPSC exploring the utility of adjuvant treatment [31].

Because patients also at stage I are at significant risk of recurrence, adjuvant therapy is often recommended for patients at all stages. The role of radiotherapy is shown in the recent Cochrane meta-analysis of four randomized studies. The addition of pelvic external beam radiotherapy to surgery reduced by 72% the risk of pelvic recurrence with no evidence of reduction in the risk of recurrence or distant metastases or the risk of death [32-33]. The subgroup analysis showed that this treatment was associated with a trend toward reducing the risk of death in patients with multiple risk factors, such as the grade and stage IC. In advanced stages more studies have shown the important role of chemotherapy.

GOG 177 was the first phase III study about chemotherapy in advanced or recurrent endometrial cancer that showed a survival advantage. Paclitaxel-doxorubicin-cisplatin proved to be better than doxorubicin-cisplatin, but the toxicity of the three-drug regimen has precluded general acceptance. Paclitaxel-carboplatin has given high response rates in endometrial cancer and is widely used, despite the lack of evidence based on randomised studies [34]. GOG 122 was a pivotal randomised study that compared doxorubicin-cisplatin with whole abdominal radiotherapy in advanced optimally operated endometrial cancer and showed that chemotherapy with doxorubicin-cisplatin results in superior survival.

In terms of recurrences, data are: 109 (54%) of 202 patients treated with whole abdominal irradiation (WAI) recurred 13%, 16%, and 22%, in the pelvis, abdominal, and extra-abdominal regions, respectively. Chemotherapy reduces extra-abdominal recurrences only from 22% to 18% [35].

In the randomized PORTEC (Post Operative Radiation Therapy in Endometrial Cancer) study, which enrolled 715 patients at intermediate-risk, the addition of adjuvant pelvic external beam radiotherapy reduced the loco-regional recurrence (4% vs. 14%, $p<0.001$) and increased the (25% vs. 6%, $p<0.0001$) compared with surgery alone, while deaths from cancer (9% vs. 6%), 5-yrs survival (81% vs. 85%) and actuarial survival to 8 years (71% vs. 77%) were unchanged.

Vaginal brachytherapy alone was used as post-operative treatment in patients with low-risk disease (stage IB, grade 1-2) and in those with intermediate or high-risk disease (stage I grade 3, or stage IC) but with histologically negative lymph nodes.

A more recent update of this study showed that, despite its efficacy in reducing loco-regional recurrence, External beam radiation therapy (EBRT) should be avoided in patients with low and intermediate-risk endometrial cancer because of long term toxicity [36-37].

A phase III study of the Nordic Society of Gynecological Oncology (NSGO) and the European Organization for Research and Treatment of Cancer (EORTC) trial comparing adjuvant pelvic EBRT with or without vaginal brachytherapy (44 Gy) versus the same radiotherapy preceded or followed by four cycles of platinum-based chemotherapy with different regimens (cisplatin 50 mg/m^2 + doxorubicin 50 mg/m^2 or epirubicin 75 mg/m^2; paclitaxel 175 mg/m^2 + epirubicin 60 mg/m^2 + carboplatin AUC 5; paclitaxel 175 mg/m^2 + carboplatin AUC 5-6) in 372 patients with endometrial cancer stage I-IIIC high-risk showed an improved survival in CTRT group.

High-risk patients were defined as those patients with serous or clear cell histology or undifferentiated or those with endometrioid histology but with grade 3 and/or deep myometrial invasion and/or non-diploid DNA. After a median follow-up of 3.5 years, the hazard ratio (HR) for progression-free survival was 0.58 (95%CI 0.34-0.99, $p=0.046$) in favor of combined treatment, progression-free survival at 5 years was 82% versus 75% [38].

The significance of the sequential or concurrent chemo-radiotherapy is now under investigation in a randomized trial called PORTEC 3 which includes patients with high-risk endometrioid carcinoma (stage IB grade 3 with LVSI, stage IC grade G3, stage II grade 3, stage IIIA, stage IIIC) and patients with papillary serous or clear cell carcinoma in stage IB-

III. Patients are randomized to receive EBRT alone or with concurrent cisplatin (50 mg/m^2 days 1 and 22) and followed by chemotherapy with 4 cycles of carboplatin AUC 5 and paclitaxel 175 mg/m^2.

Table 2. Studies on chemotherapy treatment in UPSC/endometrial cancer

Study	Phase	Stage	CT Regimen	Survival
GOG 177	III	Advanced, Recurrence	DOX, CDDP vs. DOX, CDDP, TAX	
GOG 122	Pivotal	III-IV	DOX, CDDP + RT vs. RT	CT: + 24 months
Susumu et al.	III	Intermediate, high-risk	CYCLO, DOXO vs. RT	No difference
GOG 209	III	III-IV	CBDCA, TAX vs. DTX, CYCLO, EPIDOX	PFI 5.3 vs. 8.3 mos, OS 15.3 vs. 12.3 mos p=0.037
NSGO/EORTC		I-III, high-risk	Various CT regimens + RT vs. RT	PFS 82% vs. 75%
PORTEC 3	III	I-III, high-risk	CTRT vs. RT	Ongoing

CBDCA: carboplatin
CDDP: cisplatin
CT: chemotherapy
CYCLO: cyclophosphamide
DOX: doxorubicin
DTX: docetaxel
EPIDOX: epirubicin
RT: radiotherapy
TAX.: paclitaxel

All studies described seems to show a benefit in terms of PFI and OS in patients defined as high risk included UPSC treated with combination of chemotherapy cisplatinum-taxane based stage IB-IV plus or minus radiotherapy. PORTEC 3 will be able to answer to this question.

Conclusion

Serous endometrial intraepithelial carcinoma is a precursor and often co-exist with invasive serous invasive carcinoma. P53 is often mutated and UPSC is not part of BRCA 1 and BRCA2 syndromes, literature report only few cases.

UPSC is a rare disease with aggressive biological features and with tendency to spread outside the pelvis. Surgical approach is optimal cytoreduction performed with hysterectomy with bilateral salpingoophorectomy, pelvic and para-aortic lymphadenectomy and peritoneal washing, therefore it should consider to perform omentectomy and peritoneal biopsies Due to its aggressive phenotype is indicated adjuvant chemotherapy and radiotherapy even in early stages.

References

[1] American Cancer Society. Cancer facts and figures 2009. Atlanta: *American Cancer Society*; 2009.

[2] Hendrickson, M; Ross, J; Eifel, P; Martinez, A; Kenpson, R. Uterine papillary serous carcinoma: a highly malignant form of endometrial adenocarcinoma. *Am. J. Surg. Pathol.* 1982;6:93-108.

[3] Bokhman, JV. Two Pathogenetic types of endometrial cancer. *Gynecol. Oncol.* 1983;15:10-7.

[4] Kelly, MG; O'Malley, DM; Hui, P; McAlpine, J; Yu, H; Rutherford, TJ; et al. Improved survival in surgical stage I patients with uterine papillary serous carcinoma treated with adjuvant platinum-based chemotherapy. *Gynecol. Oncol.* 2005;8:353-9.

[5] Wilson, TO; Podratz, KC; Gaffey, TA; Malkasian, GD Jr; O'Brien, PC; Naessens, JM. Evaluation of unfavorable histologic subtype in endometrial adenocarcinoma. *Am. J. Obstet. Gynecol.* 1990;162:418-23.

[6] Christopherson, WM. The significance of the pathologic findings in endometrial cancer. *Clin. Obstet. Gynaecol.* 1986;13:673-93.

[7] Chen, JL; Trost, DC; Wilkinson, EJ. Endometrial papillary adenocarcinomas: two clinicopathological types. *Int. J. Gynecol. Pathol.* 1985;4:279-88.

[8] Sherman, ME; Bitterman, P; Rosenshein, NB; Delgado, G; Kurman, RJ. Uterine serous carcinoma. A morphologically diverse neoplasm with unifying clincopathological features. *Am. J. Surg. Pathol.* 1992;16:600-10.

[9] Sharon, X; Li, MD; Setsuko, KC; Liang, C; Shaopo, Z; Yi, Z; et al. Endometrial galandular dysplasia: a putative precursos lesion of uterine papillary serous carcinoma. partII: molecular features. *Int. J. Surg. Pathol.* 2004;12:319-31.

[10] Lax, SF; Kendall, B; Tashiro, H; Slebos, RJ; Hedrick, L. The frequency of p53; K-ras mutations and microsatellite instability differs in uterine endometrioid and serous carcinoma: evidence of distinct molecular genetic pathways. *Cancer* 2000;88-814-24.

[11] Tashiro, H; Isacson, C; Levine, R; Kurman, RJ; Cho, KR; Hedrick, L. p53 gene mutations are common in uterine serous carcinoma and occur early in their pathogenesis. *Am. J. Pathol.* 1997;150:177-85.

[12] Lavie, O; Ben-Arie, A; Segev Y; Faro, J; Barak, F; Haya, N; eet al. BRCA germline mutations in women with uterine serous carcinoma-still debate. *Int. J. Gynecol. Cancer* 2010;20:1531-4.

[13] Biron-Shental, T; Drucker, L; Altara, M; Bernheim, J; Fishman, A. High incidence of BRCA 1-2 germline mutations; previous breast cancer and familial cancer history in jewish patients with ugterine serous papillary carcinoma. *Eur. J. Surg. Oncol.* 2006;32:1097-100.

[14] Goshen, R; Chu, W; Elit, L; Pal, T; Hakimi, J; Ackerman, I; et al. is uterine papillary serous adenocarcinoma a manifestation of the hereditary breast ovarian cancer syndrome? *Gynecol. Oncol.* 2000; 79:477.

[15] Kwon, JS; Lenehan, J; Carey, M; Ainsworth, P. Prolonged surival among women with germline mutations and advanced endometrial cancer: a case series. *Int. J. Gynecol. Cancer* 2008;18:546-9.

[16] Lavie, O; Ben-Arie, A; Philip, A; Rennert, G; Cohen, Y; Feiner, B; et al. BRCA2 germline mutation in a women with uterine serous papillary carcinoma- case report. *Gynecol. Oncol.* 2005;99:486-8.
[17] Levine, DA; Lin, O; Barakat, RR; Robson, ME; McDermott, D; Cohen, L; et al. Risk of endometrial carcinoma associated with BRCA mutation. *Gynecol. Oncol.* 2001;80: 395-8.
[18] Hornereich, G; Beller, U; Lavie, O; Renbaum, P; Cohen, Y; Levy-Lahad, E. Is uterine serous papillary carcinoma a BRCA1 related disease? Case report and review of the literature. *Gynecol. Oncol.* 1999;75:300-4.
[19] Bandera, CA; Muto, MG; Schorge, JO; Berkowitz, RS; Rubin, SC; Mok, SC. BRCA1 gene mutations in women with papillary serous carcinoma of the peritoneum. *Obstet. Gynecol.* 1998;92:596-600.
[20] Duggan, BD; Felix, JC; Muderspach, LI; Tougeman, D; Zang, J; Shibata, D. Microsatellite instability in sporadic endometrial carcinoma. *J. Natl. Cancer Inst.* 1994;86:1216-21.
[21] Catasus, L; Machin, P.; Matias-Gulu, X; Prat, J. Microsatellite instability in endometrial carcinoma clinicopathologic correlatios in a series of 42 cases. *Hum. Pathol.* 1998;29:1160-4.
[22] An HJ; Knim Kl; Kim JY et al. Microsatellite instability in endometriod type endometrial adenocarcinoma is associated with poor prognostic indicators. *Am. J. Surg. Pathol.* 2007;31:846-53.
[23] Catasus, L; Gallardo, A; Prat, J. Molecular genetics of endometrial carcinoma. *Diagnostic Histopat* 2009;15:554-63.
[24] Boruta, DM; Gehrig, PA. Management of womwn with uterine papillary serous cancer: a Society of Gynecolgic Oncology (SGO) review. *Gynecol. Oncol.* 2009;115:142-53.
[25] Chan, JK; Cheung, MK. Therapeutic role of lymph node resection in endometrial cancer a study of 12333 patients. *Cancer* 2006;107(8):1823-30.
[26] Thomas, MB; Mariani, A; Cliby, WA; Keeney, GL. Role of cytoreduction in stage III and IV uterine papillary serpus carcinoma. *Gynecol. Oncol.* 2007;107:190-3.
[27] Karpas, CM; Bridge, MF. Endometrial adenocarcinoma with psammomatous bodies. *Am. J. Obstet. Gynecol.* 1963;87:935-43.
[28] Chan, JK; Loizzi, V; Youssef, M. Significance of comprehensive surgical staging in noninvasive papillary serous carcinoma of endometrium *Gynecol. Oncol.* 2003;90: 181-5.
[29] Geisler, JP; Geisler, HE; Melton, ME; Wiemann, MC. What staging surgery should be performed on patients with uterine papillary serous carcinoma. *Gynecol. Oncol.* 1999;74:465-7.
[30] Gehrig, PA; Van Lee, L; Fowler, WC Jr. The role of omentectomy during the surgical staging of uterine serous carcinoma. *Int. J. Gynecol. Cancer* 2003;13:212-5.
[31] Fader, AN; Drake, RD; O'Malley, D; Heidi, E; Gibbons, MS; Warner, KH; et al. Platinum/Taxan–based chemotherapy with or without radiation therapy favorably impacts survival outcomes in stage I uterine papillary serous carcinoma. *Cancer* 2009;15:2119-26.
[32] Kong, A; Johnson, N; Cornes, P; Simera, I; Collingwood, M; Williams, C; et al. Adjuvant radiotherapy for stage I endometrial cancer. *Cochrane Database Syst. Rev.* 2007;2:CD003916.

[33] Hogberg, T. Adjuvant chemotherapy in endometrial carcinoma: overview of randomised trials. *Clin. Oncol.* 2008;20:463-9.

[34] Randall, ME; Filiaci, VL; Muss, H; Spirtos, NM; Mannel, RS; WC Jr; et al. Randomized phase III trial of whole-abdominal irradiation versus doxorubicin and cisplatin chemotherapy in advanced. *J. Clin. Oncol.* 2006;24:365-44.

[35] Fleming, GF; Brunetto, VL; Cella, D; Look, KY; Reid, GC; Munkarah, AR; et al. Phase III trial of doxorubicin plus cisplatin with or without paclitaxel plus filgrastim in advanced endometrial carcinoma: a Gynecologic Oncology Group Study. *J. Clin. Oncol.* 2004;22:2159-66.

[36] Susumu, N; Sagae, S; Udagawa, Y; Niwa, K; Kuramoto, H; Satoh, S; et al; Japanese Gynecologic Oncology Group. Randomized phase III trial of pelvic radiotherapy versus cisplatin-based combined chemotherapy in patients with intermediate- and high-risk endometrial cancer: a Japanese Gynecologic Oncology Group study. *Gynecol. Oncol.* 2008;108:226-33.

[37] Nout, RA; van de Poll-Franse, LV; Lybeert, ML; Wárlám-Rodenhuis, CC; Jobsen, JJ; Mens, JW; et al. Long-term outcome and quality of life of patients with endometrial carcinoma treated with or without pelvic radiotherapy in the post operative radiation therapy in endometrial carcinoma 1 (PORTEC-1) trial. *J. Clin. Oncol.* 2011;29: 1692-700.

[38] Hogberg, T; Rosenberg, P; Kristensen, G; de Oliveira, CF; de Pont Christensen, R; Sorbe, B; et al. A randomized phase-III study on adjuvant treatment with radiation (RT) ± chemotherapy (CT) in early-stage high-risk endometrial cancer (NSGO-EC-9501/ EORTC 55991). *J. Clin. Oncol.* 2007;25:5503.

In: Endometrial Cancer: Prevention, Diagnosis and Treatment ISBN: 978-1-62257-740-8
Editor: Stefano Greggi

Chapter XIII

How to Select Patients to Adjuvant Radiotherapy?

Alessandro Colombo*[*], *Simona Sacco and Romerai D'Amico
Radiotherapy, "Alessandro Manzoni" Hospital, Lecco, Italy

Abstract

The endometrial cancer is the most common gynecological cancer, and the treatment of choice is the surgery. The addiction of an adjuvant treatment is related to different risk factors.

In recent years the indication for adjuvant therapy for endometrial cancer has undergone significant changes. This occurred following the publication of several controlled clinical studies related to different patient populations. Radiation therapy has always proved effective in improving local control, without having an impact on overall survival, resulting in an increase of late toxicity. On the other hand, chemotherapy appears to reduce the incidence of distant metastases but once again without increasing the survival.

The current trend is to reduce the impact of adjuvant therapy in low-risk tumors, favoring the observation or vaginal brachytherapy. In tumors at higher risk is increasingly being considered the association between radiation therapy and chemotherapy. Participation in controlled clinical trials is strongly recommended. In the absence of a shared standard of care, it becomes even more important to involve the patient in the therapeutic choice.

Introduction

The endometrial cancer is the most common gynecological cancer in industrialized countries. The treatment of choice is the surgery (total hysterectomy and bilateral salpingo-

[*] E-mail address: a.colombo@ospedale.lecco.it.

oophorectomy with or without lymphadenectomy), that must be performed whenever possible.

Based on the presence of different prognostic factors (stage of disease, type of histology, histologic grade, deep myometrial infiltration, detection of involvement of vascular spaces, nodal involvement), patients are divided into risk classes (Table 1).

The classification reported is the one proposed in 1988 by the International Federation of Gynecology and Obstetrics. The published studies refer in fact to this and not to that updated in 2009.

In about half of patients the disease presents a low-risk category (FIGO stage 1988 IA-IB, G1-2) while the other half is evenly distributed among patients at intermediate-risk (IA-IB, G3; IC-IIA, G1-2) and high-risk (all other stages). Adjuvant therapy is an open question, and was usually represented by radiotherapy. Until a few years ago radiotherapy as external beam radiation (EBRT), brachytherapy (BT) or as combination of these, was applied almost systematically in all patients with intermediate or high risk and often in the low risk group. The recent publication of several controlled clinical studies has opened new perspectives on these issues.

Table 1. Distribution of risk classes in endometrial cancer

Class of Risk	FIGO Stage 2009	FIGO Stage 1988	Grade	Histology
Low	IA	IA-IB-IIA(MI<50%)	1-2	E
Intermediate	IB	IC-IIA(MI>50%)	1-2	E
	IA	IA-IB	3	E
High	IB	IC-IIA(MI>50%)	3	E
	II-III-IV	IIB-III-IV	1-2-3	E
	IA-IB	IA-IB-IC	-	PS / CC

Legend. E: endometrioid; CC: clear cell; MI: myometrial invasion; PS: papillary-serous.

Low-Risk Group (Stage IA-IB, G1-2; IIA, Myometrial Invasion < 50%, G1-2)

The standard does not require any additional treatment after surgery, particularly given the high probability of recovery of a relapse that in about 70% of cases occurs in the vagina, with a probability of disease control at 5 years by about 50-70% [1,2]. A controlled clinical study published in 2009 by Sorbe, comparing observations versus vaginal BT in this category of patients, confirms that there are not significant differences between the two groups in terms of local control (96.9% observation, 98.8% brachytherapy), overall survival and toxicity, however moderate in both groups [3].

Intermediate-Risk Group (IA-B G3; IC, G1-2; IIA, Myometrial Invasion > 50%, G1-2)

In this population there are major problems due to the heterogeneity of the population. In the literature five controlled clinical studies have been published on the role of adjuvant therapy for this group of cancers. EBRT demonstrated a significant impact on local control of disease, but only in some subgroups showed a trend towards improved overall survival.

The trial published in 1980 by Aalders comparing adjuvant BT (60 Gy) combined with RT (44 Gy) to the same vaginal BT in 540 patients with stage I, showed a significant increase in local control (98.1% vs. 93.1%) as an advantage in terms of overall survival was present only in the subgroup of patients with deep myometrial invasion and tumor G3; this study shows that the lymph vascular spaces infiltration (LVSI) is an important prognostic factor with a significantly higher mortality rate in patients with this feature [4].

Broadly similar results are shown in the important study PORTEC-1 (pelvic RT vs. observation in 714 patients stage IB, G2-3; IC, G1-2), with a reduced risk of local recurrence from 14% to 5%, but no advantage on overall survival. The authors concluded that postoperative radiotherapy is not indicated in patients with stage 1 endometrial carcinoma below 60 years and patients with G2 tumours with superficial invasion [5].

An evaluation of the late toxic effects shows that there is a significant difference between the two groups with the overall toxicity of 26% for the radiotherapy group compared with 4% for the no further treatment arm. In addition all G3-4 toxicities (3%) were recorded in the radiation therapy group [6].

These results are confirmed by a re-evaluation with follow up of 15 years, in which the multivariate analysis confirms the prognostic significance of high/intermediate-risk (HIR) criteria for treatment selection (G3, age > 60 years and myometrial invasion > 50%). A trend for long-term risk of secondary cancers was also detected.

Therefore it is confirmed that EBRT should be avoided in patients with low/intermediate-risk endometrial cancer [7]. In this study were not included patients with stage IC G3 tumors, although they were still registered. An analysis of these 99 patients, published in 2004 showed that in this group, all underwent adjuvant pelvic RT, the rate of local control and survival at 5 years were significantly lower than those of the arm of the study PORTEC RT-1 (respectively 86% vs. 97% and 58% vs. 81%). This confirms that patients with stage IC, G3 endometrial carcinoma are at high risk of local relapse, early distant spread and endometrial carcinoma-related death.

To improve survival for this patient group more aggressive adjuvant therapy should be tested in randomized clinical trials, to improve the prognosis for these patients [8].

In the GOG 99 trial of 390 patients, with a design similar to the previous, there was a significant reduction of pelvic recurrence rate in RT arm (1.7 vs. 12%), more evident in the subgroup of patients defined as high intermediate risk category according to the following risk factors: increasing age, moderate to poorly differentiated tumor grade, presence of LVSI, and outer-third myometrial invasion. From the results of that analysis a subgroup of patients with HIR was defined as: patients older than 70 years with only one of the other risk factors, patients aged 50 years or more with any two of the other risk factors, or any age with all three of the other risk factors. The difference in OS between the two arms (95.8 vs.92.6%) showed a trend in favour of radiation therapy without reaching statistical significance. It should however be noted that in about half of the deceased patients the cause was not related to endometrial cancer [9].

This study was criticized because large majority of patients were in the low-risk class (58% stage IB, 82% grade 1 or 2, 41% under 60 years). Moreover because the study was closed to patient accrual more than 8 years before the publication of the paper (in 1995), is not clear why are taken into account the 2 year local control rates and 4 year survival rates: in fact, late relapses are not rare, even though most of these occurs in the first 24 months [10,11].

In the study of non-inferiority PORTEC-2, 427 patients in high or intermediate risk class (age > 60 years, stage IC G1-2, or stage IIA IBG3 G1-2 with myometrial invasion < 50%) were randomized between the vaginal BT and EBRT: despite a modest but significant increase in pelvic recurrence in the BT arm (3.6% vs. 0.3%), the rates of distant metastases, disease-free and overall survival were similar.

The conclusion is that vaginal BT is effective in ensuring vaginal control, with fewer gastrointestinal toxic effects than with EBRT (G1-2 12.6% vs. 53.8%) so vaginal BT should be considered the treatment of choice in high intermediate risk endometrial cancer, due to less toxicity and improved quality of life [12].

These results were confirmed in a Sweden clinical trial published in 2011, in which 527 patients medium-risk endometrial carcinomas (FIGO surgical stage I; endometrioid histological type; presence of one of the following risk factors: FIGO G3, myometrial infiltration > 50%, DNA aneuploidy; nuclear grade 1-2, pathologically negative lymph nodes, negative abdominal cytology) were randomly assigned to vaginal BT plus EBRT (arm A) or to the same BT (arm B).

Less vaginal recurrences were diagnosed in the combined treatment arm (1.9% vs. 2.7%). Five-year locoregional relapse rates were 1.5% after EBRT plus vaginal BT and 5% after vaginal irradiation alone. No difference in terms of overall survival rates was detected nor for endometrial cancer-related death. Combined radiotherapy was well tolerated, with serious (G3) late side effects of less than 2%. However, there was a significant difference in favour of vaginal BT alone in terms of cumulative toxicity.

Combined RT should be probably better for cases with two or more high-risk factors. Vaginal BT alone should be the adjuvant treatment option in the other cases [13].

Recently have been published the results of the study of ASTEC-NCIC on 1408 patients with stage IB G3, IC-IIA, randomly allocated to hysterectomy and bilateral salpingo-oophorectomy, peritoneal washings, and palpation of para-aortic nodes versus standard surgery plus lymphadenectomy [14]. After surgery, according to the presence of risk factors, 905 patients were randomized to observation or to EBRT with a dose of 40-46 Gy to the pelvis; BT was allowed according to the Centre's policy for stage I or IIA women randomization arm. Primary outcome measure was overall survival, and all analyses were by intention to treat.

After a median follow-up of 58 months, there was no evidence that overall survival with external beam radiotherapy was better than observation (84% in both groups).There was a lower incidence of local recurrences in the RT arm with a 5-year cumulative incidence rate of 6.1% in the observation group and 3.2% in the EBRT group. The severe late toxicity was higher in the RT arm (8% vs. 3%)

This study presents some problems because BT has been administered in more than half of patients in each arm, then only 92% of patients in the RT arm carried out the treatment and of these 18% received a lower dose of 40 Gy. A meta-analysis considering the data of PORTEC-1 GOG 99, and ASTEC-NCIC confirmed, however, no significant impact on survival of RT [15].

In conclusion, for patients with cancer at intermediate risk or high-intermediate risk, radiation brings an advantage in terms of local control, even if they are small and not without complications, while no significant impact on survival is detected.

High-Risk Group (IC, G3; IIB; III; IVA)

Five other prospective randomized studies take into account patients with locally advanced disease.

In the study sponsored by the Italian National Research Council, published in 2006, 345 patients with stages IC G3, II G3 (myometrial invasion > 50%) and III, submitted to hysterectomy and bilateral salpingo-oophorectomy with or without pelvic lymphadenectomy, were randomized between pelvic RT (45 Gy) and chemotherapy exclusive (cisplatin, CDDP, cyclophosphamide, CTX, and adriamycin, ADM, for 5 cycles). With a median survival of 95.5 months this study has not shown any difference in terms of 7 year DFS (56 vs. 60%) and OS (62%) between the two arms. In patients undergoing RT was achieved better local control of disease, while those treated with chemotherapy showed a lower rate of distant metastasis. Both treatments were well tolerated [16].

On a population of 384 patients, with characteristics quite similar to that of the previous study (IC-IIIC FIGO stage endometrial carcinoma with deeper than 50% myometrial invasion), the trial of the Japanese Gynecologic Oncology Group (JGOG), included a randomization between pelvic RT (45-50 Gy) and chemotherapy (CDDP, CTX and ADM for at least 3 courses). Also in this case no significant difference for DFS (83.5 vs. 81.8%) or OS (85.3 vs. 86.7%) was detected. Was noted, however, that patients at high intermediate risk (stage IC patients over age 70 years or having G3 endometrioid adenocarcinoma or stage II or IIIA positive cytology with deeper than 50% myometrial invasion in the corpus) had a better result in the chemotherapy arm, but the authors recognize that the validity of this subset analysis is limited. G3 and G4 toxicities were experienced in 1.6% (3/193) of the pelvic radiation therapy and 4.7% (9/192) of the CAP groups [17].

The Finnish study of 156 patients IA-IIIA-B and IC G3 published in 2008, with a randomization between RT alone and the same RT associated with 3 cycles of CDDP, ADM and CTX, does not demonstrate significant differences in overall survival, disease-free (84.7% in the RT group, 82.1% in the chemo-RT) and local control of disease. Curiously, the rate of distant metastases was higher in patients in the chemo-RT arm (20.2 vs. 13.8). In conclusion, there would be no benefit from adding chemotherapy to radiotherapy in this series. It should be noted, however, that only one third of patients had G3 disease and that only about 60% of the patients had infiltration of the outer half of myometrium [18].

At the 2007 ASCO Annual Meeting were presented the results of the study NSGO-EC-9501/EORTC 55991, which assigned 367 patients with stage I-IIIC (with sufficiently high risk of micrometastases) to a pelvic RT (44 Gy) associated or not to BT or to the same RT given before or after 4 cycles of CT with CDDP and ADM. With a median follow-up of 3.5 years, the PFS was significantly greater in the chemotherapy arm, although 27% of patients had not received a complete chemotherapy [19].

Recently, data from 383 patients in the study NSGO-EC-9501/EORTC 55991 were collected and analyzed together with those enrolled in the ILIADE III - MANGO (157 patients). In total 540 patients are examined (534 of these evaluable) with stage I-IIIC (all with high risk of micrometastases) assigned to a pelvic RT (44-50 Gy) with or without a vaginal brachytherapy or to the same RT given before or after 4 cycles of CT with ADM or CDDP and carboplatin, CBDCA and taxol, TXL. From this analysis it appears that the cause-specific survival was significantly greater in the chemo-radiation arm (p=0.01), while for absolute survival, there would be only a trend (p=0.07). It should be noted that published data can be criticized, given the variety of treatments administered, and the collection incomplete of certain data: for example, in the 15% of the patients the histological grade of the disease is unknown and for the 46% of the population is not known whether has been carried a lymphadenectomy [20].

The GOG 122 trial compares whole abdominal irradiation (WAI) and chemotherapy in 396 patients with stages III and IV with any histological type, with residual disease less than 2 cm. The arm RT planned WAI 30 Gy / 20 fractions plus a pelvic boost of 15 Gy / 8 fractions, while the CT consisted of CDDP + ADM for 8 cycles every 3 weeks. The differences in favor of the chemotherapy arm are significant both in terms of DFS (50 vs. 38%) and OS (55 vs. 42%), as was to be expected given the low doses of radiotherapy and histological features and distribution of the disease. Toxicity was greater in the CT arm. It should be stressed that this cannot be considered an adjuvant therapy study in the strict sense, given the possible presence of macroscopic residual disease [21].

In case of illness at high risk of metastases the chemotherapy should be considered as associated with radiotherapy as a therapy exclusive, although only in this study an advantage is showed for this treatment in terms of overall survival compared with a sub-optimal radiotherapy.

Conclusion

In light of the foregoing, it can be concluded that at present the only standard supported by adequate levels of evidence is the clinical and instrumental monitoring and therapy to tumor recurrence in low-risk class. For patients with intermediate risk disease category options are represented by brachytherapy, external radiation therapy and observation (in particular for the class of low-intermediate risk). In any case we may affirm that in patients with the disease in high intermediate and high risk class chemotherapy may contribute to improve survival, while radiotherapy helps to reduce the risk of local recurrence, so probably the patients in these classes may benefit from an integration of radiotherapy and chemotherapy (Table 2).

These findings deserve to be confirmed in large population studies and careful selection of patients, and they will move towards new studies that combine the two methods both as concurrent or sequential treatment.

The ongoing PORTEC 3 study is comparing radiotherapy with the concomitant and sequential use of chemotherapy and radiotherapy in patients with endometrioid stage I grade 3, stage II-III and any stage serous and clear cell carcinomas. There are two recruiting GOG trials (249 and 258) comparing combined chemotherapy and radiotherapy to radiotherapy alone or chemotherapy alone.

In selecting an adjuvant treatment, if there are no precise indications based on evidence, it is essential to adequately inform the patient, presenting risks and benefits of different options. Should not be forgotten that the improvement of local control of disease is an important result: recurrence, in fact, results usually in more aggressive and toxic therapies with respect to adjuvant treatment, and has a very negative psychological impact.

Table 2. Adjuvant treatment in endometrial cancer

FIGO Stage	Adjuvant Treatment	
I	IA G1-2	Observation
	IA G3 IB G1-2	Observation or vaginal BT - if negative prognostic factor*: consider pelvic RT and/or adjunctive CT
	IB G3	Pelvic RT - if negative prognostic factor*: consider combination of RT and CT
II	Pelvic RT and vaginal BT - if G1, MI<50%, no LVSI and complete surgical staging: consider BT alone - - if negative prognostic factor*: CT ± RT	
III-IV	CT - if close surgical margins or parametrial invasion: consider RT (± BT) - if positive nodes: CT-RT - if metastatic disease: palliative CT-RT	

Legend. BT: brachytherapy; CT: chemotherapy; LVSI: lymph vascular space involvement; MI: myometrial invasion; RT: radiotherapy.

* G3, MI, LVSI, cervical glandular involvement, incomplete surgical staging, age > 60 years.

References

[1] Jhingran A, Burke TW, Eifel PJ. Definitive radiotherapy for patients with isolated vaginal recurrence of endometrial carcinoma after hysterectomy, *Int. J. Radiat. Oncol. Biol. Phys.*, 56:1366–1372, 2003.

[2] Creutzberg CL, van Putten WLJ, Koper PC, Lybeert MLM, Jobsen JJ, Wàrlàm-Rodenhuis CC, De Winter KAJ, Lutgens LCHW, van den Bergh ACM, van der Steen-Banasik E, Beerman E, van Lent M for the PORTEC Study Group. Survival after relapse in patients with endometrial cancer: results from a randomized trial. *Gynecol. Oncol.* 89: 201–209, 2003.

[3] Sorbe B, Nordström B, Mäenpää J, Kuhelj J, Kuhelj D, Okkan S, Delaloye JF, Frankendal B, Intravaginal brachytherapy in FIGO stage I low-risk endometrial cancer: a controlled randomized study. *Int. J. Gynecol. Cancer*;19:873-878, 2009.

[4] Aalders J, Abeler V, Kolstad P, Onsrud M. Postoperative external irradiation and prognostic parameters in stage I endometrial carcinoma: clinical and histopathologic study of 540 patients. *Obstet. Gynecol.* 1980; 56: 419-427.

[5] Creutzberg CL, van Putten WL, Koper PC, Lybeert ML, Jobsen JJ, Warlam-Rodenhuis CC, et al. Surgery and postoperative radiotherapy versus surgery alone for patients with stage-1 endometrial carcinoma: multicentre randomised trial. PORTEC Study Group. Post Operative Radiation Therapy in Endometrial Carcinoma. *Lancet;* 355: 1404-1411, 2000.

[6] Creutzberg CL, van Putten WL, Koper PC et al. The morbidity of treatment for patients with Stage I endometrial cancer: results from a randomized trial. Int. J. Radiat. Oncol. Biol. Phys. 2001;51:1246–55.
[7] Creutzberg CL, Nout RA, , Lybeert MLM et al., Fifteen-year radiotherapy outcomes of the randomized PORTEC-1 trial for endometrial carcinoma. *Int. J. Radiat. Oncol. Biol. Phys.*, 81:631–638, 2011.
[8] Creutzberg CL, van Putten WL, Warlam-Rodenhuis CC, van den Bergh AC, de Winter KA, Koper PC, et al. Outcome of high-risk stage IC, grade 3, compared with stage I endometrial carcinoma patients: the Postoperative Radiation Therapy in Endometrial Carcinoma Trial. *J. Clin. Oncol.*, 22:1234–41, 2004.
[9] Roberts JA, Brunetto VL, Zaino RJ, Spirtos NM, Bloss JD, Pearlman A, Maiman MA, Bell JG. A phase III trial of surgery with or without adjunctive external pelvic radiation therapy in intermediate risk endometrial adenocarcinoma: a Gynecologic Oncology Group study. *Gynecol. Oncol.*; 92: 744-751,2004.
[10] Creutzberg CL, GOG-99: ending the controversy regarding pelvic radiotherapy for endometrial carcinoma? *Gynecol. Oncol.* 92:740–743 , 2004.
[11] Berman ML, Adjuvant radiotherapy following properly staged endometrial cancer: what role? *Gynecol. Oncol.* 92:737-739, 2004.
[12] Nout RA, Smit VT, Putter H, Jürgenliemk-Schulz IM, Jobsen JJ, Lutgens LC, van der Steen-Banasik EM, Mens JW, Slot A, Kroese MC, van Bunningen BN, Ansink AC, van Putten WL, Creutzberg CL; Vaginal brachytherapy versus pelvic external beam radiotherapy for patients with endometrial cancer of high-intermediate risk (PORTEC-2): an open-label, non-inferiority, randomised trial. *Lancet.* 375:816-23, 2010.
[13] Sorbe B, Horvath G, Andersson H, Boman K, Lundgren C, Pettersson B, External pelvic and vaginal irradiation versus vaginal irradiation alone as postoperative therapy in medium-risk endometrial carcinoma—a prospective randomized study. *Int. J. Radiat. Oncol. Biol. Phys*, e-pub 2011.
[14] Kitchener H, Swart A, Qian W, Amos C, Parmar MK, Study group ASTEC. Efficacy of systematic pelvic lymphadenectomy in endometrial cancer (MRC ASTEC trial): a randomised study. *Lancet;*373:125–36. 2009.
[15] ASTEC/EN.5 Study Group, Blake P, Swart AM, Orton J, Kitchener H, Whelan T, Lukka H, Eisenhauer E, Bacon M, Tu D, Parmar MK, Amos C, Murray C, Qian W. Adjuvant external beam radiotherapy in the treatment of endometrial cancer (MRC ASTEC and NCIC CTG EN.5 randomised trials): pooled trial results, systematic review, and meta-analysis. *Lancet*; 373:137-46, 2009.
[16] Maggi R, Lissoni A, Spina A, Melpignano M, Zola P, Favalli G, Colombo A and Fossati R Adjuvant chemotherapy vs radiotherapy in high-risk endometrial carcinoma: results of a randomised trial. *British Journal of Cancer*; 95, 266–271, 2006.
[17] Susumu N, Sagae S, Udagawa Y, Niwa K, Kuramoto H, Satoh S, Kudo R; Randomized phase III trial of pelvic radiotherapy versus cisplatin-based combined chemotherapy in patients with intermediate- and high-risk endometrial cancer: a Japanese Gynecologic Oncology Group study. *Gynecol. Oncol..;*108:226-33, 2008.
[18] Kuoppala T, Mäenpää J, Tomas E, Puistola U, Salmi T, Grenman S, Lehtovirta P, Fors M, Luukkaala T, Sipilä P, Surgically staged high-risk endometrial cancer: randomized study of adjuvant radiotherapy alone vs. sequential chemo-radiotherapy. *Gynecol Oncol.* 110:190-5, 2008.

[19] Hogberg T, Rosenberg P, Kristensen G, de Oliveira CF, de Pont Christensen R, Sorbe B, Lundgren C, Salmi T, Andersson H, Reed NS. A randomized phase-III study on adjuvant treatment with radiation (RT) ± chemotherapy (CT) in early-stage high-risk endometrial cancer (NSGO-EC-9501/EORTC 55991). *J. Clin. Oncol.*, 2007 *ASCO Annual Meeting Proceedings* 25, (18S): 5503, 2007.

[20] Hogberg T, Signorelli M, Freire de Oliveira C, Fossati R , Lissoni AA, Sorbe B, Andersson H, Grenman S, Lundgren, Rosenberg P, Boman K, Tholander B, Scambia G, Reed N, Cormio G, Tognon G, Clarke J, Sawicki T, Zola P and KristensenG. Sequential adjuvant chemotherapy and radiotherapy in endometrial cancer – Results from two randomised studies *Eur. J. Cancer*. 46: 2422-2431, 2010.

[21] Randall ME, Filiaci VL, Muss H, Spirtos NM, Mannel RS, Fowler J, Thigpen JT, Benda JA. Randomized phase III trial of whole-abdominal irradiation versus doxorubicin and cisplatin chemotherapy in advanced endometrial carcinoma: a Gynecologic Oncology Group study. *J. Clin. Oncol.;* 24:36-44, 2006.

In: Endometrial Cancer: Prevention, Diagnosis and Treatment ISBN: 978-1-62257-740-8
Editor: Stefano Greggi

Chapter XIV

Chemotherapy in the Adjuvant and Advanced-Recurrent Settings

Sandro Pignata*[*], *Carmela Pisano, Sabrina Chiara Cecere, Francesca Esposito, Davide Leopardo, Giovanni Salvatore Bruni and Gaetano Facchini

Medical Oncology, National Cancer Institute "G. Pascale," Naples, Italy

Abstract

Endometrial cancer is a highly curable malignancy when it presents as uterine-confined disease, but the prognosis for metastatic or recurrent endometrial cancer is poor. For those patients which are diagnosed at an early stage, surgery alone may be adequate for cure and clinical outcome is often favorable, with approximately 90% of cases surviving at 5 years. However, after primary diagnosis and treatment, roughly 30-40% of patients with stage III and IV are expected to recur within the following 5 years. Adjuvant treatment for endometrial cancer is not yet clearly defined. FIGO Stage I-III endometrial cancer patients, usually undergo surgery and some of them are offered adjuvant treatment based on risk assessment. Grade, age, stage are considered all independent risk factor for recurrence. Radiotherapy (RT) has been considered the adjuvant therapy of choice for decades, being able to reduce local recurrence rate and improving progression free survival, but without any impact on overall survival. In the last two decades, a shift toward the use of more systemic chemotherapy (CT) in addition or instead of radiation has occurred, although few prospective studies have been performed in this field.

On the other end the median survival of women with recurrent or metastatic endometrial cancer is only approximately 12 months. Hormonal therapy, most commonly with progestins, benefits a small group of patients. Cytotoxic chemotherapy is indicated as frontline treatment for the majority of women with metastatic or recurrent disease. Combination chemotherapy typically produces quite high response rates, although combination regimens have not always improved survival historically. Recently, a GOG

[*] E-mail address: s.pignata@istitutotumori.na.it.

randomized trial compared doxorubicin plus cisplatin to the triplet of doxorubicin, cisplatin and paclitaxel and it was found that the addition of paclitaxel significantly improved response rate, progression-free survival, and overall survival although at the price of significant toxicity.

Introduction

Endometrial cancer is the most common malignancy of the female genital tract; the crude incidence of endometrial carcinoma in the European Union is estimated to be 16 cases/100,000 women/year (range 13-24) with a mortality rate of 4-5 cases/100,000/year [1].

For those patients which are diagnosed at an early stage, surgery alone may be adequate for cure and clinical outcome is often favorable, with approximately 90% of cases surviving at 5 years. Nevertheless, approximately 16% of cases are identified with either stage III or IV disease [2] with a 5-year survival rates ranging from 30-89% and 0-10% [3], respectively. Moreover, after primary diagnosis and treatment, roughly 30-40% of patients with stage III and IV are expected to recur within the following 5 years [3]. Early stage endometrial cancer is categorize in 3 different risk categories for recurrence. FIGO stage, grading, and age are considered the most important prognostic factors for recurrence. FIGO stage I, grade 1 cancers are considered at low risk for recurrence and are usually treated only by surgery. The presence of grade 3, and the deep invasion of the myometrium define a category of patients at high risk for relapse and in these patients an adjuvant treatment is usually prescribed. Also elderly patients have a poorer prognosis compared to their younger counterpart. Histology also offers prognostic information; compared to the endometrioid histotype, serous papillary and clear cell are associated to an increased risk of recurrence, although their optimal adjuvant treatment has not been clearly established.

Chemotherapy as Adjuvant Therapy

Adjuvant treatment for endometrial cancer is not yet clearly defined. FIGO Stage I-III endometrial cancer patients, usually undergo surgery and some of them are offered adjuvant treatment based on risk assessment. Grade, age, stage are all independent risk factors for recurrence and are usually considered for the choice of the adjuvant therapy [4].

Radiotherapy (RT) has been considered the adjuvant therapy of choice for decades, being able to reduce local recurrence rate and improving progression free survival, but without any impact on overall survival [5]. In the last two decades, a shift toward the use of more systemic chemotherapy (CT) in addition or instead of radiation has occurred, although few prospective studies have been performed in this field. A shift from external beam radiotherapy (EBRT) to the use of brachytherapy (BT) has also occurred in the last years based on randomized trial showing equal efficacy and a better toxicity profile.

Few randomized trials [6-8] (Table 1) in patients with high-risk endometrial cancer have investigated the role of CT compared to RT as adjuvant therapy in endometrial cancer. The GOG 122 study [6], comparing abdominal irradiation versus CT has shown a significant improvement in PFS and OS in favor of the systemic treatment. However, this trial included also patients with FIGO stage IV (27%), although with optimal residual disease after surgery. In this study, the pattern of recurrence was different, with CT more efficient then abdominal irradiation in reducing distant recurrences (10% vs. 19%), at the cost of a higher pelvic failure rate (18 vs. 13%). A Japanese randomized study compared pelvic RT with cisplatin-based CT in patients with intermediate/high-risk endometrial cancer. No statistically significant difference was found in the whole study population, while both PFS and overall survival were significantly better for patients assigned to CT in the subgroup characterized by higher risk [7]. On the other hand, superiority for adjuvant CT over RT alone was not confirmed in an Italian trial [8] in which 345 women with high-risk resected endometrial cancer (IC-III, 65% stage III) were randomly assigned to six cycles of CAP (cisplatin, doxorubicin and cyclophosphamide) or RT (45 to 50 Gy) following surgery.

Table 1. Trials with radiotherapy versus chemotherapy in high-risk endometrial cancer

Trial	FIGO Stage	Treatment Arms	5-yrs PFS	5-yrs OS
GOG 122	III-IV (RD≤2cm)	WAI vs. Adjuvant CT (AP)	42 vs. 38%	53 vs. 42%
Japanese GOG study	IC-III	Adjuvant PRT vs. Adjuvant CT (CAP)	83.5% vs. 81.8%	85.3% vs. 86.7%
Maggi, et al.	IC, G3 II, G3, MI>50% III	PRT vs. Adjuvant CT (CAP)	63 vs. 60%	69 vs. 66%

Legend. AP: doxorubicin and cisplatin; CAP: cyclophosphamide, doxorubicin and cisplatin; CT: chemotherapy; MI: myometrial invasion; PRT: pelvic radiotherapy; RD: residual disease; WAI: whole-abdominal irradiation.

The lower rate of distant metastatic relapses found in these trials in patients treated with CT may support the hypothesis of the usefulness of a combined approach with CT and RT, given concurrently or sequentially.

Few trials have evaluated the role of CT in addition to RT in endometrial cancer, and the studies were performed in a mixed population of high risk patients including stage III; only few randomized trials have been performed and most data come from phase II or retrospective studies that suggest encouraging OS and PFS data for the combined modality [9-18] (Table 2). The largest randomized phase III trial addressing this question is the NSGO-EC-9501/EORTC 55991 [17] study that randomized 372 patients with high-risk endometrial cancer (stage I to IIIC, grade 3, deep myometrial invasion, DNA non-diploidy, serous, clear-cell, or anaplastic histology) to receive either EBRT with or without vaginal BT, or RT plus sequential platinum-based CT. In the final analysis [17], there was a significant 36% reduction in the rate of relapse or death with the combined therapy (HR 0.64, 95%CI 0.41-0.99, p=0.04), and the difference favoring RT-CT was significant also for Cancer Specific Survival with HR 0.51 (95%CI 0.28-0.90, p=0.02); on the other hand, no significant difference was identified in the OS. However, in this trial only the 1.6% of the entire study population was affected by stage III endometrial cancer. On the other side, the addition of CT.

Table 2. Multimodal approaches: comparison between chemotherapy or radiotherapy alone and combined treatment

Trial	Disease	Treatment Arms	RR	5-yrs DFS	5-yrs OS
Hoskins et al.	Group 1 Primarily advanced non-PSC	CT (CBDCA AUC 5-7, PTX 175 mg/m^2, 1q28) + RT	78%	n/a	2% (3yrs)
	Group 2 Primarily advanced PSC	CT (CBDCA AUC 5-7, PTX 175 mg/m^2, 1q28) + RT	60%		39%
	Group 3 Recurrent non-PSC	CT (CBDCA AUC 5-7, PTX 175 mg/m^2, 1q28)	56%		43%
	Group 4 Recurrent PSC	CT (CBDCA AUC 5-7, PTX 175 mg/m^2, 1q28)	50%		n/a
Lupe et al.	FIGO Stage III-IV	Adjuvant CT (PTX 175mg/m^2, CBDCA 350 mg/m^2, 1q21) → PRT (45Gy) → 2 cycles of CT	n/a	n/a	55% (2yrs)
		Para-aortic RT and/or VBT added at the discretion of the treating physician			55%
RTOG 9708	FIGO Stage IC, G2-3 IIA-B III	PRT (45Gy / 25 fractions) + CDDP 50mg/m^2 1q28 → VBT → 4 courses of CDDP 50 mg/m^2, PTX 175 mg/m^2 (at 4-week intervals following completion of RT)	n/a	81% (4yrs)	85% (4yrs)

Trial	Disease	Treatment Arms	RR	5-yrs DFS	5-yrs OS
Secord et al.	FIGO Stage III-IV	Adjuvant CT* altretamine Adjuvant RT Concomitant CT-RT * CAP, TAP, CP, single-agent CDDP	n/a	19% 59% 62%	33% 70% 79% (3yrs)
Kuoppala et al.	FIGO Stage IA-B, G3 IC-IIIA	Arm 1: RT alone (56Gy) Arm 2: RT + CDDP 50mg/m^2, EPI 60mg/m^2, CYC 500mg/m^2	n/a	18 (mos) 25 (mos)	85% 82%

Legend. BT: brachytherapy; CAP: cyclophosphamide, doxorubicin and cisplatin; CBDCA: carboplatin; CDDP: cisplatin; CP: cyclophosphamide and cisplatin; CT: chemotherapy; CYC: cyclophosphamide; EPI: epirubicin; PRT: pelvic radiotherapy; PSC: papillary serous cancer; PTX: paclitaxel; RT: radiotherapy; TAP: paclitaxel, doxorubicin and cisplatin; VBT: vaginal brachytherapy.

to adjuvant RT failed to improve overall survival or recurrence free interval in a randomized Finnish trial, in which 156 patients with high-risk disease (stage I-IIIA) were randomly assigned to adjuvant RT alone or RT combined with three courses of cisplatin, epirubicin and cyclophosfamide [18].

More advanced stages have been enrolled in the MANGO-ILIADE III trial [19], in which more than 60% of patients were III stage disease; in this study patients were randomly allocated to adjuvant CT (doxorubicin 60 mg/m^2 plus cisplatin 50 mg/m^2, every 3 weeks for three cycles) with or without sequential RT. The final data, recently published, pointed in the same direction of NSGO-EC-9501/EORTC55991 but without reaching a statistically significant difference between control and study arms. Differently, when pooling the data from both studies there was a highly significant difference favoring RT-CT [19], when considering both PFS (HR 0.63, 95%CI 0.41-0.99, p=0.009) and CSS (HR 0.55, 95%CI 0.35-0.88, p=0.01). The question of the role of CT in high risk-advanced stage of endometrial cancer is now the subject of a large multinational randomized phase III trial, the PORTEC 3, comparing RT alone with RT, concurrent CT and sequential CT in high risk endometrial cancer. This trial is ongoing and the results will not be available for a number of years [20]. Recently, a retrospective study from our group [21] showed in a cohort of patients with stage III endometrial cancer the combine sequential treatment of CT and RT was more effective than CT or RT alone. Prospective phase III trial are ongoing to clarify the role of combined CT and RT in this setting.

Chemotherapy in Advanced Disease

Patients with advanced or recurrent disease have a worse prognosis, and results obtained with systemic therapy are far from being impressive. Treatment of advanced endometrial cancer remains a difficult task for the oncologist due to both the small number of studies performed and the absence of a clear indication of the best therapeutic option to adopt in a population of patients that are often elderly and have associated comorbidities. In fact, many patients with endometrial cancer are obese with significant co-morbidity such as diabetes mellitus and ischemic heart disease, which can restrict treatment options.

Therapy for recurrent or metastatic endometrial cancer is palliative. Unfortunately, the 5-year survival of patients with recurrent or metastatic endometrial cancer remains poor, with median survival times of less than a year in most Gynecologic Oncology Group (GOG) trials. Although reported response rates (RRs) of the most active systemic CT have been as high as 70% in this setting, the median duration of such responses remains short, from 4 to 8 months [22].

Chemotherapy and hormonal therapy are the mainstays of treatment for advanced disease, except for rare cases amenable to surgery or RT such as isolated vaginal recurrences or solitary pulmonary metastases. Hormonal therapy with progestins may be effective for patients whose tumors are estrogen and progesterone receptor-positive (more common with low-grade tumors), but it is relatively ineffective for receptor-poor tumors. Among patients with advanced endometrial cancer treated with medroxyprogesterone acetate on a GOG trial (GOG 81), 37% of patients whose tumors were progesterone receptor-positive responded compared with 8% of women whose cancers were progesterone receptor-negative [23,24].

Women whose tumors have low levels of progesterone-receptor expression tend to have higher-grade histology. CT then becomes the cornerstone of treatment. Other trials have evaluated the role of tamoxifene or of a sequential approach with progestins and tamoxifene, showing activity on receptor-positive patients.

Early studies used single CT agents with modest response rates and remission durations of 4-6 months were seen. Combinations of two or more drugs have been employed, but the general perception is that these patients tolerate CT less well than comparable patients with breast or ovarian cancers [22].

Combination CT typically produces higher response rates than single-agent therapy, but it tends to produce more toxicity, and the effect on survival of combination therapy versus sequential single-agent therapy remains uncertain in most metastatic solid tumors. Recent systematic reviews of randomized clinical trials show that there is a limited body of evidence available to help clinicians make decisions about the best CT regimen to be used in advanced or recurrent endometrial cancer [25,26]. Doxorubicin, with or without cisplatin, has long been considered the standard regimen for treating advanced or recurrent endometrial carcinoma. Single agent CT with doxorubicin has achieved RRs in the range of 17-25% [27]. When cisplatin was combined with doxorubicin, two randomized trials demonstrated improved responses with the combination. Absolute RRs increased from 25 to 42% in one study [29] and from 17 to 43% in the other trial [30]. Unfortunately, neither trial showed improved survival. The only randomized trial (GOG 177) showing a survival advantage evaluated the addition of paclitaxel to cisplatin plus doxorubicin, but the three-drug arm was definitely more toxic, requiring filgrastim support and causing a significant increase in thrombocytopenia and neurotoxicity [29]. GOG 177, which accrued patients between 1998 and 2000, randomized them to doxorubicin 45 mg/m^2 and cisplatin 50 mg/m^2 on day 1 followed by paclitaxel 160 mg/m^2 on day 2 (TAP) with G-CSF support or AP. TAP produced a statistically significant improvement in RRs (57% vs. 34%), PFS (median, 8.3 vs. 5.3 months), and OS (median, 15.3 vs. 12.3 months) compared with AP.

Randomized studies in advanced endometrial cancer have been recently reviewed by the Cochrane [31]. Eleven studies were identified. The quality of the 11 identified RCTs of cytotoxic CT in advanced or recurrent endometrial adenocarcinoma randomly assigning 2,288 women was somewhat variable. Response rates varied between RCTs, with the worst rates in the most heavily pre-treated patients [31]. In a number of trials, combination therapy led to a higher response than single-agent treatment or other combinations [31], but with the exception of Fleming et al. [30], this better response rate did not translate into better PFS or OS, at least at the individual trial level. A meta-analysis of the six trials that compared more intense CT combinations indicates that more intense CT significantly improves the median PFS, but not OS. This is, however, at the expense of increased grade 3/4 toxicity. It should be noted that a number of these trials pre-date the routine use of the type-3 serotonin receptor (5-HT3) antagonists and the rate of grade 3 and 4 vomiting may be higher than what one would expect in current practice. Across these six trials, the results are fairly consistent and no one regimen appears superior to another in improving PFS and OS.

Thus, the only RCT that reported a significant improvement in PFS and OS was the GOG 177 that compared doxorubicin, cisplatin and paclitaxel versus doxorubicin and cisplatin [30], with the benefit associated with the paclitaxel-containing arm. Grade 3 or 4 thrombocytopenia and neurological toxicity, however, were also significantly greater and there were five treatment-related deaths with the paclitaxel arm. Clinicians therefore have to consider whether the modest survival gain of the order of 3 months justifies the toxicity of a three-drug combination in the individual patient.

Table 3. Combination chemotherapy trials

Trial	Year	Chemoterapy Regimen	n	RR	Median OS (months)
EORTC 55872	2003	DOX 60mg/m^2 d1q28	87	17%	7
		DOX 60mg/m^2 + CDDP 50mg/m^2 d1q28	90	43%	9
GOG 107	2004	DOX 60mg/m2 d1q21	150	25%	9.0
		DOX 60mg/m^2 + CDDP 50mg/m^2 d1q21	131	42%	6.7
GOG 48	1994	DOX 60mg/m^2 d1q21	132	22%	6.7
		DOX 60mg/m^2 + CYC 500mg/m^2 d1q21	144	30%	7.3
GOG 177	2004	DOX 60mg/m^2 d1 + CDDP 50mg/m^2 d1q21	129	34%	12.3
		DOX 45mg/m^2 + CDDP 50mg/m^2 + PTX 160mg/m^2 d1q21 + G-CSF	134	57%	15.3

Legend. CDDP: cisplatin; CYC: cyclophosphamide; DOX: doxorubicin; G-CSF: granulocyte colony-stimulating factor; PTX: paclitaxel.

The optimal CT regimen to be used is not yet established, but there is wide experience in other tumors with the use of carboplatin and paclitaxel together, and this combination merits consideration in endometrial cancer as well as carboplatin and liposomal doxorubicin for which more limited data exist. A trial is ongoing within the GOG group comparing carboplatin/paclitaxel with the triplet regimen of carboplatin/paclitaxel/doxorubicin [32].

References

[1] Jemal, A; Murray, T; Ward, E; et al. Cancer statistics; 2005. *CA Cancer J Clin* 2005;55:10-30.

[2] Werner, HMJ; Trovik, J; Marcickiewicz, J; et al. Revision of FIGO surgical staging in 2009 for endometrial cancer validates to improve risk stratification. *Gynecol Oncol* 2011 Nov 17. [Epub ahead of print]

[3] Scheithauer, HR; Schulz, DS; Belka, C. Endometrial cancer-reduce to the minimum. A new paradigm for adjuvant treatments? *Radiat Oncol* 2011;6:164.

[4] Colombo, N; Preti, E; Landoni, F; et al. ESMO Guidelines Working Group Endometrial cancer: ESMO Clinical Practice Guidelines for diagnosis, treatment and follow-up. *Ann Oncol* 2011;22(Suppl6):vi35-9.

[5] Smith, RS; Kapp, DS; Chen, Q; et al. Treatment of high-risk uterine cancer with whole abdomino-pelvic radiation therapy. *Int J Radiat Oncol Biol Phys* 2000;48:767-78.
[6] Randall, ME; Filiaci, VL; Muss, H; et al. Randomized phase III trial of whole abdominal irradiation versus doxorubicin and cisplatin chemotherapy in advanced endometrial carcinoma: a Gynecologic Oncology Group study. *J Clin Oncol* 2006;24:36-44.
[7] Susumu, N; Sagae, S; Udagawa, Y; et al. Randomized phase III trial of pelvic radiotherapy versus cisplatin-based combined chemotherapy in patients with intermediate-and high-risk endometrial cancer: a Japanese Gynecologic Oncology Group study. *Gynecol Oncol* 2008;108:226-33.
[8] Maggi, R; Lissoni, A; Spina, F; et al. Adjuvant chemotherapy vs radiotherapy in high-risk endometrial carcinoma: results of a randomized trial. *Br J Cancer* 2006;95:266-71.
[9] Hoskins, PJ; Swenerton, KD; Pike, JA; et al. Paclitaxel and carboplatin, alone or with irradiation, in advanced or recurrent endometrial cancer: a phase II study. *J Clin Oncol* 2001;19:4048-53.
[10] Greven, K; Winter, K; Underhill, K; et al. Final analysis of RTOG 9708: adjuvant postoperative irradiation combined with cisplatin/paclitaxel chemotherapy following surgery for patients with high-risk endometrial cancer. *Gynecol Oncol* 2006;103:155-9.
[11] Lupe, K; Kwon, J; D'Souza, D; et al. Adjuvant paclitaxel and carboplatin chemotherapy with involved field radiation in advanced endometrial cancer: a sequential approach. *Int J Radiat Oncol Biol Phys* 2007;67:110-6.
[12] Secord, AA; Havrilesky, LJ; Bae-Jump, V; et al. The role of multi-modality adjuvant chemotherapy and radiation in women with advanced stage endometrial cancer. *Gynecol Oncol* 2007;107:285-91.
[13] Kuoppala, T; Mäenpää, J; Tomas, E; et al. Surgically staged high-risk endometrial cancer: randomized study of adjuvant radiotherapy alone vs. sequential chemo-radiotherapy. *Gynecol Oncol* 2008;110:190-5.
[14] Fowler, JM; Brady, WE; Grigsby, PW; et al. Sequential chemotherapy and irradiation in advanced stage endometrial cancer: a Gynecologic Oncology Group phase I trial of doxorubicin-cisplatin followed by whole abdomen irradiation. *Gynecol Oncol* 2009;112:553-7.
[15] Secord, AA; Havrilesky, LJ; O'Malley, DM; et al. A multicenter evaluation of sequential multimodality therapy and clinical outcome for the treatment of advanced endometrial cancer. *Gynecol Oncol* 2009;114:442-7.
[16] De Marzi, P; Frigerio, L; Cipriani, S; et al. Adjuvant treatment with concomitant radiotherapy and chemotherapy in high-risk endometrial cancer: a clinical experience. *Gynecol Oncol* 2010;116:408-12.
[17] Hogberg, T; Rosenberg, P; Kristensen, G; et al. A randomized phase-III study on adjuvant treatment with radiation (RT)±chemotherapy (CT) in early stage high-risk endometrial cancer (NSGO-EC-9501/EORTC 55991). *J Clin Oncol* 2007;25:5503.
[18] Kuoppalaa, T; Mäenpääa, J; Tomasa, E; et al. Surgically staged high-risk endometrial cancer: Randomized study of adjuvant radiotherapy alone vs. sequential chemo-radiotherapy. *Gynecol Oncol* 2008;110:190-5.
[19] Hogberg, T; Signorelli, M; De Oliveira, CF; et al. Sequential adjuvant chemotherapy and radiotherapy in endometrial cancer-Results from two randomised studies. *Eur J Cancer* 2010;46:2422-31.

[20] National Cancer Institute. PORTEC 3:
[21] http://clinicaltrials.gov/ct2/show/NCT00411138.
[22] Marchetti, C; Pisano, C; Pignata, S; et al. Use of adjuvant therapy in patients with FIGO stage III endometrial carcinoma: a multicenter retrospective study. *Oncology* 2011;81:104-12.
[23] Obel, JC; Friberg, G; Fleming, GF; et al. Chemotherapy in Endometrial Cancer. *Clin Adv Hematol Oncol* 2006;4:459-68.
[24] Thigpen, JT; Brady, MF; Alvarez, RD; et al. Oral medroxyprogesterone acetate in the treatment of advanced or recurrent endometrial carcinoma: a dose-response study by the Gynecologic Oncology Group. *J Clin Oncol* 1999;17:1736-44.
[25] Iwai, K; Fukuda, K; Hachisuga, T; et al. Prognostic significance of progesterone receptor immunohistochemistry for lymph node metastases in endometrial carcinoma. *Gynecol Oncol* 1999;72:351-9.
[26] Polyzos, NP; Pavlidis, N; Paraskevaidis, E; et al. Randomized evidence for chemotherapy and hormonal therapy regimens for advanced endometrial cancer: an overview of survival data. *Eur J Cancer* 2006;42:319-26.
[27] Carey, MS; Gawlik, C; Fung-Kee-Fung, M; et al. Systematic review of systemic therapy for advanced or recurrent endometrial cancer. Cancer Care Ontario Practice Guidelines Initiative Gynecology Cancer Disease Site Group. *Gynecol Oncol* 2006;101:158-67.
[28] Thigpen, JT; Blessing, JA; DiSaia, PJ; et al. Randomize comparison of doxorubicin versus doxorubicin and cyclophosphamyde in advanced or recurrent endometrial cancer: a Gynecologic Oncology Group study. *J Clin Oncol* 1994;12:1408-14.
[29] Thigpen, JT; Brady, MF; Homesley, HD; et al. A phase III trial of doxorubicin with or without cisplatin: a Gynecologic Oncology Group study. *J Clin Oncol* 2004;22:3902-8.
[30] Aapro, MS; Van Wijk, FH; Bolis, G; et al. Doxorubicine versus doxorubicin and cisplatin in advanced endometrial cancer: definitive results by a randomized study (55872) of the EORTC gynecologic cancer group. *Ann Oncol* 2003;14:441-8.
[31] Fleming, GF; Brunetto, VL; Cella, D; et al. Phase III Trial of Doxorubicin Plus Cisplatin With or Without Paclitaxel Plus Filgrastim in Advanced Endometrial Carcinoma: A Gynecologic Oncology Group Study. *J Clin Oncol* 2004;22:2159-66.
[32] Johnson, N; Bryant, A; Miles, T; et al. Adjuvant chemotherapy for endometrial cancer after hysterectomy. Cochrane Database Syst Rev. *Cochrane Database Syst Rev* 2011;5:CD003175.
[33] National Cancer Institute, GOG-209: http://www.cancer.gov/search/ViewClinicalTrials.aspx?cdrid=305940&protocolsearchid=4206096&version=healthprofessional.

In: Endometrial Cancer: Prevention, Diagnosis and Treatment ISBN: 978-1-62257-740-8
Editor: Stefano Greggi

Chapter XV

Follow-Up Criteria: Background and Procedures

Paolo Zola*[*], *Stefania Perotto, Elisa Piovano and Luca Fuso
Obstetrics and Gynecology, University of Turin, Italy

Abstract

Endometrial cancer represents the most common gynecologic malignancy after breast cancer. The overall recurrence rate is 13% and correlates with prognostic factors of the primary tumor. The anatomic sites of endometrial cancer relapse are mostly equivalently distributed between local (pelvic) and distant (abdominal and chest). Most endometrial cancer recurrences are symptomatic, even if vaginal vault relapses represent a particular setting of a more frequently asymptomatic disease. Most of endometrial cancer recurrences occur within 3 years since diagnosis of primary tumor. Long term surveillance programs are mainly addressed to the early detection of the recurrence, the rationale of follow-up being that an earlier diagnosis of relapse correlates with lower morbidity and mortality rates. Adjunctive objectives of routine follow-up are identification of treatment complications and detection of possible second tumors associated with endometrial cancer. Although guidelines recommend minimalist follow-up, there is a wide variability in gynecological oncology practice. No rationale is available today for any particular follow-up protocol; follow-up procedures should probably be tailored according to different prognostic factors; only physical examination, including pelvic-rectal examination, showed some utility in detecting recurrence.

In this setting TOTEM trial is ongoing in Italy: this RCT randomizes patients to a minimalist or intensive follow-up to compare the effect of the two regimens on 5-years overall survival.

[*] E-mail address: paolo.zola@unito.it.

Background

Cancer treatment accounts for a considerable percentage of the total global healthcare disbursement [1] and a substantial amount of it is considered to be imputable to follow-up procedures.

The term "follow-up", in Oncology, refers to a group of pre-scheduled medical tests and procedures settled up to identify disease relapses at a pre-clinical stage. The overall goal of follow-up is to timely identify disease recurrence amenable to treatment, with the aim of extending survival or improving patients' quality of life [2]. This concept of long-term monitoring assumes that an early diagnosis may reduce patient's morbidity and mortality.

The planning of follow-up care is based on many concerns including the type and stage of cancer, the aggressiveness of the cancer cells, technological options for detecting and treating relapses, the need to make the patient feel safe.

The proper setting of a follow-up program has to balance among the needs of clinicians, patients and Health Care System.

The clinician plans systematic visits with the aim of evaluate performance status of patients, discover complications of primary treatment (often a combination of integrated modalities) and to detect recurrent disease in advance in order to plan lifesaving therapies. Other objectives of routine follow-up are the detection of second tumors and providing support and counseling to patients and families [3]. At the same time the interest of the physician is focused on finding the most suitable program of follow-up for each patient (time interval between controls, diagnostic tests) [4-6].

The patient wants to receive reassurances about her health status, to reduce the anxiety and depression related to the diagnosis and the treatment of the neoplasia. Psycho-oncological and sexuality concerns should be addressed during the visit and psychotherapeutic treatment facilities should be suggested.

The Health System Administrators have their major interest in assessing the effectiveness of diagnostic and therapeutic procedures, monitoring complications due to treatment, limiting costs.

During the last few years evidence-based medicine (EBM) gained increasing acknowledgment and became a useful instrument to manage problems related to containment of resource pressure [3]. Moreover, in the near future, medical decisions will need to be made in an explicit and clear way, with decisional pathways available to everyone interested. In addition, physicians will need to produce and describe the scientific evidence that supports and drives their own decisions.

If we use the EBM instrument to go throught gynecological cancers we discover a critical lack of randomized clinical trials about follow-up strategies for all these patients (with the exception of breast cancer). As a consequence of this low level of available evidence, in the common practice a wide variability exists in the approach to the follow-up care of gynecological cancers [4,7-15]. Considerable differences exist among the policies of surveillance adopted by different Institutions and even among the policies adopted by different physicians working in the same Institution.

This variability has been detected both internationally [16] than in Italy, through a retrospective multicentric study [17]. Furthermore, the data collected in "A Piedmont Regional Oncology Network Study" showed that much of the unexplained variability in the follow-up for gynecological malignancies is attributable to different habits of centers belonging to the cancer network, independently of the clinical characteristics of the patients [18].

The follow-up policies include two main types of regimens. The first could be defined as "minimalist" (clinical examination associated with rare medical tests) and the second as "intensive" (clinical examination, imaging and markers).

Recurrence

Recurrence is defined as a pathologically documented disease after a disease-free interval of 3 or more months, whereas persistence of disease is defined as the presence of disease within 3 months from the end of primary treatment. The overall recurrence rate is 13% [19]. Endometrial cancer relapses are mostly uniformly distributed between local (pelvis 32%, vaginal vault 17%) and distant sites (abdomen and chest 51.2%) [20-23].

70% of endometrial cancer recurrences occur within 3 years from primary diagnosis [24-26].

Recurrence can be asymptomatic and then being identified with routine clinical and/or imaging evaluations such as physical examination, chest X-rays, abdominal and or pelvic ultrasonography (US), computed tomography (CT) scan and positron emission tomography (PET). Recurrence is defined as symptomatic when the patient reports symptoms during follow-up visit or symptoms determine an anticipation of the visit. 70% of endometrial cancer recurrences are associated with symptoms. Nonetheless vaginal vault recurrences are more frequently asymptomatic than other sites recurrences [27].

While primary endometrial cancer is characterized by a relatively good prognosis, the outcome of recurrent patients is poor. Disease-free interval after recurrence treatment is less than 1 year in 45% of the cases and more than 5 years in only 12% of the cases. The overall 5- and 10-years survival rates after recurrence are 26% and 22%, respectively [27-29].

Follow-up Procedures

Pap-smear

Available literature shows that citologic examination of vaginal vault does not contribute in the diagnosis of endometrial cancer relapse. Nonetheless this test is often routine at follow-up consultation. Only two studies continue to recommend pap smear testing; the rationale is the possibility of diagnosing a potentially curable relapse in the upper vagina [29,30].

Ultrasound Imaging

Morice et al performed annual routine US of the abdomen, which resulted in the detection of one asymptomatic relapse along the aorta among the 351 patients followed up, representing 4% of the asymptomatic relapse cases [11].

Another study performed US imaging 4 times per year for the first 2 years and twice per year for the remaining time of follow-up and detected 3 relapses in 133 patients, add up to 13% of the asymptomatic relapse cases detected [31].

X-rays

Ten follow-up programs of the 14 studies included in Fung-Kee-Fung review's [19] used thorax X-rays. Most of the studies used X-rays annually. Lung X-rays detected between 0 and 54% of asymptomatic relapse cases.

CT Scan

Only one study systematically performed annual CT scan as part of a follow-up plan [31]. This detected 5 relapse cases, constituting 38% of the asymptomatic relapse cases detected; similar to X-rays, the relapse is detected at a time where no effective treatment is available. Any study therefore recommends routinely using of CT.

PET and MRI

Any literature study has assessed the effects of systemically magnetic resonance imaging (MRI) and PET/CT scan to detect a relapse of endometrial cancer. American College of Radiology suggests PET/TC scan in in patients with clinically suspected recurrence.

American College of Radiology (ACR) Appropriateness Criteria 2010
Post-therapy evaluation in patients with clinically suspected recurrence

Radiologic Procedure	Procedure Rating	Comments
FDG-PET skull base to mid-thigh and CT abdomen and pelvis with or without contrast	9	A diagnostic quality CT examination is performed.
MRI pelvis with or without contrast	8	If FDG-PET is not performed. MRI of pelvis without and with contrast is preferred.
CT pelvis with contrast	8	If FDG-PET is not performed.
MRI abdomen with or without contrast	8	If FDG-PET is not performed. MRI of abdomen without and with contrast is preferred.
CT abdomen with contrast	7	If FDG-PET or MRI of abdomen is not performed or unavailable.
CT chest with or without contrast	6	Very appropriate for patients with more advanced stage disease or high-risk histology. CT chest with contrast is better to assess hilar node.
X-ray chest	4	May be appropriate if chest CT and FDG-PET is not performed or unavailable.

Rating Scale. 1,2,3: usually not appropriate; 4,5,6: may be appropriate; 7,8,9: usually appropriate

Concerning endometrial cancer follow-up, the following sources are available in the literature: two clinical practice guidelines published in 2011 [32,33], two clinical practice guidelines published in 2010 [34,35] and three systematic reviews: one conducted by Fung-Kee-Fung et al. at Ontario University and by the Ottawa Regional Cancer Centre in 2006 [19] that included in its analysis 16 retrospective studies and two systematics reviews; another one conducted by Lajer et al. at the Copenhagen Institute for Health services research in 2010 [36] that include the same 14 studies and a nationwide questionnaire survey and another review published by Sartori et al. in 2010 [37].

In Italy a randomized clinical trial (TOTEM trial) is ongoing (NCT00916708) and randomizes endometrial cancer patients to minimalist or intensive follow up.

Available guidelines give heterogeneous suggestions and recommendations that are based on limited or inconsistent scientific evidence (level B) and sometimes on consensus and expert opinion (level C).

Although the evidence from retrospective studies is limited, some compelling issues may contribute to improving daily practice while waiting for results of the ongoing randomized controlled trial on endometrial cancer follow-up.

The first issue is that patients treated for an endometrial cancer are at a relatively low risk of recurrence (overall recurrence rate across the studies is 13% and in patients at low risk is 1-3%). Second, most relapses occur in women with bad prognostic factors within 3 years from the end of the primary treatment. Lastly, most endometrial cancer recurrences are symptomatic, even if vaginal vault relapses are a particular setting for more frequently asymptomatic disease [37].

Therefore most of patients do not relapse, and those who do are often symptomatic, suggesting that recurrences can be detected regardless of follow-up strategy.

During the follow-up evaluation, patient should be encouraged to recognize the signs and symptoms of recurrent disease, such as pain, bleeding, swelling, nausea or vomiting, appetite decrease or weight loss, dizziness or blackouts, coughing or shortness of breath, a new mass or skin lesions.

An appropriate follow-up schedule should reflect prognostic factors, with few follow-up visits for patients with a favorable profile, compared with cases with one or more unfavorable prognostic factors.

Sartori et al [37] report an high percentage of distant metastases with an unfavorable prognosis unrelated to the timing of recurrence detection: this raises the question of whether early diagnosis by follow-up would really result in a survival benefit.

Gynecological evaluation, on the other hand, is fundamental during routine follow-up visits to detect vaginal vault recurrences, which are both frequent and often asymptomatic and which represent the most curable recurrent lesions. It is recommended that all patients being followed up by a health care professional who is knowledgeable about the natural history of the disease, and who is comfortable performing speculum and pelvic exams, in order to diagnose or detect a local recurrence [19].

Finally, the epidemiological observation that most recurrences occur within 3 years after the primary treatment supports the common trend to stop intensive follow-up after the fifth year.

The psychological impact of follow-up programs must be taken into account as well in the global feasibility definition of such programs. Psychosocial support is very important for cancer survivors but to date, it has not been objectively assessed [38].

In conclusion, no rationale (examination sensitivity/ sensibility, cost-effectiveness, or patient survival benefit) is available today for any particular follow-up protocol. No reliable differences in survival are detected between patients with symptomatic or asymptomatic recurrences (in particular for distant recurrences), and there are no differences in patient outcomes in the type of follow-up regimen used. Only a physical examination including pelvic-rectal examination proved effective in detecting recurrence. Other routine tests such as Pap smear, chest x-ray, abdomen ultrasound, CT scan, and CA-125 should not be routinely used in follow-up programs [37].

The general objective of TOTEM randomized clinical trial is to compare the effect of the two follow-up regimens (minimalist and intensive programs) on 5-year overall survival.

The secondary objectives are to quantify the intensive program possibility to advance the diagnosis comparing to minimalist program, to evaluate the differences in terms of complications, rates of recurrences, second primary tumors and maybe other diseases, to assess the accuracy of the two schemes of follow-up in diagnosing the relapse of disease in asymptomatic patients, to describe the compliance to different follow-up programs, to evaluate quality of life and patients satisfaction about the two strategies of follow-up and to evaluate the cost-effectiveness and the cost-utility of the two regimens.

Inclusion criteria are: patients treated surgically for endometrial cancer in complete clinical remission; no previous or concurrent neoplasia (with the exception of carcinoma in situ of the cervix and basalioma of the skin); other concomitant RCT may be allowed in the absence of any restriction concerning follow-up; obtaining a written informed consensus before randomization; age > 18 years.

Minimalist follow-up regimen (Arm 1) – low-risk

Procedures	**Months since randomization**														
	0	**4**	**6**	**8**	**12**	**16**	**18**	**20**	**24**	**30**	**36**	**42**	**48**	**54**	**60**
Visit	X		X		X		X		X	X	X	X	X	X	X
QoL Questionnaire	X		X		X				X		X		X		X

Intensive follow-up regimen (Arm 2) – low-risk

Procedures	**Months since randomization**														
	0	**4**	**6**	**8**	**12**	**16**	**18**	**20**	**24**	**30**	**36**	**42**	**48**	**54**	**60**
Visit	X	X		X	X	X		X	X	X	X	X	X	X	X
Pap smear					X				X		X		X		X
CT chest, abdomen, pelvis					X				X						
QoL Questionnaire	X	X			X				X		X		X		X

Minimalist follow-up regimen (Arm 1) – high-risk

Procedures	Months since randomization														
	0	**4**	**6**	**8**	**12**	**16**	**18**	**20**	**24**	**30**	**36**	**42**	**48**	**54**	**60**
Visit	X	X		X	X	X		X	X	X	X	X	X	X	X
CT chest, abdomen, pelvis					X				X						
QoL Questionnaire	X	X			X				X		X		X		X

Intensive follow-up regimen (Arm 2) – high-risk

Procedures	Months since randomization														
	0	**4**	**6**	**8**	**12**	**16**	**20**	**24**	**28**	**32**	**36**	**42**	**48**	**54**	**60**
Visit	X	X		X	X	X	X	X	X	X	X	X	X	X	X
CA125		X		X	X	X	X	X	X	X	X	X	X	X	X
Transabdominal & -vaginal US		X		X		X	X		X	X		X		X	
Pap smear					X			X			X		X		X
CT chest, abdomen, pelvis					X			X			X		X		X
QoL Questionnaire	X	X			X			X			X		X		X

Patients are firstly stratified according to their risk level of recurrence in 2 groups. In the group 1 there are the patients at low risk of recurrence (stage IA G1 and stage IA G2); in the group 2 there are the patients at high risk of recurrence (≥ stage IA G3).

Patients are then randomized to two regimens of follow-up: minimalist (Arm 1) and intensive (Arm 2).

In presence of symptoms or signs suggesting a relapse or in case of abnormal examinations, the patients leaves the trial and the clinician prescribes all medical tests and examinations required.

References

[1] Brown, ML; Riey, GF; Schussler, N; Etzioni, R. Estimating health care costs related to cancer treatment from SEER Medicare data. *Med Care* 2002;40:104-17.

[2] Grogan, M; Rangan, A; Gebski, V; Boyges, J. The value of follow-up of patients with early breast cancer treated with conservative surgery and radiation therapy. *Breast* 2002;11:163-9.

[3] Muir, JA; Gray, J. Evidence-based health care: how to make health policy and management decisions. London: Churchill Livingstone; 1999.
[4] Morice, P. Value of routine follow-up procedures for patients with stage I/II cervical cancer treated with combined surgery-radiation therapy. *Ann Oncol* 2004;15:218-23.
[5] Von Georgy, R; Schubert, K; Grant, P; Munstedt, K. Post therapy survellance and after-care in ovarian cancer. *Eur J Obstet Gynecol Reprod Biol* 2004;114:228-33.
[6] Sackett, D. Evidence-based medicine: what it is and what it isn't. *BMJ* 1996;312:371-2.
[7] Richert-Boe, KE. Heterogeneity of cancer surveillance practices among medical oncologists in Washington and Oregon. *Cancer* 1995;75:2605-12.
[8] Loomer, L; Brockschmidt, JK; Muss, HB; Saylor, G. Postoperative follow-up of patients with early breast cancer. Pattern of care among clinical oncologist and a review of the literature. *Cancer* 1991;67:55-60.
[9] Vernava, A; Longo, W; Virgo, K; Coplin, MA; Wade, TP; Johnson, FE. Current follow-up strategies after resection of colon cancer. Results of a survey of members of the American Society of colon and rectal Surgeons. *Dis Colon Rectum* 1994;37:573-82.
[10] Foster, MF; Hill, J; Leaper, DJ. Follow-up after colorectal cancer, recurrent practice in Wales and southwest England. *Int J Colorectal Dis* 1987;2:118-9.
[11] Morice, P; Levy-Piedbois, C; Ajaj, S; Pautier, P; Haie-Meder, C; Lhomme, C; et al. Value and cost evaluation of routin follow-up for patients with clinical stag I/II endometrial cancer. *Eur J Cancer* 2001;37:895-90.
[12] Agboola, OO; Grunfeld, E; Coyle, D; Perry, GA. Cost and benefits of routine follow-up after curative treatment for endometrial cancer. *CMAJ* 1997;157:879-86.
[13] Tjalma, WA; van Dam, PA; Makar, AP; Cruickshank, DJ. The clinical value and cost-effectiveness of follow-up in endometrial cancer patients. *Int J Gynecol Cancer* 2004;14:931-7.
[14] Bodurka-Bevers, D; Morris, M; Eifel, PJ; Levenback, C; Bavers, MW; Lucas, KR; et al. Post-therapy surveillance of women with cervical cancer: an outcomes analysis. *Gynecol Oncol* 2000;78:187-93.
[15] Bristow, RE; Purinton, SC; Santillan, A; Diaz-Montes, TP; Gardner, GJ; Giuntoli, RL. Cost-effectiveness of routine vaginal cytology for endometrial cancer surveillance. *Gynecol Oncol* 2006;103:709-13.
[16] Favalli, G. International survey on follow-up. Unpublished data, 2000.
[17] Zola, P; Fuso, L; Mazzola, S; Piovano, E; Perotto, S; Gadducci, A; et al. Could follow-up different modalities play a role in asymptomatic cervical cancer relapses diagnosis? An Italian multicenter retrospective analysis. *Gynecol Oncol* 2007;107(Suppl):150-4.
[18] Fuso, L; Evangelista, A; Pagano, E; Piovano, E; Perotto, S; Mazzola, S; et al. Variation in Gynecological oncology follow-up practice: attributable to cancer centers or to patient characteristics? A Piedmont Regional Oncology Network Study. *Tumori* 2011;97:551-8.
[19] Fung-Kee-Fung, M; Dodge, J; Elit, L; Lukka, H; Chambers, A; Oliver, T; and the Gynecology Cancer Disease Site Group. Follow-up after primary therapy for endometrial cancer: a clinical practice guideline. Program in Evidence-Based Care, Cancer Care Ontario, 2006.
[20] Keys, HM, Roberts, JA, Brunetto, VL, Zaino, RJ, Spirtos, NM, Bloss, JD; et al. A phase III trial of surgery with or without adjunctive external pelvic radiation therapy in

intermediate risk endometrial carcinoma: A Gynecologic Oncology Group Study. *Gynecol Oncol* 2004;92:744-51.

[21] Creutzberg, CL; van Putten, WL; Koper, PC; Lybeert, ML; Jobsen, JJ; Wárlám-Rodenhuis, CC; et al. Surgery and postoperative radiotherapy versus surgery alone for patients with stage I endometrial carcinoma: multicentre randomised trial PORTEC study group. Post Operative Radiation Therapy in Endometrial Carcinoma. *Lancet* 2000; 335:1404-1411.

[22] Aalders, J; Abeler, V; Kolstad, P. Recurrent adenocarcinoma of the endometrium: a clinical and histopathological study of 379 patients. *Gynecol Oncol* 1984;17:85-103.

[23] Piver, S; Yazgi, R; Blumenson, L; Tsukada, Y. A prospective trial comparing hysterectomy; hysterectomy plus vaginal radium and uterine radium plus hysterectomy in stage I endometrial carcinoma. *Obstet Gynecol* 1979;54:85-9.

[24] Menczer, J. Endometrial carcinoma. Is routine intensive periodic follow-up of value? *Eur J Gynecol Oncol* 2000;21:461-5.

[25] Boronow, RC; Morrow, CP; Creasman, WT; Disaia, PJ; Silverberg, SG; Miller, A; et al. Surgical staging in endometrial cancer: clinical pathology finding a prospective study. *Obstet Gynecol* 1984;63:825-32.

[26] Wylie, J; Irwin, C; Pintilie, M; Levin, W; Manchul, L; Milosevic, M; et al. Results of radical radiotherapy for recurrent endometrial cancer. *Gynecol Oncol* 2000;77:66-72.

[27] Sartori, E; Laface, B; Gadducci, A; Maggino, T; Zola, P; Landoni, F; et al. Factors influencing survival in endometrial cancer relapsing patients: a Cooperation Task Force study. *Int J Gynecol Cancer* 2003;13:458-65.

[28] Salvesen, HB; Akslen, LA; Irvesen, T; Irvesen, OE. Recurrence of endometrial carcinoma and the valueof routine follow-up. *Br J Obstet Gynecol* 1997;104:1302-7.

[29] Podczasky, E; Kaminsky, P; Gurski, K; MacNeill, C; Stryker, JA; Singapuri, K; et al. Detection and patterns of treatment failure in 300 consecutive cases of “early” endometrial cancer after primary surgery. *Gynecol Oncol* 1992;47:323-7.

[30] Gordon, AF; Owen, P; Chien, PFW; Duncan, ID. A critical evaluation of follow-up of women treated for endometrial adenocarcinoma. *J Obstet Gynecol* 1997;17:386-9.

[31] Gadducci, A; Cosio, S; Fanucchi, A; Cristofani, R; Genazzani, AR. An intensive follow-up does not change survival of patients with clinical stage I endometrial cancer. *Anticancer Res* 2000;20:1977-84.

[32] Colombo, N; Preti, E; Landoni, F; Carinelli, S; Colombo, A; Marini, C; et al; ESMO Guidelines Working Group. Endometrial cancer: ESMO Clinical Practice Guidelines for diagnosis; treatment and follow-up. *Ann Oncol* 2011;22(Suppl6):35-9.

[33] Querleu, D; Planchamp, F; Narducci, F; Morice, P; Joly, F; Genestie, C; et al. Clinical practice guidelines for the management of patients with endometrial cancer in France: recommendations of the Institut National du Cancer and the Société Française d'Oncologie Gynécologique. *Int J Gynecol Cancer* 2011;21:945-50.

[34] American College of Radiology (ACR). ACR Appropriateness Criteria pretreatment evaluation and follow-up of endometrial cancer of the uterus. Online publication, 2010.

[35] Agency for Healthcare Research and Quality. National Guidelines Clearinghouse. Online publication, 2010

[36] Lajer H, Jensen MB, Kilsmark J, Albaek J, Svane D, Mirza MR, Geertsen PF, Reerman D, Hansen K, Milter MC, Mogensen O. The value of gynecologic cancer follow-up: evidence-based ignorance? Int J Gynecol Cancer. 2010 Nov;20(8):1307-20. Review.

[37] Sartori E, Pasinetti B, Chiudinelli F, Gadducci A, Landoni F, Maggino T, Piovano E, Zola P. Surveillance procedures for patients treated for endometrial cancer: a review of the literature. Int J Gynecol Cancer. 2010 Aug;20(6):985-92. Review.

[38] Berchuck, A; Anspach, C; Evans, AC; Soper, JT; Rodriguez, GC; Dodge, R; et al. Postsurgical surveillance of patients with FIGO stage I-II endometrial adenocarcinoma. *Gynecol Oncol* 1995;59:20-4.

Index

A

B

C

D

E

F

G

H

I

L

M

N

O

P

T

U

V

W

Y